D0464711

FEB 0 3 2003

COPING WITH STRESS

COPING WITH STRESS

EFFECTIVE PEOPLE AND PROCESSES

Edited by
C. R. Snyder

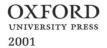

UNIVERSITY PRESS

2001

OXFORD

UNIVERSITY PRESS

Oxford   New York
Athens   Auckland   Bangkok   Bogotá   Buenos Aires   Calcutta
Cape Town   Chennai   Dar es Salaam   Delhi   Florence   Hong Kong   Istanbul
Karachi   Kuala Lumpur   Madrid   Melbourne   Mexico City   Mumbai   Nairobi
Paris   São Paulo   Shanghai   Singapore   Taipei   Toky   Toronto   Warsaw

and associated companies in
Berlin   Ibadan

Copyright © 2001 by Oxford University Press

Published by Oxford University Press, Inc.
198 Madison Avenue, New York, New York 10016

Oxford is a registered trademark of Oxford University Press

All rights reserved. No part of this publication may be reproduced,
stored in a retrieval system or transmitted, in any form or by any means,
electronic, mechanical, photocopying, recording or otherwise,
without the prior permission of Oxford University Press.

Library of Congress Cataloging-in-Publication Data
Coping with stress : effective people and processes / edited by C.R. Snyder.
    p.   cm.
    Includes bibliographical references and indexes.
    ISBN 0-19-513044-8
    1. Adjustment (Psychology)   2. Stress (Psychology)   I. Snyder, C. R.
BF335.S69   2001
155.2'4—dc21   00-041644

1 2 3 4 5 6 7 8 9

Printed in the United States of America
on acid-free paper

To Drew and Staci and
Tyler and Teresa and
other single-parent coping teams

Foreword

As I was reading *Coping with Stress*, I kept thinking that this book should be in everyone's survival kit for life in the twenty-first century. In the preface, Snyder reminds us of the comment by the baseball player, Yogi Berra, who said, "The future ain't what it used to be." Humans will face major challenges in this new century. This book is exciting because it teaches us how we can effectively meet these challenges. The chapters in this book, taken together, provide theory and research that show us how to "cope" adaptively with the big and small challenges of life. Indeed, the biggest challenge of all, our certain death, is confronted in the chapter on terror management theory. Snyder and the contributing authors do an outstanding job of presenting cutting-edge theory and research about the coping process. They take an interdisciplinary approach and utilize concepts and methods from social, personality, clinical, cognitive, lifespan, and cross-cultural psychology to illuminate the coping process and how it can go wrong. Snyder and Pulvers do a masterful job of providing conceptual continuity across the contributions with their beginning and concluding chapters. I never will be able to think about work on coping again without having the image of Snyder's "coping machine" flood my mind! The message of this book is optimistic. Each of us *can* become a better coping machine. The theory and research in this book provide blueprints for building better coping machines.

Lyn Y. Abramson

Preface

As we are about to begin the twenty-first century, understanding the processes of coping with stress, as well as the people who are facile at such coping, seems rather daunting. When Alvin Toffler published *Future Shock* in 1971, he argued persuasively, at least to me, that change was occurring at an ever-accelerating pace. Furthermore, despite the already enormous impacts of the personal computer and internet in the year 2000, I believe that we have seen only a small sample of their ultimate influences on our culture in general, and science in particular (see Toffler, 1981). As baseball catcher turned philosopher Yogi Berra has told us, "The future ain't what it used to be." There is much wisdom in Yogi's words. We will be facing new and ever-changing stressors in our attempts to cope in the fast-paced society of the coming decades. If we do not cope, we will be unable to find our place and get somewhere in that future, much like the car driver poised on the entry ramp of a super highway trying to find an opening in the flow of traffic where there is none. I say these things not to alarm, nor, of course, am I the first to talk this way—for centuries writers have warily described the wonders lurking "out there" in the future.

As I cast my thoughts toward those tomorrows, I am drawn back to what my Grandpa Gus used to tell me about the "old days." Everyone probably has an elder who has recounted similar tales of yesteryear. Without going into details, those "good old days" don't seem so good to me. They were very difficult for the majority, and horrific for a sizable minority of our ancestors. And the stressors they faced stagger the imagination—lacking food and shelter, fighting world wars, and being open to the ravages of contagious diseases. Looking back, the stressors may seem more barbaric than the ones we face today. We owe this in large part to the continual advances in science, technology, medicine, food production, governance, and economic circumstances, to name but a few of the forces driving progress in our civilization.

So, is it the case that we are experiencing very little stress, especially in comparison to our ancestors? I think not, because stress is relative to the latest temporal context, and there *always have been* and *always will be* events that cause psychological pain, events that shake the very foundations of our beings. We still do not get out of this life journey without facing deaths—those of our loved ones and our own. Furthermore, for many fellow citizens in our "modern" world, the list of stressors still includes starvation, terrible living circumstances, illnesses, and diseases with chronic, high levels of suffering. Undeniably, therefore, stressors keep rolling in like waves onto the psychological shores of humanity. The other day I saw a car in our quiet college town with a bumper sticker that aptly captures this point. In bold print, it asked, "OK, what PROBLEM is NEXT?"

Although we may resonate to this bumper sticker question, we are not defenseless to all these stressors. Indeed, in varying degrees, humans are adept at responding to stressors by *coping*. Understanding such capabilities is humbling in that I am truly amazed at the coping feats of some people; moreover, coping is fascinating because it comes in so many forms. Thus, I long have been seduced by both the processes and individual differences in coping. *Coping* and *copers*, how could a social scientist not be drawn to these topics?

In editing this volume, I continue my quest to better understand the coping process. Additionally, I sought to showcase the insights of experts who have devoted major portions of their careers trying to unlocking the secrets of "their" particular coping topics. Moreover, I wanted to select coping topics that were at once important and intriguing. In the ensuing pages, you can draw your own conclusions as to whether my goals have been met.

I greatly appreciate my editors at Oxford, Joan Bossert and Catherine Carlin for having an interest in what hopefully will become a movement— positive psychology. They repeatedly supported my writing projects aimed at unveiling and understanding the strengths in people. I also would like to thank my authors for being superb *and* punctual scholars—a rare combination indeed. To Lyn Abramson, whose ideas have advanced immeasurably the study of coping, goes a full dose of thanks for taking about 10 seconds to accept my invitation to write the foreword for this volume. My assistants in the Clinical Psychology Program in the Department of Psychology at the University of Kansas—Martha Dickinson and later Bonnie Shaffer—have helped at various stages in seeing to it that this project came to fruition. Likewise, my colleagues—faculty members and graduate students—in the Clinical Psychology Program at Kansas have supported me daily in both word and deed. To my family, I once again owe a debt of gratitude for letting me hole myself up in my office at home in order to get this latest book completed. Lastly, I would like to thank the people who, in the very conduct of their lives, have provided me with glimpses of everyday coping heroics. Many were students and colleagues, others were psychotherapy clients, some were patients in hospitals, and yet others were persons who have been participants in my research program. To my delight, I also have found such people in my family. There obviously is much to learn about this topic, but the fact that there are superb copers among us should provide hope about our possible effectiveness in dealing with the vicissitudes of life.

C. R. S.
Lawrence, Kansas

References

Toffler, A. (1971). *Future shock*. New York: Bantam Doubleday Dell.
Toffler, A. (1981). *The third wave: The classic study of tomorrow*. New York: Bantam Doubleday Dell.

Contents

Contributors

Edward C. Chang, Assistant Professor, Department of Psychology, University of Michigan, Ann Arbor

W. Keith Dooley, Doctoral Student, Graduate Training Program in Life-Span Developmental Psychology, Department of Psychology, The University of Georgia

Joseph R. Ferrari, Associate Professor, Department of Psychology, DePaul University, Chicago

Jeff Greenberg, Professor, Department of Psychology, University of Arizona, Tucson

Nancy A. Hamilton, Assistant Professor, Department of Psychology, Southern Methodist University, Dallas

Rick E. Ingram, Professor, Department of Psychology, Southern Methodist University, Dallas

Anita E. Kelly, Associate Professor and Director, Graduate Training Program in Clinical and Counseling Psychology, Department of Psychology, University of Notre Dame

Herbert M. Lefcourt, Distinguished Professor Emeritus, Department of Psychology, University of Waterloo, Waterloo, Ontario

Heidi Levitt, Assistant Professor, Clinical Psychology Program, Department of Psychology, University of Memphis

Michael E. McCullough, Director of Research, National Institute for Healthcare Research, Rockville, Maryland

Robert A. Neimeyer, Professor, Clinical Psychology Program, Department of Psychology, University of Memphis

Kenneth I. Pargament, Professor and Director of Clinical Training, Department of Psychology, Bowling Green State University

Margaret M. Poloma, Professor, Department of Sociology, University of Akron

Kimberley Mann Pulvers, Doctoral Student, Graduate Training Program in Clinical Psychology, Department of Psychology, University of Kansas, Lawrence

Tom Pyszczynski, Professor, Department of Psychology, University of Colorado, Colorado Springs

James M. Sandy, Instructor, Health Psychology Training Program, Ferkauf Graduate School of Psychology and Albert Einstein College of Medicine of Yeshiva University

C. R. Snyder, Professor and Director, Graduate Training Program in Clinical Psychology, Department of Psychology, University of Kansas, Lawrence

Sheldon Solomon, Professor, Department of Psychology, Skidmore College, Saratoga Springs

Eric Strachan, Doctoral Student, Graduate Program in Clinical Psychology, University of Nebraska, Lincoln

Nalini Tarakeshwar, Doctoral Student, Graduate Program in Clinical Psychology Program, Department of Psychology, Bowling Green State University

Redford B. Williams, Professor of Psychiatry and Behavioral Sciences, Professor of Medicine, Professor of Psychology, and Director of the Behavioral Medicine Research Center at Duke University Medical Center

Virginia P. Williams, President, Williams LifeSkills, Inc.

Gail M. Williamson, Professor and Chair, Life-Span Developmental Psychology, Department of Psychology, The University of Georgia

Thomas Ashby Wills, Professor, Health Psychology Training Program, Ferkauf Graduate School of Psychology and Albert Einstein College of Medicine of Yeshiva University

COPING WITH STRESS

1

Dr. Seuss,
the Coping Machine, and
"Oh, the Places You'll Go"

C. R. Snyder
Kimberley Mann Pulvers

Why Dr. Seuss?

In thinking about your childhood, or the childhoods of your children or grandchildren, chances are that you are familiar with Dr. Seuss "children's" books. These books were authored by Theodor Seuss Geisel (1904–1991) and were rich with coping themes in which the protagonist deals with problems. These problems, of course, were some of the very impediments that children would meet in their adult years.[1] Thus, Dr. Seuss may have been one of the major children's book authors who offered early instruction about the coping process. Seuss brought his coping themes to life with rich, imaginary characters and machines that could handle whatever impediments they encountered. Even today, the Seuss heritage conjures memorable words and pictures, and we wish to borrow such spark to enliven this chapter on the coping construct.

Our goal in this chapter is to present a model of coping that has broad applications. To accomplish this, in the first section, we describe previous definitions of coping, along with our own. Then, in the second section, we present a schematic for understanding our model of coping and describe the nature of appraisal-like processes involved in stressors that impact subsequent coping. In the third section, we explore individual differences in people (the "coping machines") that can moderate coping responses to a stressor. In the fourth section, we explicate the responses that are, in varying degrees, effective according to our model. Finally, we provide a brief conclusion.

Definition of Coping

Coping has become a central concept in psychology, as well as working its way into the lexicon of society more generally. For the average person, coping represents a description of what must be done to keep his or her life at a reasonably high level of satisfaction. Thus, coping may involve a variety of thoughts, emotions, and actions.

As psychologists have studied coping in the last two decades, it has become an increasingly complex construct. It is seen as the effortful attempt to deal with stressors that are beyond the "normal" range of functioning, with the purpose of reducing the negative impacts of those stressors. For many scholars, the coping thoughts, feelings, and actions are characterized by two important qualifiers: (1) they involve purposeful, effortful, and conscious actions; and (2) they occur in response to "big" events, that is, events that shake the customary senses of stability or threaten to undermine the usual activities of people. Additionally, coping is typically not a single response, but a series of responses, initiated and repeated as necessary to handle the remaining, continued, or transformed nature of the stressor. There also are those researchers who emphasize either the personality *or* situational factors as having the primary influence on coping. Our view is that both personality *and* situational factors are *interactively* implicated in coping. To complicate matters further, how people appraise (or interpret) a stressor has been introduced as crucial for deriving a more precise understanding of the coping process. Indeed, a float representing coping in a parade displaying the grand ideas of psychology would have a multifaceted, Dr. Seuss–like appearance that would simultaneously amaze and delight and yet defy understanding for many people. Our goal in this chapter is to provide a model of coping that is as succinct as possible and yet attends to the complexities that must be considered in this evolving field.

For our purposes, *coping reflects thinking, feeling, or acting so as to preserve a satisfied psychological state when it is threatened*. We would note that this definition differs from two of the qualifiers that previously have been placed upon the coping process by several scholars. First, let's consider the view that coping must involve purposeful, conscious, and effortful actions. Purposeful, yes we would agree, in the sense that the individual is responding to a stressor *for a reason*—to reduce its noxiousness. The conscious and effortful parameters seem unduly constraining, however. The generally accepted view is that only those adaptive processes involving effort should be conceived as falling under the rubric of coping (1). The difficulty with this provision, however, lies in its vagueness. Who is to define what is "effortful?" At what point does any motivated behavior reach the threshold of being effortful? Furthermore, at times, doing the very least necessary—what is sometimes called the minimalist perspective—is the most productive level of effort. Turning to consciousness issues, we see no necessity to yoke total awareness to the coping concept (for views in support of the importance of consciousness in coping, see references 2, 3,

4, 5, and 6). Additionally, as has been the case in the history of psychology, the term "consciousness" is plagued by ambiguity. Consciousness as judged by whom? And what is it? Again, we have difficulty in the implied all or none nature of such consciousness. In point of fact, there is some evidence that we engage in cognitive coping *without* awareness (7); moreover, *we fairly often purposefully engage in coping activities that are below our level of awareness* (8, 9, 10). In our view, that an adaptive behavior has become automatized via repetition does not negate its coping properties. Also, the stipulation of coping as necessarily conscious delimits the applications of this important construct (see 11).

Costa, Somerfield, and McCrae (12) have reasoned that "progress has been hampered . . . by the assumption that stress and coping are special processes, governed by their own laws, and lying outside the normal range of human adaptation. By contrast, we have come to see stress and coping as an intrinsic part of the fabric of action and experience" (p. 44). We agree and thus have reformulated a definition of coping that accentuates a natural, everyday process that is at the heart of our lives—from development through all of our adult years.

Coping Machines: Individual Differences Variables

Each person has built a particular "coping machine." Dr. Seuss, no doubt, would produce a whimsical rendering of this machine, perhaps one similar to that shown in the left side of Figure 1.1. Admittedly, we had fun in crafting such a "coping machine," but we also present it as an image to vivify the point that each person brings his or her set of characteristics to form a "vehicle" for dealing with whatever stressors may be encountered. In this section, we will describe the psychological motivation and personality dimensions that shape such "coping machines."

As we have written elsewhere (13), the history of coping over the last three decades has shifted from an emphasis on situational (see capstone exemplar, 14) to individual differences factors. The "individual differences approach rests on the assumption that there are important dimensions of personhood along which people can be rated or measured, and that such information is critical for understanding their subsequent coping adventures" (13, p. 13). Or, in statistical parlance, such individual differences variables *moderate* the nature of the subsequent stress and coping activities.

Scholars already are calling for the measurement of both weaknesses and, as importantly, the strengths of people (15, 16, 17, 18). Moreover, suggestions have been made regarding the personality variables that may serve as potential moderators of stress (19). Some of the individual differences variables that have been examined in regard to their moderating influences on coping include optimism (20), learned optimism (21), hope (22), mastery (23), locus of control (24), self-efficacy (25, 26), neuroticism, extraversion,

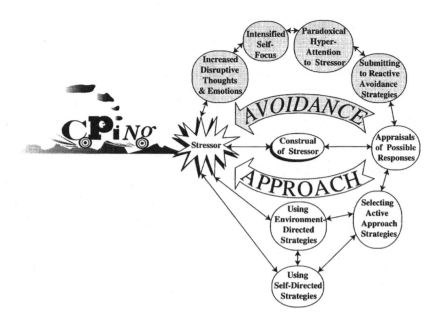

Figure 1.1. The approach and avoidance interactive steps in the stress and coping sequential model.

openness to experience, agreeableness, and conscientiousness (the five-factor model; 12, 27), emotional intelligence (28), problem-solving (29), self-esteem (30), depression (31), social support (32), forgiveness (33), hostility (34), humor (35), and perceived control (36). Many of these variables serve as positive moderators and others as negative moderators, and they are grouped accordingly in Table 1.1.

As a general principle, the positive moderators should yield their beneficial influences through approach coping, whereas the negative moderators should lead to their detrimental influences by avoidance coping (we will discuss approach and avoidance coping in more detail subsequently). Unfortunately, little research has been conducted in regard to the relative overlap and proportions of variance of these individual differences variables in moderating the stress and coping process (2). Thus, at this point in time, we can only speculate about the contributions of each individual differences variable in moderating the stress and coping process.

Beyond the aforementioned *psychological* individual differences factors, there are differences among people in their socioeconomic status, intelligence, education, financial resources, marital/relationship status, age, race, gender, and physical health (37). For example, racial differences in coping with pain appear—Irish-Americans minimizing their pain and persons of Jewish and Italian decent openly expressing their pains (38). One of the views in literature is that men supposedly are prone to use problem-focused strategies, whereas women use emotion-focused ones (39). It is the

Table 1.1 Individual Differences Variables Moderating the Coping Process, Names of Measuring Instruments, and References for Each Measure

Variable Name	Name of Measuring Instrument	Reference
Positive Moderators		
Control	Desirability of Control Scale	127
Emotional Intelligence	Multidimensional Emotional Intelligence	128
Hope[b]	Hope Scale	129
Humor	Situational Humor Response Questionnaire	130
Optimism	Life Orientation Test—Revised	131
Learned Optimism[c]	Attributional Style Questionnaire	132
Locus of Control	Internal-External Locus of Control Scale	133
Mastery	"Kind of Person" Implicit Theory Scale	134
Problem Solving	Problem Solving Inventory	135
Self-Efficacy	Self-Efficacy Scale	136
Self-Esteem[d]	Self-Esteem Scale	137
Social Support	Social Support Questionnaire	138
Negative Moderators		
Depression	Beck Depression Inventory	139
Hopelessness	Hopelessness Scale	140
Hostility	Hostile Automatic Thoughts Scale	141
Positive and Negative Moderators		
Five-Factor Model[a]	Revised NEO Five-Factor Inventory	142

[a] Taps neuroticism, extraversion, openness to experience, agreeableness, and conscientiousness.
[b] This is for adults. See 143 for the Children's Hope Scale.
[c] This is for adults. See 144 for the Children's Attributional Style Questionnaire.
[d] This scale is a state one, although instructions note that the set can be a trait one.

case, however, that researchers sometimes do not find support for this conclusion (40). Moreover, whatever researchers may have found previously about men or women being more disposed toward problem- or emotion-focused coping, such conclusions would be clouded by their use of confounded emotion-focused coping measures (see later discussion). Generally, of these nonpsychological "resources," the more beneficial ones appear to be higher socioeconomic status (41, 42, 43), higher income (44, 45), and better physical health (46).

To state that there are many human individual differences is unremarkable in and of itself, but what is important is how these individual differences prime people to react differently—to take different routes—as they encounter the inevitable stressors in their life journeys. To put it simply, some individuals (coping machines in an automobile analogy) are better able to get to their desired destinations. Thus, a coping machine with one or more of the following "options" (taken from Table 1.1) should work better: *high*: desired control (located within oneself rather than outside), emotional intelligence, hope, humor, mastery, optimism, problem solving, self-efficacy, self-esteem, social support, extraversion, openness to experience, forgiveness, agreeableness, conscientiousness, socioeconomic status, income, education, and physical health; and *low*: depression, neuroticism, hopelessness, and hostility. Now that we have an idea of what types of coping machines may fare better, we next turn to the various appraisal-based dimensions of stressors.

Appraisal-Based Dimensions of Stressors

For our present purposes, we would direct your attention to that portion of Figure 1.1 which lies directly ahead of the coping machine—the stressor. It is important to describe the appraisal-like characteristics of such stressors because they influence the nature of the coping responses. There are several parameters along which stressors can be "weighted," with some being less and others being appraised as more stressful (for a review of these issues, see 1, 2, 41, 47, 48, 49, and 50).

First, we would suggest that stressors that are related to more important life arenas should have more appraisal impact. For example, an undergraduate student trying to gain admission to a selective graduate program would interpret a C grade in a course as being more stressful than would a retired person taking the course for personal enjoyment.

Second, a stressor that portends to have an impact on several rather than just one aspect of one's life should be more disturbing. For example, a job loss could impact the family, where one lives, what one thinks of oneself, how one spends time, etc.

Third, stressors that are likely to continue over time should capture our coping efforts in the short and long term. For example, a severe, chronic back injury demands our coping efforts in the present *and into the foreseeable future* (51).

Fourth, stressors of greater severity should require more coping. We would hasten to note, however, that stressors of seemingly lesser severity also can elicit coping. A stressor needs only to be of sufficient severity so that the person responds to it (either below or beyond awareness). This position that "small" stressors can elicit coping responses differs from the view held by some scholars that coping *only occurs in response to stressors of major severity* (for review, see 12). This latter assumption, in our estimation, suffers from some flaws. Briefly, at what point does a stressor become appraised as being "severe"? And how consistent is this "severe" stressor notion with what people actually nominate as the stressors in their lives? The answer to this latter question is "Not very." More specifically, people describe stressors as including rather ordinary events such as raising a teenage son or being treated rudely by an acquaintance (52). Additionally, the major instrument for measuring stressors, the Social Readjustment Rating Questionnaire (53), contains items that do not seem very severe in their stressfulness—e.g., vacations and holidays. We also would note that several coping researchers already have abandoned their foci on major, stressful life events in favor of daily hassles and chronic strains (e.g., 54, 55, 56, 57). Therefore, our position is that stressors of varying severities (including seemingly less severe ones) may necessitate coping, but that the more severe stressors elicit more profound needs for coping.[2]

Fifth, stressors can vary in ambiguity, with some being more and others less ambiguous to appraise (see 1, 2, 41). We would suggest that increasingly less ambiguity should make a stressor more perceptually obvious and, in turn, more threatening.

Sixth, stressors may differ in the degree to which they seem to be amenable to one's control (see 41, 58, 59, 60). As stressors are appraised as being more under the control of the person dealing with them, they also should be less threatening.

Although we have presented six parameters that should impact how stressors are viewed *across people*, we strongly believe that the most productive approach to understanding a stressor is to understand *how it is construed by the individual*. This view is at the heart of the influential theory of coping advocated by Lazarus and Folkman (1). Any given stressor simply cannot have veridical reality across people because the "same" stressor will not be interpreted by two persons in the same manner. As such, a stressor is a unique and phenomenological personal matter that is driven by the individual differences variables that we have described previously. For example, a person who is very high in hope will view being diagnosed with cancer, or the death of a loved one, much differently than a low-hope person (51, 61, 62, 63). Or, because of a particular previous history with a given stressor, the person will interpret it differently than the person lacking such a previous history. Because of this extremely person-specific meaning of any given stressor, we would repeat our earlier point that a stressor does not need to be large to elicit a coping response. Rather it only needs to be of sufficient "weight" that the person responds to it (either below or beyond awareness), and it is to the topic of response alternatives that we now turn.

Oh, the Places You'll Go

In the children's book *Oh, the Places You'll Go*, Geisel (64) gives us glimpses of the many roads we will travel in life. So, when taking to the road and encountering obstacles that reflect varying degrees of stress, how will our metaphorical "coping machine" react? We will take this coping journey stage by stage, along one of two major pathways to coping—avoidance and approach.

Which Coping Path?

At the risk of oversimplifying matters, according to research findings, our coping adventures generally take one of two routes—avoidance or approach. This avoidance-approach idea is not a new one, in that it appeared in early psychoanalytic theories of defense (65), as well as the behavioral (66) and phenomenological (67) research pertaining to conflict, and the health psychology context more recently (68, 69). Perhaps most germane to our present model is an *American Psychologist* article by Roth and Cohen that appeared in 1986 (59). These authors make a cogent argument for linking the coping process with the avoidance-approach systems and note 14 separate midrange coping theories that are based on this dichotomy. More recently, Moos and Schaefer (70) reason that the avoidance-approach idea is central to their coping model. Given this widespread theoretical advocacy of the avoidance-approach dimension, it should come as no surprise that this distinction has emerged as the highest order factor in the Coping Strategies Inventory (71).

A further distinction worth mentioning is that avoidance or approach coping behaviors can occur at either the covert, within-person level, or at the more overt level (72). In our model, most of the coping activities along either an avoidance or approach route (see circled stages in Figure 1.1) occur at an internal, mental, and emotional locus. At times, however, the coping activities naturally will become overt and visible. For our subsequent exposition of the coping stages, we assume that the activity is occurring at an internal, within-person level, unless we indicate otherwise.

The Avoidance Route

The "Avoidance" counterclockwise path can be seen in the top portion of Figure 1.1. As a brief preview of the effectiveness of this avoidance coping pathway, based on our review of the relevant research literature, we conclude—with a few important exceptions that we will discuss—that avoidance is *not* adaptive (see 70). In many instances, the use of avoidance coping makes matters worse for the person trying to deal with a stressor. In this section, we will describe what happens at each stage of the avoidance coping process shown in the middle to upper counterclockwise cycle of Figure 1.1.

Construal of Stressor   As shown in Figure 1.1, there is a left to right feedforward flow as the stressor necessitates a construal. Construal reflects an individual's particular mental representation regarding the "factual" nature of the stressor (73). "Factual" is in quotation marks to highlight our belief that the experience of a stressor is a distinctly individual matter that varies from person to person and, as such, there is no one true construal of a given stressor. A major aspect of this construal reflects the person's first overall judgment concerning how serious the stressor may be and what is at stake. This evaluation is similar to what Lazarus and Folkman (1) have called primary appraisal.

For a stressor to even be considered as requiring coping, we would argue that the person must construe the stressor as having personal relevance (otherwise, the event is not a stressor to that person). Richard Lazarus previously has arrived at a similar view of the appraisal process (74). As an example of this personal relevance issue, a large drop in the stock market may be highly relevant to a person who has a huge equity portfolio, but it may be totally irrelevant to a young grade school teacher who has no stocks. Perhaps another vivid means of making this point is to consider one's reactions to the tragedies (earthquakes, tornadoes, hurricanes, bombings, etc.) that are the common fare of television news shows. Although there certainly may be empathy for the victims in some far distant state or land, we do not view these events as personally relevant stressors, nor as being threatening ones to us (for naturalistic and laboratory corroboration, see 75). Therefore, for our present purposes in describing the avoidance path, we assume that the stressor is relevant to the individual.

If a stressor is of an extremely severe and weighty magnitude such that it threatens one's actual physical existence (e.g., automobile accident, rape, etc.), the individual may react with what has been called "denial numbness" (76, 77). In terms of Figure 1.1, it can be seen that there is a right to left feedback as the construal arrow returns to the stressor. Although there is evidence that denial can be effective in the short term, when retained for long durations, denial appears to be associated with less resistance to disease and immunocompetence (78, 79, 80, 81). Therefore, the pattern in the avoidance path coping is to continue the denial process, and this "head in the sand" tendency epitomizes avoidance.

Furthermore, the construal process will be influenced by relevant individual differences variables (in a manner similar to what we wrote earlier about the influence of individual differences on the appraisal experience of the stressor). For example, a low- as compared to a highly optimistic person may become more distraught and prone to shock and denial when having a heart attack (82). More generally, more pessimism (i.e., increasingly less optimism) appears to moderate the impact of a stressor, in that the pessimistic people may make catastrophizing construals by overreacting and overestimating the severity of stressors (83).

Appraisals of Possible Responses   Assuming that the construals have not resulted in total, denial-like blockages, people then proceed in a feed forward left-to-right direction to appraising their possible subsequent responses to the stressors *as they perceive them* (see Figure 1.1). This stage is analogous to what Lazarus and Folkman (1) have called secondary appraisal, or one's beliefs about what one can do in a given situation. Additionally, this appraisal of possible responses stage, as well as the subsequent stages in our model, bear likenesses to two other evaluation-like components espoused by Folkman and Lazarus—problem-focused coping potential = environment-directed strategies, and emotion-focused coping potential = self-directed strategies (1, 84, 85).

This appraisal of possible responses also allows the protagonist to consider any resources—physical or psychological—that she may bring to bear on the given stressor. In this regard, *the person succumbing to the avoidance path perceives that he does not have any productive resources* and, indeed, may possess counterproductive individual characteristics that contribute to a sense of not being able to deal effectively with the stressor. In emotion-focused coping potential, the person on the avoidance path perceives that he will be unable to regulate his emotions effectively in the face of the given stressor. That is to say, he has a very real concern that *he will be controlled by his emotions.*

Before leaving this appraisal section, we would note that such appraisal is conceived by some coping scholars as being conscious, effortful, accessible to self-report, and involving a fairly large amount of time. Our view, to the contrary, is that in many instances such appraisals are below conscious awareness, relatively automatic and seemingly effortless, difficult to recount verbally, and very fast in a temporal sense. Other researchers also support these latter views (1, 86, 87, 88, 89). Finally, we would highlight the fact that the appraisals of possible responses stage (for the person on the avoidance path) feed *back* so as to reify the earlier construal of the stressor as being overwhelming or extremely taxing.[3]

Submitting to Reactive Avoidance Strategies   The next stage is the submission to the inevitability of avoidance coping strategies. It is the logical extension of the person's earlier construal of the stressor as being overwhelming, as well as the inability to find any active, potentially stressor-reducing assets in one's personal repertoire. Lacking alternatives, the person's seeming only other prerogative is an unresisting acquiescence to a default avoidance set of responses. As can be discerned in Figure 1.1, having yielded to the avoidance path, this conclusion can feed back to the earlier stages so as to reinforce the power of the stressor over the individual. Having settled on the avoidance track, as we will see in the next section, "what is out of sight is *not* out of mind" for most people.

Paradoxical Hyperattention to Stressor   In a classic 1987 experiment, Wegner, Schneider, Carter, and White (90) examined what happens when people are instructed "to not think about a white bear." Try as they might, such research participants thought even more about the white bear. Indeed, white bear thoughts became captivating—the underlying principle being that attempted avoidance or suppression of thoughts about a given stimulus results in even greater cognitive attention to that stimulus (91). *The impli-*

cation for our presently described protagonist who is to trying to avoid thinking about the stressor is that, in all likelihood, he thinks even more about that stressor.[4] Thinking more and more about the stressor, there are both counterproductive feed forward implications that we will explore subsequently, but also feed back processing to solidify the earlier malevolent and looming attributions associated with that stressor. Therefore, contrary to becoming a useful self-regulatory approach for coping with stressors, cognitive avoidance often backfires and makes the stressor even more problematic (92).

Intensified Self-Focus   Experiencing the stressor ever more vividly, persons using avoidant coping begin to think about how poorly they are handling matters. In what is called the "illusion of transparency," such persons become convinced that others are paying exceptional attention to them, their failures, and their inabilities to avoid ruminating about stressors (93, 94). Furthermore, if such a person has any physical problems, the self-focus appears to heighten the awareness of any related symptoms (95). As with the other stages we have described in the avoidance path, self-focus serves to feed back and forward to increase counterproductive thinking.

Increased Disruptive Thoughts and Emotions   It also appears that self-focus amplifies any negative self-referential thoughts and feelings (see for review, 96). By this point, the person not only *cannot avoid thinking about the stressor and himself or herself, but also is flooded with negative, disruptive thoughts about the self.* The negative self-directed thoughts and feelings are rampant, and it is no longer just a matter of dealing with the stressor, but yet other stressors that are created by the protagonist's reactions become part of "the problem."

Actions Related to Stressor After Going Through First Iteration of Avoidance Coping   "Well, hell, here I am still stewing about this problem, and it seems even bigger and more difficult now! I feel awful . . ." This is one possible example of the internal self-talk of a person who has *undergone* the avoidance coping track. "Undergone" is italicized to emphasize that the person feels as if she is a passive pawn who is pummeled about by her negative and counterproductive thoughts and emotions. Despite trying not to attend to the problem, it only seems to get larger and gain strength in holding her under its influence. Caught in a cycle of negative construal and appraisal of possible responses, hyperattention to the stressor, accentuated self-focus, and disruptive thoughts and emotions, our avoidance coper is similar to a small child on a merry-go-round who feels dizzy, sick, dizzier and sicker, and yet cannot jump off. Far from being a "merry"-go-round for the avoidance coper, this carousel seems more like torment.

The Approach Route

Starting with the stressor, the clockwise path of the approach cycle can be seen in the bottom portion of Figure 1.1. Our discussion in some of these approach stages will be briefer than for the avoidance path because some of the processes are the same, but opposite in direction.

Construal of Stressor   At the start of the approach sequence, the individual construes the stressor so as to lessen its aversive, threatening qualities (see previous footnote 3). Janoff-Bulman (97, 98), for example, describes this denial process as being adaptive, in that it protects the person from becoming overwhelmed and totally dysfunctional. That is to say, the denial process gives the person some "psychological breathing space" so as to potentially come to terms with the impact of the stressor. This denial is adaptive in the short-run in that it allows persons to gradually reduce their arousal so as to begin working on a more long-term manner of coping. Denial also seems to work for some short-term stressors such as angina, pain, blood donation, noise, and uncomfortable medical procedures (80, 81, 99). This short-term denial can occur as part of the approach sequence, *but it should be emphasized that the approach coping individual soon moves out of the denial stage and begins to recognize and deal effectively with the stressor.*

The approach construal also is likely to be moderated by one or more of the individual differences variables so that the appraised magnitude of the stressor is lessened. Also, the person with an approach relative to the avoidance construal is less likely to reflect a sense of surprise. That is to say, the stressor may be anticipated more frequently in approach coping (for discussion of proactive coping, see 100).

Appraisals of Possible Responses   Having defined the perceived nature of the objective stressor in the construal stage, the next stage involves the appraisals of possible responses that the person can make. As we noted previously, this stage is similar to Lazarus and Folkman's (1) secondary appraisal, or the beliefs about what one can do in the context of a particular stressor.

Also as noted earlier, this appraisal stage in our model is similar to problem-focused coping potential and emotion-focused coping potential (1, 84, 85). For problem-focused coping potential, the person on the approach route concludes that she can act effectively to address the challenges posed by the stressor. An example here of the action-oriented, affirming self-talk would be, "I can do something to cope with this situation." For emotion-focused coping potential, the persons on the approach path perceive that they can manage whatever emotions may appear in responding to the stressor. Cumulatively, in regard to problem- and emotion-focused coping potential, the approach appraisal is started with an affirming and powerful self-referential thought that "I can . . ."

The appraisal of possible responses enables the person to perform a mental assay of any resources—both physical and psychological—that he may have to apply to the given stressor. From the approach perspective, there is a wealth of individual differences factors that have helped the person in the past which often abound, and the person should see them as being available again in the latest coping episode (see Table 1.1 for such psychological individual differences variables). Thus, the approach pathway often is traversed by persons who have had previous successes at coping with similar stressors. The associated self-talk in this instance is, "I have been here before and handled it OK." As such, the recall of previously similar and successful coping experiences enhances the hope for dealing efficaciously with the latest stressor (62, 63, 101).

Lastly, as can be discerned in Figure 1.1, the approach appraisal of the possible responses stage feeds *back* to support the earlier construal of the stressor as being of manageable magnitude. That is to say, with the arsenal of previously effective approach-coping responses in mind, the individual concludes that she can contain the size of the stressor in a construal sense.

Selecting Active Approach Strategies   Of importance in this approach scenario, it should be noted that there is an active rather than a reactive quality to approach coping thinking—the approach coper will *act* on the stressor. As such, our approach coper must select one or more coping strategies to implement. Unlike the avoidance coper who at this stage has no options and experiences and is left with the avoidance strategy as the only one available, the approach coper can select from options and choose the temporal ordering in which to apply his or her strategies.

Based on available research, it would appear that problem-focused coping ("using environment-directed strategies" in our model) is the predominant selection when the stressor is appraised as being controllable by the person; when the stressor is construed as uncontrollable, however, emotion-focused coping ("using self-directed strategies" in our model) is the prevalent choice (37). As we will explain later, however, the previous emotion-focused coping scales are sufficiently confounded with outcome of such coping that one cannot infer much based on their use. Furthermore, *emotion-focused coping can be viewed as using problem-solving coping to deal with emotions that have become the stressor* (after reacting to the original eliciting stressor). In this latter sense, emotion-focused coping could be seen as a type of problem-focused coping. Therefore, we are skeptical of the previous results regarding problem- and emotion-focused coping choices for at least two reasons. A more parsimonious explanation that we believe will be borne out in subsequent coping research is that the persons on the approach path will select the strategies that best fit the types of stressors that they experience first. Thus, at times a person may be so upset that he must work on emotion-focused self-directed strategies and *then* move to problem-solving environment-focused strategies. Or, for another person experiencing the stressor, it may be likely that she will first invoke problem-solving environment-focused strategies. Again, we place the person's perception of the stressor as *the* powerful determinant in the unfolding of subsequent coping selections and uses of either environment- or self-focused strategies. Note in Figure 1.1 that the two stages of "using environment-directed strategies" and "using self-directed strategies" are positioned at a parallel temporal point in the approach path—both have equal positive coping potentials and likelihood of being used (across differing persons). We would further emphasize that, in the course of coping with a given stressor, a person may try several strategies, sometimes sequentially, sometimes concurrently. There is a flexibility to approach coping that operates throughout the process (more on this issue later).

Strategies Directed Toward Environment   The "using of environment-directed strategies" is a common active approach, and it can be seen in the bottom middle of Figure 1.1. Because this type of coping is the most widely described one in the literature, we will spend relatively little space on it here. In essence, these approaches attempt, through the efforts of the person and any other supporting persons or institutions, to act directly on the stressor so as to weaken it and diminish its dissonance-producing properties. This has been called primary control (102). The list of problem-focused, action-oriented and approach strategies is long, and the effective coper usually calls upon several strategies in his or her armamentarium. These strategies may be applied one after another or simultaneously.

The person using environment-directed strategies often has a history of successful interventions in similar stressor circumstances, as well as psychological individual differences variables that will aid as effective moderators in the implementation of the chosen strategy or strategies. Likewise, the environment-directed strategies can interact with the self-directed ones, as shown in the bidirectional line connecting them in Figure 1.1.

After using the environment-directed strategies, the person on the approach path can monitor any perceived changes in the level of the stressor and decide whether continued efforts along the same lines would be profitable, or whether adjunct or separate approach strategies need to be tried. The person on the approach coping path perseveres until a good test has been given of one strategy (51). Furthermore, this person on the approach path remains flexible in using several strategies or combinations of active environment-directed interventions.

Strategies Directed Toward Self   The active use of emotion-focused coping will serve as our exemplar of strategies directed toward the self. In this regard, emotion-focused coping traditionally has been seen as counterproductive (103; for review and critique, see 104). Following what is called the functionalist perspective, however, the *use* of one's emotions is viewed as a positive process for attaining a sense of coherence, as well as aiding in self-regulation (105, 106).

So, how was it that coping researchers, up until fairly recently, viewed emotion-focused coping as bad? Stanton and her colleagues (104, 107) have unraveled this conundrum by systematically showing that emotion-focused coping instruments often aggregate coping strategies that tap avoidance of and approach toward a stressor. A second reason that emotion-focused coping has been viewed as being counterproductive is that it has been confounded with maladjustment in the scale items (e.g., "I feel anxious *about not being able to cope*"). Thus, higher endorsement of emotional expression by necessity has also meant that scale respondents had to simultaneously endorse the view that such emotional expression was maladaptive. Stanton and her colleagues have developed and validated the Emotional Approach Coping Scale so as to remove the two aforementioned confounds (108). Subsequent research with this instrument provides preliminary support for both the existence of the emotional approach coping concept, as well as its positive relationship with stress reduction.

Unlike the avoidance path where persons experience a swell of mostly negative emotions as undesired, reactive responses to stressors, in active emotional approach coping, the person has purposefully adopted this coping style and *uses* his or her emotions rather than being controlled (i.e., used) by them (as is the case for avoidance copers). It should be noted that "using" self-directed strategies (a proxy for emotional approach) is in the active, approach lower path of our model in recognition that it is an empowering and stress-reducing approach. In the words of Greenberg (109), "if people are organized to avoid their feelings, they rob themselves of information that helps them to orient themselves in the environment and aids in problem solving" (p. 502). Such active use of emotional approach may be adaptive in that it may "(a) promote habituation to the stressor; (b) serve a signaling function to the individual; (c) engender cognitive reappraisal; (d) direct action; and (e) regulate the social environment" (107, p. 104). Lastly, as can be seen by the line connecting these two strategies in Figure 1.1, we expect self- and environment-directed strategies to relate to each other, at times providing an interactive mediational role in the ongoing approach coping response.

Actions Related to Stressor After Going Through First Iteration of Approach Coping   Unlike the avoidance coper who is trying not to think and emote in relation to the objective stressor (but as we noted earlier, nevertheless is thrust unwillingly into placing a constant focus on the stressor), the approach coper at this stage looks forward with positive anticipation to checking how his or her approach strategies have lessened the stressor. Furthermore, because approach coping often is quite effective, this comparison to the initial stressor level should be gratifying in that it often reveals progress. (For the reader who is interested in how our model relates to other self-regulation models of coping, we would recommend Carver and Scheier [110], which we believe is the best and most current of such models.)

Occasionally, the aversiveness stressor can be totally nullified in one cycle of approach coping. More typically, however, the person will have to go through a few and perhaps even very many iterations to achieve a satisfying coping resolution. In this latter vein, some stressors may necessitate years of approach coping. Additionally, with some stressors (e.g., chronic pain), it may be unrealistic to expect the stressor to totally go away, but a more reachable goal is to reduce the stressor to a manageable level.

Our model is predicated on an overall cycling of the person's thoughts and feelings through the various stages, but we do not mean to suggest that a person always moves continuously from one stage to the next, with that lock-stage cycle continuing as needed. Rather, as one can infer from the many bidirectional arrows linking the various stages in Figure 1.1, we envision that people will move back and forth between various stages and spend varying amounts of time and energy in particular stages as needed. Skipping a stage or stages also is quite possible. Thus, while the overall approach coping model is directionally clockwise in the lower half of Figure 1.1 and is counterclockwise for avoidance coping, we do *not* mean to imply that our "coping machines" travel these routes without some backtracking and detours. Indeed, the coping machines freely move back and forth in their overall coping journeys. Therefore, to make explicit what has been implicit in the exposition of our model, *we hold that the most useful means of understanding coping is to view it as a process.* In this latter regard, we share the view of coping reached by Richard Lazarus in his five-decade program of coping research (see 74).

Although many of our examples have used stressors that are of large "weight," as we noted earlier, what is more crucial is that the person perceives the stressor to be large enough to warrant coping. In our model, it is the case that there are general factors that should make a given stressor be appraised as being "bigger" across people, but the crucial process is how the stressor is perceived by a given person. Thus, *it is the perception of the stressor and the related construal phase that are the elicitors of coping in our model.*[5]

Stress-Related Growth   Before leaving this section on approach coping, we would like to address the evidence regarding the possibility that some people actually are strengthened or grow because of their having coped with a difficult life stressor (19, 111, 112, 113). Additionally, as Snyder, Tennen, Affleck, and Cheavens (114, p. 22) have noted, "Dramatic positive changes in the aftermath of adversity have been reported in the clinical literature (115), despite the contextual and interpersonal pressures *against* personal change that have been described in detail by social psychologists (e.g., 116), and people's tendencies to select social environments that homeostatically interrupt exceptional personal changes (117)."

It may be because of the increased flexibility in thinking that stress and subsequent coping may produce growth. Given the need to match a coping strategy to a particular stressor, the need to move back and forth in using the various stages of coping, and the need to learn how to monitor one's coping, it follows that increased flexibility should result. Indeed, flexibility has been touted as one of the hallmark beneficial properties of effective coping (37, 118). In discussing flexibility, those of us who do research or treatment related to coping should remain open to the likelihood that the coping strategies used in one stressful circumstance may differ substantially from those used by a person when encountering another stressor (37).

This stress-related growth is consistent with recent calls for a "positive psychology" (119, 120) or "positive social science" (121), where the foci are on the strengths of people. As part of this strength perspective, it will be important to explore the individual differences variables that actually may benefit us in the face of coping with stressors (i.e., positive moderators of stress) (122, 123). Furthermore, by using this "positive psychology" perspective, we believe that researchers will better understand the phenomenon of stress-related growth. Lastly, it is likely that approach coping processes will be at the core of future, improved models of stress and coping.

Oh, the Thinks You Can Think

To our knowledge, this *Oh, the Thinks You Can Think* book by Geisel (124) is one of his lesser-known books. As the title would imply, the children who read this book are introduced to the wonders of *what they can choose to think about as they live their lives*. This theme, coupled with the one in the book *Oh, the Places You'll Go* (64), aptly characterizes the approach route depicted in the lower portion of our coping model shown in Figure 1.1. Although some people have led lives that may predispose them to the less adaptive avoidance coping route, we would hasten to add that scholars exploring resiliency and hope (e.g., 22, 51, 125, 126) make the point that people can come out of seemingly negative childhoods very positively. While we acknowledge the impacts of environmental forces on the coping processes, the available literature also points to significant roles for cognitive and emotional reactions as driving the content of coping. Remember this latter point as you undertake research in this area, intervene to help others, or construct your own "coping machine." Thus, in the degree to which we embrace the philosophy of *Oh, the Thinks You Can Think* and can choose to keep our coping machines on the lower rather than the upper route of Figure 1.1, then we should have happier, more fulfilling journeys in life. Indeed, it is in this spirit of successful coping that we can understand the true meaning of *Oh, the Places You'll Go*.

Acknowledgment
We thank Sheryle Gallant and Annette Stanton for helpful comments.

Notes

1. Beyond the coping themes of Geisel's Dr. Seuss stories, a less-known aspect of his work is that he attempted to decrease illiteracy among Amer-

ican schoolchildren (145). In 1954, the editors of *Life* magazine reported an alarmingly high rate of illiteracy in children, and Geisel's publisher was moved by this report to ask him to write a book that would teach children over 200 words. Taking this challenge, nine months later Geisel (146) published *The Cat in the Hat*, which used 220 crucial words for reading. This book sold widely and was purchased by libraries nationwide so that literally millions of American children have read and learned from it over the years.

2. Because of page constraints, we will not provide any description of the types of stressors, other than to note that there are three: (1) blocked goal pursuits; (2) unlearned aversive stimuli, and (3) learned aversive stimuli (see 72, pp. 380–384, for a more detailed discussion).

3. In the avoidant path, however, the person may have a slight sense of challenge in regard to the stressor in both the construal and response steps, but this affirming self-referential thinking quickly becomes overwhelmed and pushed aside by the more negative thoughts. A similar point applies to our later description of the approach copers, who may have a sliver of doubt and negative self-referential thoughts, but these fade as the affirming thoughts predominate.

4. It should be noted that there may be a minority of persons who truly can block out of consciousness that which they wish to avoid. Freud called this repression, and although there is disagreement among researchers as to the existence of such a phenomenon, practicing clinicians can readily provide examples in the actions and thoughts of their clients.

5. An additional point needs to be made in regard to the construals of persons who are on either the avoiding or approval paths. Namely, such construals typically are above the level of awareness, but some may become so automatic through repetition that there is no conscious awareness.

References

1. Lazarus, R. S., & Folkman, S. (1984). *Stress, appraisal, and coping.* New York: Springer.
2. Aldwin, C. M. (1994). *Stress, coping, and development.* New York: Guilford.
3. Haan, N. (1992). The assessment of coping, defense, and stress. In L. Goldberger & S. Breznitz (Eds.), *Handbook of stress: Theoretical and clinical aspects* (2nd ed., pp. 258–273). New York: Free Press.
4. Parker, J. D. A., & Endler, N. S. (1996). Coping and defense: A historical overview. In M. Zeidner & N. S. Endler (Eds.), *Handbook of coping: Theory, research, applications* (pp. 3–23). New York: Wiley.
5. Schwarzer, R., & Schwarzer, C. (1996). A critical survey of coping instruments. In M. Zeidner & N. S. Endler (Eds.), *Handbook of coping: Theory, research, applications* (pp. 107–132). New York: Wiley.
6. Tennen, H., & Affleck, G. (1997). Social comparison as a coping process: A critical review and application to chronic pain disorders. In B. P. Buunk & F. X. Gibbons (Eds.), *Health, coping, and well-being: Perspectives from social comparison theory* (pp. 263–298). Mahwah, NJ: Lawrence Erlbaum.
7. Erdelyi, M. H. (1979). Let's not sweep repression under the rug: Toward

a cognitive psychology of repression. In J. F. Kihlstrom & F. J. Evans (Eds.), *Functional disorders of memory* (pp. 355–402). New York: Wiley.

8. Snyder, C. R., & Higgins, R. L. (1988). Excuses: Their effective role in the negotiation of reality. *Psychological Bulletin, 104,* 23–35.

9. Snyder, C. R., & Higgins, R. L. (1988). From making to being the excuse: An analysis of deception and verbal/nonverbal issues. *Journal of Nonverbal Behavior, 12,* 237–252.

10. Snyder, C. R., Higgins, R. L., & Stucky, R. J. (1983). *Excuses: Masquerades in search of grace.* New York: Wiley-Interscience.

11. Coyne, J. C., & Gottlieb, B. H. (1996). The mismeasure of coping by checklist. *Journal of Personality, 64,* 959–991.

12. Costa, P. T., Jr., Somerfield, M. R., & McCrae, R. R. (1996). Personality and coping: A reconceptualization. In M. Zeidner & N. S. Endler (Eds.), *Handbook of coping: Theory, research, and applications* (pp. 44–61). New York: Wiley.

13. Snyder, C. R., & Dinoff, B. (1999). Coping: Where have you been? In C. R. Snyder (Ed.), *Coping: The psychology of what works* (pp. 3–19). New York: Oxford University Press.

14. Mischel, W. (1968). *Personality and assessment.* New York: Wiley

15. Exner, J. E., Jr. (1998, February). *The future of the Rorschach.* Master lecture presented at the Society for Personality Assessment Annual Meeting, Boston, MA.

16. Handler, L., & Potash, H. M. (1999). Assessment of psychological health. *Journal of Personality Assessment, 72,* 181–184.

17. Lopez, S., Ciarlelli, R., Coffman, L., Stone, M., & Wyatt, L. (2000). Diagnosing for strengths: On measuring hope building blocks. In C. R. Snyder (Ed.), *Handbook of hope: Theory, research, and applications* (pp. 57–85). San Diego: Academic Press.

18. Wright, B. A. (1991). Labeling: The need for greater person-environment individuation. In C. R. Snyder & D. R. Forsyth (Eds.), *Handbook of social and clinical psychology: The health perspective* (pp. 469–487). New York: Pergamon.

19. Tedeschi, R. G., & Calhoun, L. G. (1995). *Trauma and transformation: Growing in the aftermath of suffering.* Thousand Oaks, CA: Sage.

20. Carver, C. S., & Scheier, M. F. (1999). Optimism. In C. R. Snyder (Ed.), *Coping: The psychology of what works* (pp. 182–231). New York: Oxford University Press.

21. Shatté, A. J., Reivich, K., Gillham, J., & Seligman, M. E. P. (1999). Learned optimism in children. In C. R. Snyder (Ed.), *Coping: The psychology of what works* (pp. 165–181). New York: Oxford University Press.

22. Snyder, C. R. (Ed.) (2000). *Handbook of hope: Theory, research, and applications.* San Diego, CA: Academic Press.

23. Dweck, C. S., & Sorich, L. A. (1999). Mastery-oriented thinking. In C. R. Snyder (Ed.), *Coping: The psychology of what works* (pp. 232–251). New York: Oxford University Press.

24. Roberto, K. A. (1992). Coping strategies of older women with fractures: Resources and outcomes. *Journal of Gerontology: Psychological Sciences, 47,* 21–26.

25. Bandura, A. (1997). *Self efficacy: The exercise of control.* New York: Freeman.
26. Chwalisz, K., Altmaier, E. M., & Russell, D. W. (1992). Causal attributions, self-efficacy cognitions, and coping with stress. *Journal of Social and Clinical Psychology, 11,* 377–400.
27. Watson, D., David, J. P., & Suls, J. (1999). Personality, affectivity, and coping. In C. R. Snyder (Ed.), *Coping: The psychology of what works* (pp. 119–140). New York: Oxford University Press.
28. Salovey, P., Bedell, B. T., Detweiler, J. B., & Mayer, J. D. (1999). Coping intelligently: Emotional intelligence and the coping process. In C. R. Snyder (Ed.), *Coping: The psychology of what works* (pp. 141–164). New York: Oxford University Press.
29. Heppner, P. P., & Hillerbrand, E. T. (1991). Problem-solving training implications for remedial and preventive training. In C. R. Snyder & D. R. Forsyth (Eds.), *Handbook of social and clinical psychology: The health perspective* (pp. 681–698). Elmsford, NY: Pergamon.
30. Baumeister, R. F. (Ed.). (1993). *Self-esteem: The puzzle of low self-regard.* New York: Plenum.
31. Cheavens, J. (2000). Light through the shadows: Depression and hope. In C. R. Snyder (Ed.), *Handbook of hope: Theory, research, and applications* (pp. 321–340). San Diego, CA: Academic Press.
32. Sarason, B. R., Sarason, I. G., & Pierce, G. R. (Eds.) (1990). *Social support: An interactional view.* New York: Wiley.
33. McCullough, M., Pargament, K. I., & Thoreson, C. E. (Eds.) (2000). *Forgiveness: Theory, research, and practice.* New York: Guilford.
34. Siegman, A. W., & Smith, T. W. (Eds.) (1994). *Anger, hostility, and the heart.* Hillsdale, NJ: Erlbaum.
35. Cogan, B., Cogan, D., Waltz, W., & McCue, M. (1987). Effects of laughter and relaxation on discomfort thresholds. *Journal of Behavioral Medicine, 10,* 139–144.
36. Cohen, S., & Edwards, J. R. (1989). Personality characteristics as moderators of the relationship between stress and disorder. In R. W. J. Neufeld (Ed.), *Advances in the investigation of psychological stress* (pp. 235–283). New York: Wiley.
37. Lazarus, R. S. (1999). Coping. In R. S. Lazarus, *Stress and emotion: A new synthesis* (pp. 101–125). New York: Springer.
38. Zborowski, M. (1952). Cultural components in responses to pain. *Journal of Social Issues, 8,* 16–30.
39. L'Abate, L. (1992). A theory of family competence and coping. In B. C. Carpenter (Ed.), *Personal coping: Theory, research, and applications* (pp. 199–217). Westport, CT: Praeger.
40. Thoits, P. A. (1991). Gender differences in coping with emotional stress. In J. Eckenrode (Ed.), *The social context of coping* (pp. 107–138). New York: Plenum.
41. Dohrenwend, B. P. (1998). Theoretical integration. In B. P. Dohrenwend (Ed.), *Adversity, stress, and psychopathology* (pp. 539–555). New York: Oxford University Press.
42. Pearlin, L. I. (1989). The sociological study of stress. *Journal of Health and Social Behavior, 30,* 241–256.

43. Wills, T. A., & Depaulo, B. M. (1991). Interpersonal analysis of the help-seeking process. In C. R. Snyder & D. R. Forsyth (Eds.), *Handbook of social and clinical psychology: The health perspective* (pp. 350–375). Elmsford, NY: Pergamon.
44. Diener, E. (1984). Subjective well-being. *Psychological Bulletin, 95*, 542–575.
45. Veroff, J. B., Douvan, E., & Kulka, R. A. (1981). *The inner American: A self-portrait from 1957 to 1976*. New York: Basic Books.
46. Williamson, G. M., Parmelee, P. A., & Shaffer D. R. (Eds.) (2000) *Physical illness and depression in older adults: A handbook of theory, research, and practice*. New York: Plenum.
47. Epstein, S. (1982). Conflict and stress. In I. Goldberger and S. Breznitz (Eds.), *Handbook of stress: Theoretical and clinical aspects* (pp. 49–60). New York: Free Press.
48. Pearlin, L. I. (1993). The social contexts of stress. In L. Goldberger & S. Breznitz (Eds.), *Handbook of stress: Theoretical and clinical aspects* (pp. 303–315). New York: Free Press.
49. Paterson, R. J., & Neufeld, R. W. J. (1987). Clear danger: Situational determinants of the appraisal of threat. *Psychological Bulletin, 101* (3), 404–416.
50. Wheaton, B. (1996). The domains and boundaries of stress concepts. In H. B. Kaplan (Ed.), *Psychosocial stress: Perspectives on structure, theory, life-course, and methods* (pp. 29–70). New York: Academic Press.
51. Snyder, C. R. (1994). *The psychology of hope: You can get there from here*. New York: Free Press.
52. McCrae, R. R. (1984). Situational determinants of coping responses: Loss, threat, and challenge. *Journal of Personality and Social Psychology, 46*, 919–928.
53. Holmes, T. H., & Rahe, R. H. (1967). The social readjustment scale. *Journal of Psychosomatic Research, 11*, 213–218.
54. DeLongis, A., Coyne, J. C., Dakof, G., Folkman, S., & Lazarus, R. S. (1982). Relationship of daily hassles, uplifts, and major life events to health status. *Health Psychology, 1*, 119–136.
55. Kanner, A. D., Coyne, J. C., Schaefer, C., & Lazarus, R. S. (1981). Comparison of two modes of stress measurement: Daily hassles and uplifts versus major life events. *Journal of Behavioral Medicine, 4*, 1–39.
56. Lepore, S. J., Palsane, M. N., & Evans, G. W. (1991). Daily hassles and chronic strains: A hierarchy of stressors? *Social Science and Medicine, 33*, 1029–1036.
57. Neale, J. M., Hooley, J. M., Jandorf, L., & Stone, A. A. (1999). Daily life events and mood. In C. R. Snyder & C. E. Ford (Eds.), *Coping with negative life events: Clinical and social psychological perspectives* (pp. 161–189). New York: Plenum.
58. Mattlin, J., Wethington, E., & Kessler, R. C. (1990). Situational determinants of coping and coping effectiveness. *Journal of Health and Social Behavior, 31*, 103–122.
59. Roth, S., & Cohen, L. J. (1986). Approach, avoidance, and coping with stress. *American Psychologist, 41*, 813–819.

60. Vitaliano, P. P., DeWolfe, D. J., Maiuro, R. D., Russo, J., & Katon, W. (1990). Appraisal changeability of a stressor as a modifier of the relationship between coping and depression: A test of the hypothesis of fit. *Journal of Personality and Social Psychology, 59*, 582–592.

61. Irving, L. M., Snyder, C. R., & Crowson Jr., J. J. (1998). Hope and the negotiation of cancer facts by college students. *Journal of Personality, 66*, 198–214.

62. Snyder, C. R. (1998). A case for hope in pain, loss, and suffering. In J. H. Harvey, J. Omarzu, & E. Miller (Eds.), *Perspectives on loss: A sourcebook* (pp. 63–79). Washington, DC: Taylor & Francis.

63. Snyder, C. R. (In press). The hope mandala: Coping with the loss of a loved one. In Jane Gillham (Ed.), *Optimism and hope*. Radnor, PA: Templeton Foundation/Washington, DC: American Psychological Association.

64. Geisel, T. (1990). *Oh, the places you'll go*. New York: Random House.

65. Freud, S. (1957). Instincts and their vicissitudes. In J. Strachey (Ed.), *Standard edition of the complete psychological works of Sigmund Freud* (pp. 111–142). London: Hogarth. (Originally published in 1915.)

66. Miller, N. E. (1944). Experimental studies of conflict. In J. McV.Hunt (Ed.), *Personality and the behavior disorders* (Vol. 1, pp. 431–465). New York: Ronald Press.

67. Lewin, K. (1951). *Field theory in social science*. New York: Harper & Row.

68. Carver, C. S., & Scheier, M. F. (1993). Vigilant and avoidant coping in two patient samples. In H. W. Krohne (Ed.), *Attention and avoidance: Strategies in coping with aversiveness* (pp. 295–320). Seattle: Hogrefe & Huber.

69. Carver, C. S., & Scheier, M. F. (1994). Situational coping and coping dispositions in a stressful transaction. *Journal of Personality and Social Psychology, 66*, 184–195.

70. Moos, R. H., & Schaefer, J. A. (1993). Coping resources and process: Current concepts and measures. In L. Goldberger & S. Breznitz (Eds.), *Handbook of stress: Theoretical and clinical aspects* (pp. 234–257). New York: Free Press.

71. Tobin, D. L., Holroyd, K. A., Reynolds, R. V., & Wigal, J. K. (1989). The hierarchical factor structure of the Coping Strategies Inventory. *Cognitive Therapy and Research, 13*, 343–361.

72. Houston, B. K. (1987). Stress and coping. In C. R. Snyder & C. E. Ford (Eds.), *Coping with negative life events: Clinical and social psychological perspectives* (pp. 373–399). New York: Plenum.

73. Smith, C. A. (1991). The self, appraisal, and coping. In C. R. Snyder & D. R. Forsyth (Eds.), *Handbook of social and clinical psychology: The health perspective* (pp. 116–137). Elmsford, NY: Pergamon.

74. Lazarus, R. S. (1998). *Fifty years of the research and theory of R. S. Lazarus: An analysis of historical and perennial issues*. Mahwah, NJ: Erlbaum

75. Heath, L. (1984). Impact of newspaper crime reports on fear of crime: Multimethodological investigation. *Journal of Personality and Social Psychology, 47*, 263–276.

76. Horowitz, M. (1976). *Stress response syndromes*. New York: Free Press.

77. Horowitz, M. (1990). A model of mourning: Change in schemas of self and other. *Journal of American Psychoanalytic Association, 38*, 297–324.

78. Jamner, L. D., Schwartz, G. E., & Leigh, H. (1988). The relationship between repressive and defensive coping styles and monocyte, eosinophile, and serum glucose levels: Support for the opioid peptide hypothesis of repression. *Psychosomatic Medicine, 50*, 567–575.

79. Levine, J., Warrenburg, S., Kerns, R., Schwartz, G., Delaney, R., Fontanta, A., Gradman, A., Smith, S., Allen, S., & Cascione, R. (1987). The role of denial in recovery from coronary heart disease. *Psychosomatic Medicine, 49*, 109–117.

80. Mullen, B., & Suls, J. (1982). The effectiveness of attention and rejection as coping styles. *Journal of Psychosomatic Research, 26*, 43–49.

81. Suls, J., & Fletcher, B. (1985). The relative efficacy of avoidant and nonavoidant coping strategies: A meta-analysis. *Health Psychology, 4*, 249–288.

82. Scheier, M. F., Matthews, K. A., Owens, J. F., Magovern, G. J., Lefebvre, R. C., & Carver, C. (1989). Dispositional optimism and recovery from coronary artery bypass surgery: The beneficial effects on physical and psychological well-being. *Journal of Personality and Social Psychology, 57*, 1024–1040.

83. Peterson, C., & Moon, C. H. (1999). Coping with catastrophes and catastrophizing. In C. R. Snyder (Ed.), *Coping: The psychology of what works* (pp. 252–278). New York: Oxford University Press.

84. Folkman, S., & Lazarus, R. S. (1985). If it changes it must be a process: Study of emotion and coping during three stages of a college examination. *Journal of Personality and Social Psychology, 48*, 150–170.

85. Folkman, S., Lazarus, R. S., Dunkel-Schetter, C., DeLongis, A., & Gruen, R. J. (1986). The dynamics of a stressful encounter: Cognitive appraisal, coping, and encounter outcomes. *Journal of Personality and Social Psychology, 50*, 992–1003.

86. Lazarus, R. S. (1966). *Psychological stress and the coping process.* New York: McGraw-Hill.

87. Lazarus, R. S. (1982). Thoughts on the relations between emotion and cognition. *American Psychologist, 37*, 1019–1024.

88. Lazarus, R. S. (1984). On the primacy of cognition. *American Psychologist, 39*, 124–129.

89. Lazarus, R. S., & Smith, C. A. (1988). Knowledge and appraisal in the cognition-emotion relationship. *Cognition and Emotion, 2*, 281–300.

90. Wegner, D. M., Schneider, D. J., Carter, S. R., & White, T. L. (1987). Paradoxical effects of thought suppression. *Journal of Personality and Social Psychology, 53*, 5–13.

91. Wegner, D. M. (1994). Ironic processes of mental control. *Psychological Review, 101*, 34–52.

92. Dale, K. L., & Baumeister, R. F. (1999). Self-regulatory psychopathology. In R. M. Kowalski & M. R. Leary (Eds.), *The social psychology of emotional and behavioral problems* (pp. 139–166). Washington, DC: American Psychological Association.

93. Gilovich, T., Kruger, J., & Savitsky, K. (1999). Everyday egocentrism and everyday interpersonal problems. In R. M. Kowalski & M. R. Leary

MALASPINA UNIVERSITY-COLLEGE LIBRARY

(Eds.), *The social psychology of emotional and behavioral problems* (pp. 69–95). Washington, DC: American Psychological Association.

94. Gilovich, T., Savitsky, K., & Medvec, V. H. (1998). The illusion of transparency: Biased assessments of others' ability to read our emotional states. *Journal of Personality and Social Psychology, 75*, 332–346.

95. Pennebaker, J. W., & Lightner, J. M. (1980). Competition of internal and external information in an exercise situation. *Journal of Personality and Social Psychology, 39*, 165–174.

96. Pyszczynski, T., Hamilton, J. C., Greenberg, J., & Becker, S. E. (1991). Self-awareness and psychological dysfunction. In C. R. Snyder & D. R. Forsyth (Eds.), *Handbook of social and clinical psychology: The health perspective* (pp. 138–157). Elmsford, NY: Pergamon.

97. Janoff-Bulman, R. (1992). *Shattered assumptions: Towards a new psychology of trauma.* New York: Free Press.

98. Janoff-Bulman, R. (1999). Rebuilding shattered assumptions after traumatic life events: Coping processes and outcomes. In C. R. Snyder (Ed.), *Coping: The psychology of what works* (pp. 305–323). New York: Oxford University Press.

99. Levenson, J. L., Kay, R., Monteferrante, J., & Herman, M. V. (1984). Denial predicts favorable outcome in unstable angina pectoris. *Psychosomatic Medicine, 46*, 25–32.

100. Aspinwall, L. G., & Taylor, S. E. (1997). A stitch in time: Self-regulation and proactive coping. *Psychological Bulletin, 121*, 417–436.

101. Snyder, C. R., McDermott, D., Cook, W., & Rapoff, M. (1997). *Hope for the journey: Helping children through the good times and the bad.* Boulder, CO, San Francisco, CA: Westview/HarperCollins.

102. Rothbaum, F., Weisz, J., & Snyder, S. (1982). Changing the world and changing the self: A two-process model of perceived control. *Journal of Personality and Social Psychology, 42*, 5–37.

103. Pearlin, L. I., & Schooler, C. (1978). The structure of coping. *Journal of Health and Social Behavior, 19*, 2–21.

104. Stanton, A. L., Danoff-Burg, S., Cameron, C. L., & Ellis, A. P. (1994). Coping through emotional approach: Problems of conceptualization and confounding. *Journal of Personality and Social Psychology, 66*, 350–362.

105. Bretherton, I., Fritz, J., Zahn-Waxler, C., & Ridgeway, D. (1986). Learning to talk about emotions: A functionalist perspective. *Child Development, 57*, 529–548.

106. Campos, B., Campos, R. G., & Barrett, K. (1989). Emergent themes in the study of emotional development and emotion regulation. *Developmental Psychology, 25*, 393–402.

107. Stanton, A. L., & Franz, R. (1999). Focusing on emotion: An adaptive coping strategy? In C. R. Snyder (Ed.), *Coping: The psychology of what works* (pp. 90–118). New York: Oxford University Press.

108. Stanton, A. L., Kirk, S. B., Cameron, C. L., & Danoff-Burg, S. (in press). Coping through emotional approach: Scale construction and validation. *Journal of Personality and Social Psychology.*

109. Greenberg, L. S. (1993). Emotion and change processes in psychotherapy. In M. Lewis & J. M. Haviland (Eds.), *Handbook of emotions* (pp. 499–508). New York: Guilford.

110. Carver, C. S., & Scheier, M. F. (1998). *On the self-regulation of behavior.* New York: Cambridge University Press.

111. Ickovics, J. R., & Park, C. L. (1998). Paradigm shift: Why a focus on health is important. *Journal of Social Issues, 54,* 237–244.

112. O'Leary, V. E. (1998). Strength in the face of adversity: Individual and social thriving. *Journal of Social Issues, 54,* 425–446.

113. Tedeschi, R., & Calhoun, L. (1996). The post-traumatic growth inventory: Measuring the positive legacy of trauma. *Journal of Traumatic Stress, 9,* 455–471.

114. Snyder, C. R., Tennen, H., Affleck, G., & Cheavens, J. (2000). Social, personality, clinical, and health psychology tributaries: The merging of a scholarly "river of dreams." *Personality and Social Psychology Review, 4,* 16–29.

115. Herman, J. L. (1992). *Trauma and recovery: The aftermath of violence from domestic abuse to political terror.* New York: Basic Books.

116. Baumeister, R. F. (1994). The crystallization of discontent in the process of major life change. In T. F. Heatherton & J. L. Weinberger, (Eds.), *Can personality change?* (pp. 281–297). Washington, DC: American Psychological Association.

117. Watzlawick, P., Weakland, J. H., & Fisch, R. (1974). *Change: Principles of problem formulation and problem resolution.* New York: Norton.

118. Snyder, C. R. (1999). Coping: Where are you going? In C. R. Snyder (Ed.), *Coping: The psychology of what works* (pp. 324–333). New York: Oxford University Press.

119. McCullough, M., & Snyder, C. R. (2000). Classical sources of human strength: Revisiting an old home and building a new one. *Journal of Social and Clinical Psychology, 19,* 1–10.

120. Snyder, C. R., & McCullough, M. (2000). A positive psychology field of dreams: "If you build it, they will come . . .". *Journal of Social and Clinical Psychology, 19,* 1–10.

121. Seligman, M. E. P. (1998). Positive social science. *American Psychological Association Monitor, 29 (4),* 2, 5.

122. Gould, S. J. (1993). *Eight little piggies: Reflections on natural history.* New York: W. W. Norton.

123. Lifton, R. J. (1993). *The protean self: Human resilience in an age of fragmentation.* New York: Basic Books.

124. Geisel, T. (1974). *Oh, the thinks you can think.* New York: Random House.

125. Werner, E. E. (1984). Resilient children. *Young Children,* November, 68–72.

126. Werner, E. E., & Smith, R. S. (1982). *Vulnerable but invincible: A study of resilient children.* New York: McGraw-Hill.

127. Burger, J. M., & Cooper, H. M. (1979). The disability of control. *Motivation and Emotion, 3,* 381–393.

128. Mayer, J. D., Salovey, P., & Caruso, D. (1997). *Emotional IQ test* [CD-ROM version]. Needham, MA: Virtual Knowledge.

129. Snyder, C. R., Harris, C., Anderson, J. R., Holleran, S. A., Irving, L. M., Sigmon, S. T., Yoshinobu, L., Gibb, J., Langelle, C., & Harney, P. (1991). The will and the ways: Development and validation of an individual-differences measure of hope. *Journal of Personality and Social Psychology, 60,* 570–585.

130. Martin, R. A., & Lefcourt, H. M. (1984). The Situational Humor Response Questionnaire: A quantitative measure of sense of humor. *Journal of Personality and Social Psychology, 47,* 145–155.

131. Scheier, M. F., Carver, C., & Bridges, M. W. (1994). Distinguishing optimism from neuroticism (and trait anxiety, self-mastery, and self-esteem): A reevaluation of the Life Orientation Test. *Journal of Personality and Social Psychology, 67,* 1063–1078.

132. Peterson, C., Semmel, A., von Baeyer, C., Abramson, L. Y., Metalsky, G. I., & Seligman, M. E. P. (1982). The Attributional Style Questionnaire. *Cognitive Therapy and Research, 6,* 287–298.

133. Rotter, J. B. (1966). Generalized expectancies for internal versus external control of reinforcement. *Psychological Monographs, 80* (1, Whole No. 609).

134. Dweck, C. S. (1999). *Self-theories: Their role in motivation, personality, and development.* Philadelphia, PA: Psychology Press.

135. Heppner, P. P., & Petersen, C. H. (1982). The development and implications of a personal problem-solving inventory. *Journal of Counseling Psychology, 29,* 66–75.

136. Sherer, M., Maddux, J. E., Mercandante, B., Prentice-Dunn, S., Jacobs, B., & Rogers, R. W. (1982). The self-efficacy scale: Construction and validation. *Psychological Reports, 51,* 663–671.

137. Heatherton, T. F., & Polivy, J. (1991). Development and validation of a scale for measuring state self-esteem. *Journal of Personality and Social Psychology, 60,* 895–910.

138. Sarason, I. G., Levine, H. M., Basham, R. B., & Sarason, B. R. (1983). Assessing social support: The Social Support Questionnaire. *Journal of Personality and Social Psychology, 44,* 127–139.

139. Beck, A. T., Ward, C. H., Mendelsohn, M., Mock, J., & Erbaugh, J. (1961). An inventory for measuring depression. *Archives of General Psychiatry, 4,* 53–63.

140. Beck, A. T., Weissman, D., Lester, D., & Texler, L. (1974). The measurement of pessimism: The Hopelessness Scale. *Journal of Consulting and Clinical Psychology, 42,* 861–865.

141. Snyder, C. R., Crowson, J. J., Jr., Houston, B. K., Kurylo, M., & Poirier, J. (1997). Assessing hostile automatic thoughts: Development and validation of the HAT Scale. *Cognitive Therapy and Research, 4,* 477–492.

142. Costa, P. T., Jr., & McCrae, R. R. (1992). *Revised NEO Personality Inventory (NEO-PI-R) and NEO Five-Factor Inventory (NEO-FFI) professional manual.* Odessa, FL: Psychological Assessment Resources.

143. Snyder, C. R., Hoza, B., Pelham, W. E., Rapoff, M., Ware, L., Danovsky, M., Highberger, L., Rubinstein, H., & Stahl, K. J. (1997). The development and validation of the Children's Hope Scale. *Journal of Pediatric Psychology, 22,* 399–421.

144. Seligman, M. E. P., Kaslow, N. J., Alloy, L. B., Peterson, C., Tanen-

baum, R., & Abramson, L. Y. (1984). Attributional style and depressive symptoms among children. *Journal of Abnormal Psychology, 93,* 235–238.

145. Morgan, N., & Morgan, J. (1995). *Dr. Seuss & Mr. Geisel: A Biography.* New York: Random House.

146. Geisel, T. (1957). *The cat in the hat.* New York: Random House.

2

Getting Things Done On Time: Conquering Procrastination

Joseph R. Ferrari

> Never put off till tomorrow what you could have done today.
>
> Anonymous Proverb

In this chapter, I first will provide a brief history of the procrastination concept. Next, I will review the prevalence of two major categories of procrastination, followed by a discussion of the reasons why people procrastinate. Lastly, keeping with the coping theme of this book, I will describe what people can do about treating this "thief of time."

A Brief History

Many people delay the start or completion of tasks, often feeling uncomfortable and anxious about the delays. This phenomenon in psychological research and clinical interventions has been labeled *procrastination*. The Romans provided the roots of the present form of the word "procrastination"—*pro* = "forward" + *crastinus* = "of tomorrow" (1). Interestingly, the Roman Emperor Marcus Aurelius warned against delaying unnecessarily. The earliest known English usage of the word "procrastination" was in 1548, where it appeared in Edward Hall's *Chronicle: The Union of Two Noble and Illustrious Families of Lancestre and York*. The term is used several times in Hall's text without pejorative connotations, reflecting the idea of "informed delay" or "wisely chosen restraint" that was popular in Roman accounts (1). The word "procrastination" was in relatively common usage by the early 1600s (1). In fact, one of the most prominent plays in English literature is the dramatic story of a procrastinator named Hamlet, who could not decide what course of action he should take to avenge his father's murder (2, 3). The negative connotations of the term, however, did not seem to emerge until the mid-1800s, at approximately the time of the industrial revolution, when the word became associated with "sinful" *sloth*. In contemporary times, procrastination has meant the negative and purposeful delaying of the start or completion of a task as a form of avoidance (1).

The Prevalence of Procrastination

Research on the prevalence of procrastination has revealed that there are *no* significant gender differences in procrastination—both men and women, boys and girls, males and females engage in task delays (1, 4). Furthermore, I believe that while everyone puts some things off on occasion (e.g., "I don't like cutting my lawn"), not everyone procrastinates all the time. Ellis and Knaus (5), and recently Knaus (6), report that between 70% and 90% of western culture college students engage in *academically related procrastination*. In the research literature, academic procrastination is associated with delaying the start or finish of reports, papers, essays, and term papers, studying for exams, registering for classes, making appointments with instructors, and turning in assignments on or before their due date (e.g., 7, 8, 9, 10).

People generally delay on some tasks but not others. For example, while a college student may delay studying for an exam or reading a text chapter, that same student probably will *not* delay going downtown with friends for social activities or getting free tickets to a campus concert by a favorite music performer. Additionally, manifesting occasional delays does *not* make a person a habitual procrastinator (see 11, 12). Instead, such persons should be labeled *situational procrastinators* because their task delays are situation-specific. Although chronic procrastinators engage in situational delays, situational procrastinators do not necessarily delay chronically across all different types of tasks (13).

Besides situational forms of procrastination, there are some procrastinators for whom frequent delays have become their way of life. Harriott and Ferrari (14), and more recently Hammer and Ferrari (15), found that approximately 20% of the normal adult population engages in frequent, *chronic procrastination*. This figure is equally applicable for both men and women. People also have self-identified themselves as tending to delay the start and completion of numerous daily tasks. For example, procrastinators report delays responding to phone messages, buying gifts and sport/concert tickets, doing the dishes, and the laundry. They don't fill the car up until the gauge is on empty; they don't restock the refrigerator until it is virtually without food; they don't make decisions on where to eat out, what movies to see, or how to dress for a social event; instead, they let others make those decisions for them. They also miss doctor's appointments and fail to pay bills on time. These persons would be labeled as *dispositional* or *chronic* procrastinators.

Different Types or Categories of Chronic Procrastination

There are different types of procrastinators. Some people wait until the last moment to start or finish a task as "thrill seeking" (1, 16). Close to the deadline, these individuals either rush around trying to gather the necessary information or they perform portions of the task. If they succeed in completing the task in time, and their performance is successful, they report experiencing a "rush"—a pleasurable sense of accomplishment ("Oh, I'm good!"). These "thrill-seeking junkies" engage in what is called arousal procrastination (1).

The other general category for chronic procrastination is what most people would identify as the common label for frequent delays—*avoidance procrastination* (1). At times, avoidance procrastination may result when encountering tasks that are perceived as unpleasant or aversive. Alternatively, the person may believe that task completion would reflect his or her self-worth, and if he or she fails or does poorly on the task, it would indicate that he or she is not a worthwhile individual. By preparing a less than well thought-out business report, for example, a midlevel manager may expose himself to other employees as a less than competent person. It is also possible that the person lacks self-confidence in his or her ability and believes that success at the task would instill high expectations for future performances on similar tasks. For instance, if a date goes well, then the partners would be obligated to see each other again and become more vulnerable through deeper self-disclosure over time. Such chronic procrastinators operate from task aversiveness, fear of failure, or fear of success, respectively.

To understand the motives for chronic procrastination, it is crucial to consider the type of procrastinator. The arousal procrastinator is motivated by a thrill-seeking or sensation-seeking motive (18)—they get a "kick" from rushing around at the last possible moment to complete the task (16). This may be a primary motive for those who shop for holiday gifts on Christmas eve (19). Rushing around and succeeding with completing a task close to a deadline must have some rewarding value. Researchers have not demonstrated this link directly, but it seems quite plausible. Unfortunately, by rushing at the last minute, chronic procrastinators may perform poorly because of their impulsivity under time pressures (20, 21). Why, then, do these people continue waiting until the last minute? Perhaps the rush is so rewarding and their success sufficiently frequent that they continue this maladaptive pattern.

Avoidance procrastinators, on the other hand, may prefer being viewed as *lacking in effort* instead of in *ability*. Ferrari, Johnson, and McCown (1) reviewed the literature and found that chronic procrastinators are very socially conscious; very concerned about their public image; very desirous of social approval; and wanting to be liked by others. Therefore, when confronted with a task on which they fear failing, they may prefer to give the impression that they are not working hard (22). Attributionally, lack of effort compared to lack of ability is less central, less threatening, and less stable to one's social and self-esteems (17).

In summary, *procrastination* is the purposive delay in starting or completing a task including making decisions. Procrastination is common to both men and women. While everyone delays at times (situational procrastination), a smaller percentage of people delay many tasks on regular bases (dispositional procrastination). Among persons who are chronic procrastinators, there are *arousal procrastinators*, people who are motivated by a desire for a thrill-seeking experience, and there are *avoidant procrastinators*, people who are motivated by fears of failure or success and task aversiveness. Interested readers wanting a further "background" understanding are directed to Ferrari et al. (1) for greater details, Ferrari and Pychyl (4) for current empirical studies, and Ferrari (23) for an encyclopedic coverage of the causes, associations, and outcomes of procrastination.

Having provided a brief overview of the prevalence, the two general types, and the reasons for procrastination, I now focus on how to treat this "thief of time."

Overview of Treatment Interventions

There are several common strategies suggested by clinical psychologists for treating procrastination (cf., 6 & 24). First, it is important to *enable the client to become aware of the causes and consequences of his or her procrastination.* Before any effective intervention is designed and implemented, the procrastinator and the therapist must identify the patterns of delay as being forms of procrastination. For instance, although procrastination tendencies may not be strongly related to obsessive-compulsive tendencies as often as believed by practitioners, they definitely are associated with passive-aggressive and anger-expressive tendencies (20, 25, 26). Knaus (6) states that procrastinators have clear "soft and hard" signs. He observes that *needless delays*, as judged by others, would constitute a hard sign of a frequent procrastinator. *Excessive excuse-making* in order to exonerate the reasons for "being late" presents a soft sign of a procrastinator. The therapist also must determine whether the delay is chronic, acute, or a recent development. Has the person been procrastinating only recently, suggesting some situational cause, or is it a pervasive pattern across settings, suggesting a lifestyle pattern? It is crucial for the client and the therapist to specify the etiology of this maladaptive pattern.

Second, it is important to determine to what degree the client *views the frequent task delays as a "personal problem."* Solomon and Rothblum (9), in their measurement of academic procrastination, always asked students whether the delay of studying, registering, or reading was a problem in their school performance. Not all students perceived their delays as being related to their performance problems. If the client does not perceive the delays as interfering with his or her life and, in fact, has not suffered any negative consequences from these delays, then it may be that his or her tendencies to procrastinate do not need much (if any) modification.

However, it is important to realize that while the client may not believe that any assistance is needed to reduce the rate of procrastination, others around that person may have different opinions. It is quite possible that the procrastinator's frequent delays impose or "force" others to suggest, start, or finish necessary tasks (27). Therefore, while the delays may not be problematic for the procrastinator, they may be problematic for those who live with the person. The perception of a client regarding the degree of impairment due to frequent procrastination must be tempered by an understanding that the client may be misreading or misrepresenting the situation.

In order to implement effective treatment of procrastination, it is likely that the therapist will need to work on a third general principle, *to change the client's personal self-statements and cognitive restructure his or her thoughts* (28). Procrastinators are excellent excuse-makers. Ferrari (19) reported that the excuses reported for delays in Christmas gift shopping depend on the type of chronic procrastinator. Arousal procrastinators claimed they waited to shop because of overextensions and numerous work commitments around the holiday season (a difficult to refute excuse because it is not readily checked by others). Avoidant procrastinators, on the other hand, stated that they were poor decision-makers, did not like shopping, and lacked the effort to shop (i.e., they made self-attributes for their delays). Moreover, Ferrari et al. (7) found that college students explained academic procrastination by saying that professors gave poor instructions and assigned boring and too frequent assignments. Based on these studies, I suggest that clients and therapists assess the types or location of attributes that procrastinators generate as reasons for their delays. If the person excessively blames outside forces ("It not my fault because . . ."; "I could have done it, but . . .": "Yes it was due, however . . ."), the helper should focus on teaching the client to recognize when and where external attributes may be contributing to the delay, versus when internal, self-related attributes may be the cause. On the other hand, if the client focuses almost exclusively on him or herself as the reason for the delay ("I'm just not good at this . . ."), the treatment will more likely be more involved—although the need for cognitive restructuring of the misattributions still is warranted.

Therapists state that to treat "yes, but" forms of excuse-making it is recommended that clients learn to enhance their levels of self-control (29, 30). Clients need to change their interpretations of the causes for events and to learn that getting tasks done in a timely manner is within their control. A different type of treatment for procrastination is Morita therapy (31, 32), where clients are taught to accept and *preserve* the adverse emotions that promote self-defeating excuses for avoiding and procrastinating. Practitioners of Morita therapy focus more on the desirable actions, rather than on self-preoccupations over the emotional reactions associated with delaying. Thus, creating cognitive reattributions regarding the reasons for delays is important and vital to an effective treatment program for procrastination.

A fourth general principle in the effective treatment of procrastination is *building self-esteem* (5, 6, 24). While the proponents of some treatment protocols may support *not* including the emotional causes or consequences for procrastination (such as in Morita therapy), there is theoretical and empirical support for including the role of affect in procrastination (e.g., 12, 13, 33). Procrastinators are both self-focused (34) and other-focused (22). They are concerned about their performance abilities *and* want to "please others" (instead of just wanting to perform well on tasks) (35). In this regard, Burka and Yuen (24) claim that procrastinators base their self-worth solely on how well they perform a task. Poor task performance reflects low self-worth and esteem. If the person never completes the task, however, then his or her self-worth is never "tested." They can convince themselves, and perhaps others, that they actually possess a higher level of ability. Such client strategies may "work" in the short run, but over time people see through them and the person does not truly stretch him or herself, "grow," and learn.

Therapists must ensure the separation of procrastination *behavior* from clients' self-perceptions of themselves as people. That is, clients must learn that self-worth or esteem do not need to be synonymous with how well they actually perform on tasks. Clients need to "own" the insight that they remain good and worthwhile people, even if a given performance is not "perfect" (6). In cases where perfection stops clients, procrastinators are being blocked from finishing tasks by fears of failure, fears of success, and a lack of confidence about future task performance. For such cases, instructing the client in relaxation exercises to treat the high levels of fear may be useful. Moreover, assessing reasons for irrational fears may be valuable (5, 28).

Treating Situation-Specific Forms of Procrastination: Behavioral and Cognitive Techniques

At this point, I will provide some concrete, hands-on techniques for treating situational forms of procrastination. In this section, I will explore treatment suggestions derived from cognitive-behavioral and social-learning clinical sources (e.g., 5, 6, 24). But first, I believe that it is important to say a few words about dispositional, chronic procrastination and behavioral, time management techniques. Chronic procrastinators tend to be present as opposed to future-oriented individuals (36). Researchers also report that chronic procrastinators tend to under- or overestimate the amount of time needed to complete projects (37). Therefore, they should benefit from time management training. Time management skills *alone*, however, are not sufficient for chronic procrastinators. Chronic procrastination is a maladaptive lifestyle with affective, behavioral, and cognitive consequences (1, 23). Thus, to tell the chronic procrastinator, "Just do it!" is like saying to the clinically depressed "Cheer-up!"—a far too simplistic approach. Industrial-organizational psychologists in corporations also maintain that time management training is not effective for all employees. Therefore, although time management training may have some benefits for chronic procrastinators, practitioners addressing such training alone cannot hope to change clients' habitual procrastinatory lifestyles.

The behavior management techniques to reduce procrastination do not work independently of each other. I next briefly describe strategies that help to reduce situational procrastination.

Time-Telling

Procrastinators are poor estimators of time. When given actual, fairly simple tasks and asked to estimate the time necessary to perform the task, they tend to underestimate how much time it will take to finish the task. Therefore, procrastinators would benefit in practicing telling time. This technique works by providing the procrastinator with varied opportunities to practice estimating how long tasks will take to complete. There is a need, however, for some external criteria against which to compare accuracy estimates. Nevertheless, the general idea is for the procrastinator to focus on time as a concept relevant to completing tasks.

Organizational Skills

Simply by misplacing things needed to perform a task effectively, some people delay task completion. Learning to be more organized is a requisite skill for procrastinators. It is important both to learn to obtain all the necessary supplies associated with completing a task and to arrange them in an orderly fashion. Procrastinators benefit from learning to prioritize, in terms of importance, the steps toward task completion and then tackling first the most important aspects.

Prompts/Reminder Notes

Related to my suggestion about organizational skills, procrastinators also can benefit from simple, physical reminder notes (e.g., Post-it notes) placed in overt locations to remind them to finish a particular task. For example, I place reminders or needed objects right by a door through which I pass. Most executives today carry appointment books and other devices (e.g., palm pilots) to organize, schedule, and remind them to perform certain tasks.

Structure the Setting to Facilitate Task Completion

Too often people do not have an established place in which to concentrate and focus exclusively on a single task. They "work" where there are too many other competing stimuli interfering with task completion. The procrastinator must find a place where s/he can focus exclusively on the target task. For example, if writing is a problem for the student, then designating a table and chair only for studying, reading, and writing will be helpful. If the person wants a snack or a break, s/he must get out of the chair, leave the table, and go some other place. At one end of my office, for example, I have a small round meeting table that I use when I need to meet with students and colleagues. I have tried to discuss important matters at my desk, but surrounded by a computer, telephone, materials on my desk, and family pictures, distractions are very likely. So, when a meeting requires concentration, I move to the roundtable and this helps me block out all other distractions. A little over a week after I introduced the table, I found that this arrangement worked well. Now, I am able to "separate" my office into the "work area" and the "meeting area." Termed "stimulus control," behavioral psychologists have known for decades that such environmental control can effectively facilitate performance. Eliminating distracters (e.g., music, TV, brothers/sisters!) can also help structure the setting to promote task completion for procrastinators (such as studying and reading).

"Bits and Pieces"

It is important to teach procrastinators not to focus on the entire task, but to focus on smaller subunits. Behavioral psychologists talk about the chain of responses needed to perform a particular target end-behavior (a process called "chaining"). In essence, the "bits and pieces" approach to time management is a type of chaining strategy because it encourages the procrastinator to focus and work one piece in the chain before moving to complete the next part of the task. It may be useful to have procrastinators briefly write out the steps needed to perform given tasks, encouraging them to complete tasks step-by-step—checking off those steps completed as a visual reward. Another good strategy involves encouraging the procrastinator to provide him or herself with self-rewards as s/he reaches major steps on the way to the final target goal.

The "5-Minute" Planner

Procrastinators tend to look at the total amount of time needed to complete a task. To counter this propensity, the person needs to break down tasks into smaller components of *time*—brief, 5-minute segments or intervals—instead of focusing on the total amount of time needed for task completion. It is a technique similar to the "bits and pieces" approach, but it focuses on the time needed to complete the steps in the sequence of task completion.

The 80% Success Rule

The procrastinator should not expect to go from "total noncompletion" to "total completion" of all tasks. Instead, it may be more realistic (and obtainable) to begin with a goal of completing at least 80% of the task. Consistent with cognitive-behavioral interventions, achieving 80% of the target task completion in this system warrants some form of reward. This reinforcer may be something the person wants, a desirable activity, or simply praise and self-assurance. It should be noted, however, that 80% of task completion is not the final goal.

The procrastinator must be encouraged (i.e., shaped) to stretch and go beyond a plateau of "almost there." Instead, major reinforcers would be based on reaching the final goal of total completion. Nevertheless, lesser reinforcers are available for reaching 80% of the task along the way toward the final goal.

Social Support for Task Completion

It is important for procrastinators to seek people who complete tasks. Such people provide positive models, whereas peers who also are fellow procrastinators only help to maintain procrastination. Building a social network that supports task completion may involve actively asking acquaintances and friends to be constructive role models. The procrastinator needs to be instructed to consider people as models who frequently "get things done" in a timely manner (who may be considered task-oriented). It is important to be associated with "doers" because they can be asked to provide praise as the procrastinator achieves task completion.

Models of Nonprocrastination

Related to the aforementioned strategy, procrastinators may benefit from seeing others who complete tasks in a timely manner and demonstrate ways that tasks can be performed effectively and efficiently. As noted previously, persons who are more effective at meeting deadlines may be role models for procrastinators. The procrastinator and the model may need to meet regularly and frequently in the initial stages of social learning. The model may also need to verbalize to the procrastinator how and when they perform interim steps toward the target goal. Keep in mind, however, that no one likes to feel belittled or incompetent. Models of nonprocrastination must be sensitive not to appear superior or "better" than the procrastinator, who already has low self-esteem.

Arrange Environmental Contingencies

Procrastinators also must learn that there are consequences for their acts. Too often the excuses made by procrastinators are readily accepted by others—after all, we all have had times when we could not meet a deadline, and the "reason" just sounds plausible. But trouble occurs when people who frequently make excuses become excessive and overly dependent on others. As a result, nonprocrastinators often must "bail out" the procrastinator by either extending the deadline or even completing the task for them. In such circumstances, the procrastinator does not learn that failing to meet deadlines is irresponsible. To facilitate this understanding it is important to have contingencies when procrastinators do not meet deadlines, although rewards are still necessary when procrastinators do achieve their goals. It must be remembered, however, that these contingencies focus on tasks, not on the person. If they associate adverse contingencies with themselves, rather than their behavior, procrastinators because of their low self-esteem are likely to experience an even greater feeling of low self-worth. It is important to stress that the failure to complete the task is the problem, and that the person is not the failure.

Summary

In sum, a set of 10 simple, concrete strategies for treating procrastination have been presented. Psychologists have identified other strategies, but further empirical validation of their effectiveness is warranted. Future researchers should evaluate carefully the strategies alone and collectively so as to ascertain the most effective individual or combined approaches. Researchers conducting such outcome studies would add greatly to the treatment of both situational and dispositional procrastination.

Addressing a "Special" Case of Situational Procrastination—Academic Tasks

Earlier in this chapter, I noted that students vary in their procrastination according to the situational form of a task. They postpone studying or writing a paper but do not procrastinate to attend a favorite concert, watch a favorite TV program, or "hang-out" with close friends. When I began my research program aimed at understanding procrastination in the late 1980s, I found scant published research, but that which did exist focused almost exclusively on treating academic procrastination. Today, researchers have broadened their foci, but we can still gleam some insight from those earlier studies on academic procrastination. I will next review that literature and the associated interventions.

Because students procrastinate so frequently (9), instructors have redesigned courses to facilitate completion of course-related materials. One such technique is the *Personal System of Instruction* (PSI), in which students are instructed to complete course materials at their own pace, and the instructor acts as a facilitator to the student (38). Using applied behavioral analysis principles, the PSI system spread rapidly across colleges and universities in the 1970s and early 1980s. While the concept was intriguing, the use of the PSI to reduce student procrastination in courses that traditionally had the structure and schedules arranged by the instructor proved to be less successful than had been hoped. For example, many students found it difficult to self-pace themselves to complete a course—quite simply, they would procrastinate (39, 40). Bijou, Morris, and Parsons (41) found that by assigning points for each unit of course work a student completed, the procrastination for handing in homework and projects was lessened in comparison to the traditional student, self-paced or instructor-paced course format.

It also has been found that students often postpone studying until just before a major exam. To encourage students to study more often, Wesp (42) implemented daily quizzes on the previous study material and found that overall grades in the course were higher through the use of daily quizzes as compared to grades in courses with traditional infrequent, major exams. Combined with a PSI structure, Wesp (42) argued that the use of frequent quizzes may greatly reduce infrequent study behavior among college students.

Another problem for college students is not completing their academic assignments. Toward this issue, Lamwers and Jazwinski (43) implemented a "course contract," in which the student and instructor agreed on contingencies for completing or not completing the various course tasks. The researchers found that the students with course contracts were more effective in meeting their deadlines than when the instructor simply imposed deadlines or used deadlines plus tokens for task completion. Perhaps having a "say" in when and how tasks are completed encourages students to become more committed to the task and to its completion.

Yet another approach for lessening procrastination is to establish a "guaranteed schedule" in conjunction with a student. Ottens (44) developed just such a schedule for overall semester assignments that was flexible in structure, rewarded task completion instead of intentions, trained students to be self-aware of procrastinating, and identified on- and off-hours for work and relaxation. The author reported that this intervention effectively treated academic procrastination by allowing better management of school-related tasks.

Finally, academic procrastination may be reduced through stress management techniques. Brown (45), for example, found that students who were overly stressed about their school assignments performed better after they had been taught stress reduction techniques such as relaxation exercises.

Most of these techniques are cognitive-behavioral in format. Researchers using such techniques also focus on specific behaviors and on *situational* procrastination. Nevertheless, methods for treating *dispositional* procrastination have been developed, and I will describe those procedures next.

Treating Chronic, Dispositional Procrastination

If the client reports consistent procrastination (across time and locale; from one task to another; and in a wide variety of situations), then treatment involving more than time management skills is needed. Although systematic clinical outcome research on treating chronic procrastination is lacking, Ferrari and his colleagues (1) have discussed approaches for treating chronic adult procrastination.

Similar to treatment strategies for situational procrastination, interventions with chronic procrastination in adults should be multidimensional. In fact, treating chronic procrastination involves some of the same components mentioned discussed previously: (1) increasing environmental cues regarding upcoming deadlines; (2) decreasing cognitions that foster impulsiveness and underestimation of task demands and time for completion; and (3) increasing self-rewards associated with task completion.

How long does it take to reduce a lifetime of habitual procrastination? That depends, but clinical psychologists Johnson and McCown of Ferrari et al.(1) found that without any other mental health or psychiatric concerns associated with the tendency to procrastinate, substantial improvements may be obtained in 12 to 25 sessions of cognitive behavioral psychotherapy. Of course, relapse rates also are high with this population. As a result, at least one-fourth of the total treatment time should be devoted to booster sessions scheduled at progressively longer intervals toward the end of therapy.

Is psychopharmacology needed? Because some forms of chronic procrastination are associated with anxiety and depression (especially in cases of arousal procrastination), medication to reduce the anxieties may be useful for some clients. But anxiolytic anti-depressive drugs do not help most procrastinators, *unless task delays are a symptom of some psychiatric disorder*. In fact, medication can yield the counterproductive effect of fostering an "I couldn't care less" attitude in procrastination clients. Consequently, it is strongly recommended that the chronic procrastinator first receive a complete battery of psychological tests to assess whether task delays are a symptom or the "root" of the person's maladjustment. Using a psychological assessment, the therapist will have a more complete picture of the person's delay tendency. The assessor should seek to determine whether the procrastination suddenly emerged without any substantial previous history (thereby suggesting an association perhaps even of a causative nature with other events), or if it has been a long-lasting, somewhat stable coping pattern. Testing definitely is warranted to answer the important questions related to history and longevity of the procrastination.

Additionally, learning to reduce one's level of stress is helpful to most people. However, caution should be exercised with procrastinators because reducing their life stressors also may further contribute to their tendencies toward not completing tasks. Therefore, it is important to ascertain prior to stress reduction training how stress impacts the client's record of task completions. Because some people become "addicted" to procrastination (especially if they experience a "rush"), stress reduction training needs to be accompanied with cognitive-behavioral therapy to promote appropriate self-statements and the acquisition of new, adaptive skills.

Some therapists also suggest psychoanalysis in the treatment of chronic procrastination (2, 3). Psychodynamic therapists attempt to uncover the unconscious roots of achievement-related event conflicts, and promote transference onto the therapist of any anger that is causing the delay tendencies. Ferrari et al. (1) recommend cognitive-behavioral and behavioral techniques for treating procrastination. If the behavior is discrete and involves a specific event or person, however, a psychodynamic framework may be beneficial in exploring the meaning of the event for the person. At this time, "good" clinical outcome research comparing treatments for procrastination has not been published. Such studies obviously are needed to help in the selection of the "empirically supported" intervention(s) for the fairly prominent problem of procrastination.

Finally, family and group therapies may be useful in treating chronic procrastination. Ferrari and Olivette (26) found that authoritarian parenting promotes the development of procrastination. Recently, Ferrari, Harriott, and Zimmerman (46) reported that chronic procrastinators claimed they had a less deep and more conflictual relationship with their father than with their mother. Thus, family therapy to ascertain what dynamics existed within the immediate household may prove to be a productive route for treatment (or at least for planning treatment and understanding the client). Also, problem-solving interventions that are designed to reduce sibling completion and sabotage or that instruct parents in ways to reward children's task completion should be incorporated into treatments of chronic procrastinators.

In addition, self-help group therapy in which clients model appropriate, successful task completion skills and provide social support to peers may be effective in reducing procrastination. On this latter point, Ferrari et al. (46) found that chronic procrastinators rely on their friends (instead of family members) when they need social support for distress. Thus, it may be that procrastinators can benefit from group intervention with friends rather than receiving guidance from a family member. Again, clinical outcome research is needed to determine which components of group and family therapy contribute to effectively reducing chronic procrastination tendencies.

Conclusions

Throughout this chapter, I have emphasized empirical findings to differentiate situational from dispositional procrastination, and how treatment protocols need to focus on these two target domains. Time management and behavioral interventions that are strictly adhered to are effective for situational procrastination, while cognitive-behavioral interventions work well to reduce dispositional, chronic procrastination. Regardless of the type of procrastination, I believe that a multifocused intervention package is needed. At this point, I believe that practitioners with a variety of techniques that can be used simultaneously will yield the best treatment outcomes for procrastination. Clinical outcome research is needed to determine which components of the intervention package are more or less effective. Until such research is done and published, using a set of interventions is the best strategy.

In summary, procrastination has affective, behavioral, and cognitive components, and labeling it simply as "laziness" is neither sufficient nor correct. The time is *now* for quality clinical research on treating the "thief of time."

Acknowledgments
This chapter was funded in part through a 1999 DePaul University Summer Research Stipend awarded to the author. Portions of the paper were presented at the first "International Meeting on Counseling the Procrastinator" (1999, August) in Toronto, Canada. The author expresses gratitude for assistance in writing this paper to Christine Jeuland, Aoife Lyons, and Corey Hammer for technical support, and C. R. Snyder, Tim Pychyl, Clarry Lay, Steve Scher, and Bill Knaus for constructive comments on the direction for writing this paper.

References

1. Ferrari, J. R., Johnson, J., & McCown, W. (1995). *Procrastination: Theory, research, and treatment.* New York: Plenum Publications.
2. Birner, L. (1993). Procrastination: Its role in transference and countertransference. *Psychoanalytic Review, 80,* 541–558.
3. Giovacchini, P. L. (1975). Productive procrastination: Technical factors in the treatment of the adolescent. In S. C. Feinstein & P. Giovacchini (Eds.), *Annual of Adolescent Psychiatry* (pp 352–370). New York: Aronson.
4. Ferrari, J. R., & Pychyl, T. (1999). *Procrastination: Current issues and future directions.* Corte Madera, CA: Select Press.
5. Ellis, A., & Knaus, W. (1977). *Overcoming procrastination.* New York: Institute for Rational Living.
6. Knauss, W. (2000). Procrastination, blame, and change. *Journal of Social Behavior and Personality, 15,* 153–166.
7. Ferrari, J. R., Keane, S., Wolfe, R., & Beck, B. (1998). The antecedents and consequences of academic excuse-making: Examining individual differences in procrastination. *Research in Higher Education, 39,* 199–215.
8. Ferrari, J. R., Wolfe, R., Wesley, J., Schoff, & Beck, B. (1995). Ego-identity and academic procrastination among university students. *Journal of College Student Development, 36,* 361–367.

9. Solomon, L., & Rothblum, E. (1984). Academic procrastination: Frequency and cognitive-behavioral correlates. *Journal of Counseling Psychology, 31*, 503–509.

10. Rothblum, E., Solomon, L., & Murakami, J. (1986). Affective, cognitive, and behavioral differences between high and low procrastinators. *Journal of Counseling Psychology, 33*, 387–394.

11. Ferrari, J. R., & Scher, S. (2000). Toward an understanding of academic and nonacademic tasks procrastinated by students. *Psychology in the Schools, 34*, 359–366.

12. Scher, S., & Ferrari, J. R. (2000). The recall of completed and noncompleted tasks through daily logs to measure procrastination. *Journal of Social Behavior and Personality, 15*, 255–265.

13. Scher, S., & Ferrari, J. R. (1999). *Procrastination: A task analysis approach.* Manuscript under review.

14. Harriott, J., & Ferrari, J. R. (1996). Prevalence of procrastination in adult samples. *Psychological Report, 78*, 611–616.

15. Hammer, C., & Ferrari, J. R. (1999). *Procrastination prevalence among adults: Midwest vs. northeast United States.* Unpublished manuscript. DePaul University, 2219 North Kenmore Avenue, Chicago, IL, 60614.

16. Ferrari, J. R. (1992b). Psychometric validation of two adult measures of procrastination: Arousal and avoidance measures. *Journal of Psychopathology and Behavioral Assessment, 14*, 97–100.

17. Snyder, C. R., Higgins, R. L., & Stucky, R. (1983). *Excuses: Masquerades in search of grace.* New York: Wiley.

18. Zuckerman, M. (1991). *Psychobiology of personality.* Cambridge, England: Cambridge University Press.

19. Ferrari, J. R. (1993a). Christmas and procrastination: Explaining lack of diligence at a "real-world" task deadline. *Personality and Individual Differences, 14*, 25–33.

20. Ferrari, J. R. (1993b). Procrastination and impulsivity: Two sides of a coin? In W. McCown, M. B. Shure, & J. Johnson (Eds.), *The impulsive client: Theory, research, and treatment* (pp. 265–271). Washington, DC: American Psychological Association.

21. Ferrari, J. R., & Specter, M. (1999). *Speed-accuracy tradeoffs by procrastinators: Effects of cognitive load and self-awareness.* Unpublished manuscript. DePaul University, 2219 North Kenmore Avenue, Chicago, IL, 60614.

22. Ferrari, J. R. (1991). Self-handicapping by procrastinators: Protecting self-esteem, social-esteem, or both? *Journal of Research in Personality, 25*, 245–261.

23. Ferrari, J. R. (1998). Procrastination. In H. Friedman (Ed.), *Encyclopedia of Mental Health, Vol. 3* (pp 281–287). San Diego, CA: Academic Press.

24. Burka, J. B., & Yuen, L. M. (1983). *Procrastination: Why you do it and what to do about it.* Reading, PA: Addison-Wesley.

25. Ferrari, J. R., & McCown, W. (1994). Procrastination tendencies among obsessive-compulsives and their relatives. *Journal of Clinical Psychology, 50*, 162–167.

26. Ferrari, J. R., & Olivette, M. (1994). Parental authority influences in the

development of female dysfunctional procrastination. *Journal of Research in Personality, 28,* 87–100.

27. Ferrari, J. R. (1994). Dysfunctional procrastination and its relationship to self-esteem, interpersonal dependency, and self-defeating behaviors. *Personality and Individual Differences, 17,* 673–679.

28. Rorer, L. G. (1983). "Deep" RET: A reformulation of some psychodynamic explanations of procrastination. *Cognitive Therapy and Research, 7,* 1–10.

29. Claiborn, C. D., Ward, S. R., & Strong, S. R. (1981). Effects of congruence between counselor interpretations and client beliefs. *Journal of Counseling Psychology, 28,* 101–109.

30. Strong, S. R., Wambach, C. A., Lopez, F. G., & Cooper, R. K. (1979). Motivational and equipping functions of interpretation in counseling. *Journal of Counseling Psychology, 26,* 98–107.

31. Ishiyama, F. I. (1990a). A Japanese perspective on client inaction: Removing attitudinal blocks through Morita therapy. *Journal of Counseling and Development, 68,* 566–570.

32. Ishiyama, F. I. (1990b). Japanese perspective on client inaction: Morita therapy. *International Journal for the Advancement of Counseling, 13,* 119–128.

33. Ferrari, J. R., & Beck, B. (1998). Affective responses before and after fraudulent excuses by academic procrastinators. *Education, 118,* 529–537.

34. Damsteegt, D. C., & Christoffersen, J. (1982). Objective self-awareness as a variable in counseling process and outcome. *Journal of Counseling Psychology, 29,* 421–424.

35. Ferrari, J. R. (1992a). Procrastinators and perfect behavior: An exploratory factor analysis of self-presentation, self-awareness, and self-handicapping components. *Journal of Research in Personality, 26,* 75–84.

36. Specter, M., & Ferrari, J. R. (2000). Time orientation perceptions among procrastinators: Focusing on the past, present, or future? *Journal of Social Behavior and Personality, 15,* 197–202.

37. Lay, C. H. (1988). The relation of procrastination and optimism to judgements of time to complete an essay and anticipation of setbacks. *Journal of Social Behavior and Personality, 3,* 210–214.

38. Keller, F. S. (1968). "Good-bye, teacher . . ." *Journal of Applied Behavior Analysis, 1,* 79–89.

39. Born, D. G., & Moore, M. C. (1978). Some belated thoughts on pacing. *Journal of Personalized Instruction, 3,* 33–36.

40. Reiser, R. A. (1984). Reducing student procrastination in a personalized system of instruction course. *Educational Curriculum and Teaching Journal, 32,* 41–49.

41. Bijou, S. W., Morris, E. K., & Parsons, J. A. (1976). A PSI course in child development with a procedure for reducing student procrastination. *Journal of Personalized Instruction, 1,* 36–40.

42. Wesp, R. (1986). Reducing procrastination through required course involvement. *Teaching of Psychology, 13,* 128–130.

43. Lamwers, L. L., & Jazwinski, C. H. (1989). A comparison of three strat-

egies to reduce student procrastination in PSI. *Teaching of Psychology,*
16, 8–12.

44. Ottens, A. J. (1982). A guaranteed scheduling technique to manage students' procrastination. *College Student Journal, 16*, 371–376.

45. Brown, R. T. (1991). Helping students confront and deal with stress and procrastination. *Journal of College Student Psychotherapy, 6*, 87–102.

46. Ferrari, J. R., Harriott, J., & Zimmerman, M. (1999). The social support networks of procrastinators: Friends or family in times of trouble? *Personality and Individual Differences*, 26, 321–334.

3

Coping and Coherence:
A Narrative Perspective on Resilience

Robert A. Neimeyer
Heidi Levitt

S ocial life abounds with the making and telling of stories. From
Sesame Street to the nightly news, and from oral traditions to
electronic media, we are constantly regaled with stories of characters, imagined or real, undertaking motivated actions toward some implicit or explicit
end. Such stories are told to instruct, inform, entertain, challenge—indeed,
the reasons for constructing and sharing narratives are nearly as diverse as
the stories themselves. On a personal level, too, our lives are saturated with
narrative exchanges, as we share accounts of our day with loved ones, relate
a troubling incident to a friend, explain our actions by placing them in a
clarifying context, or write a summary of the events of the past year to send
out with a holiday letter. Sometimes we even construct stories whose only
intended audience is ourselves, as when we record personal experiences
in narrative form in a travel log or personal diary. Our purpose in this
chapter is to reflect on this characteristically human impulse, and consider
its significance for how we cope with adverse life events. In particular, we
will draw attention to the process and structure of narrative activity and
the ways in which our attempts to formulate experience in storied terms
can "break down," compromising our ability to make sense of our past and
give direction to our future. Throughout, we will include thoughts on strategies for narrative repair that carry implications for psychotherapy in particular and coping more generally.

What Is a Narrative?

We begin with a definition of terms, distinguishing what narrative is from
what it is not. Although it is seemingly ubiquitous, narration is not the only
way of imparting symbolic order to human experience; graphic, mathe-

matical, and logical systems also provide means of representing and manipulating meanings, and yet they lack the essential features that distinguish narrative activity (1). What, then, are the special characteristics of narratives, and what implications do they carry for our understanding of coping functions? We turn to these questions next.

In its most basic form, narrative has been defined as an account in which one or more characters, each with their own intentionality, undertake a real or imagined, and mental or physical, action within the story (2). The characters in our narratives commonly include our friends, family, associates, and even enemies, whose fortes and foibles—at least from the perspective of the teller—are revealed by their actions and interactions in the story-world that we construct. A special class of storytelling consists of self-narratives or autobiographical accounts whose chief protagonist is the narrator. But whether the central character of the story is the self or another, narratives tell at least as much about their narrators as they do about the people whose experiences they purport to describe. Information about narrators is disclosed not only through their self-descriptions, but also through the manner in which storytellers selectively portray events that correspond to their motives, goals, life themes, and conflicts.

The Narrative Perspective

Narrative psychology has been gaining momentum over the last fifteen years since its inception in the 1980s (3–5). This movement is composed of cognitive scientists, developmental psychologists, clinical researchers, and psychotherapists who have found important clues in narratives about people's organizations of their experiences, as well as how such storied constructions can be reorganized in the psychotherapy process.

At the core of this approach is the belief that people give meaning to their experiences by using a storytelling structure. This understanding is in contrast to previous models of thinking rooted in rationality, logic, and, more recently, computer-programming (6). Narrative plots do not need to be organized along lines of logical or "if-then" reasoning; rather, such plots are organized along a time line, and within themes that may be shaped by idiosyncratic emotional and associational meanings. The history of our relationships, for example, often includes a conglomeration of smaller stories or "micronarratives" that we synthesize into a more encompassing life story or "macronarrative" (7). Stories at both levels, however, may include contradictory sentiments, opposing perspectives, or irrational conclusions.

For instance, if I evaluate a relationship with a friend, certain memories may suggest a very strong mutual fidelity whereas others may imply that this same person is not a friend at all. In deciding whether I would like to build my relationship with this individual, I could weave these micronarratives into a broader story about our relationship, adding contextual factors that would help me to weigh these different experiences. If my friend neglected our relationship while she was experiencing a family crisis, I might find that I could accept this neglect when contrasted with her typical attentiveness at other times. This process of constructing a macronarrative facilitates my making sense of our relationship and, in this case, may help in my decision to attribute a certain behavior to situational factors and to maintain our friendship.

Another important tenet of narrative psychology is the rejection of objectivism or foundationalism as the basis of the conceptualization of our experience (8, 9). This means that stories are not necessarily anchored in an external truth, but instead represent distinctively human constructions that reflect the social and personal perspectives of the communities and individuals who tell them. For this reason, the stories two people tell about the "same" event may differ, and yet each can yield important insights into the meanings that shape each person's perspective and responses. Consider, for example, the disparate accounts of a breakup of a long-term intimate relationship as told from the perspective of two partners. What is at issue here is not which partner is judged to be right—although this may be a crucial issue for the partners, as they try to win support for their version of the situation! Instead, we would suggest that what matters more in this scenario is how each partner configures an account of the experience that "works" for him or her in the context of his or her surrounding social system. Thus, ferreting out "the facts" usually is not relevant in this constructivist epistemology, because human realities always are considered to be ordered and formulated from a given perspective and in accordance with the cultural conventions of a given place and time. Thus, constructivists attempt to examine not only what a given story *tells*—the content of the experiences it relates—but also what it *does*, in the way that it positions the self and others in a relational field (10, 11).

What makes narrations so compelling to constructivist psychotherapists is how they impart a distinctively personal structure to a flow of events and do so in ways that are coherent with a particular model of self (12). Indeed, identity can be seen as a composite of remembered life narratives—of personal history—that together define our enduring concerns and future expectations (13–15). For instance, if the stories of my life transitions typically conclude with my deciding on the most predictable and secure course of action, I may come to define myself as someone who does not embrace change and who may plan to avoid it in the future. Furthermore, my accounts of experiences and my interpretations of these stories may gradually consolidate to form a master narrative of my life, taking on the status of an established identity when they are validated in the stories told about me by relevant others.

Narration can be seen as a basic human need. Clients in counseling often report that the telling of their stories was a crucial aspect of their therapy experience (16, 17). We relate our stories to others, both to engage in an interpersonal process that allows us to better formulate our narratives and to seek validation for our experiences. Despite our drive to communicate, we often are unable to represent our experience fully in our telling. In the process of conveying our experience, language is fundamental, constraining and molding themes in accordance with the building blocks that it provides (3, 18). Similarly, the culture in which our language and experiences are embedded can constrain our narrative construction by promoting certain culturally endorsed themes while ignoring or criticizing other possible stories (19). For example, the emphasis on American rugged individualism and self-determination may lead us to construct accounts of misfortunes that emphasize individual, rather than social responsibility for these outcomes (20).

How can an appreciation of narratives enrich our understanding of what it means to cope effectively with difficult life events? In the remainder of this chapter, we will address this question by considering the process and structure of narratives in more detail, illustrating their breakdown and repair in the context of actual case examples. By formulating coping as a narrative endeavor, we are advancing a framework in which people are viewed as "motivated storytellers" (21), an approach that helps us think in an integrated fashion about adaptation and self-change.

Narrative Process and Structure

To go beyond an intuitive understanding of stories as coping resources, it is useful to look more closely at their process and structure, at how they are told, and what they include. As we use the term, narrative *process* refers to the perspective taken by the narrator on the experience being related—whether it is being described from an internal, external, or reflexive vantage point (7). In contrast, the *structure* of the narrative refers to its essential features, including dimensions of setting, characterization, plot, theme, and fictional goal (11). We find this way of approaching coping narratives helpful because of its flexibility and applicability to informal accounts of stressful events in our day-to-day lives, to problem-focused writing in a personal journal, and to the narrative exchanges in formal helping contexts such as counseling or psychotherapy. Although communal storytelling in the form of cultural myths (22) or planned or improvisational performances (23) certainly can function as powerful coping resources, our focus will be on the more personal level of self-narratives, in which the goal is to explore, integrate, and validate the meaning of difficult life experiences. We will therefore begin with a brief consideration of narrative process and structure before applying these concepts to an illustrative self-narrative written by a young woman attempting to come to terms with a profound loss.

Narrative Process

In the process of constructing stories, we use different types of narration. The Narrative Processes theory is a model of psychotherapy process that outlines three different modes of psychotherapeutic narration: *external, internal*, and *reflexive* narrative processes (7, 24). Based upon this model, the Narrative Processes Coding System (25) has been developed for the purpose of identifying both narrative topics and processes. In this section, the understanding of narrative processes allows for a new perspective on the meaning of coping (for more information on narrative topics, see Hardke [26]. In the forthcoming sections, segments of a mock-therapy transcript will be analyzed to demonstrate types of narrative process and to provide a basis for discussing their coping properties. Although this section draws upon a psychotherapeutic context, narrative processes can be identified within most exploratory forms of communication, and this understanding can be extended easily to written journal entries, interview dialogue, or self-exploration.

External Narrative Processes   External narrative processes entail the description of an event or issue. This narrative process is labeled "external" because the narrator is focused on conveying to the audience in a clear, intelligible fashion the happenings of the story at hand. In this sense, the speaker's focus is outward. This narrative process is the form of communication that most closely corresponds with common forms of written narration, such as journalistic reporting and most fictional writing, and it concentrates heavily on the dimensions of plot, characterization, and theme as described subsequently. Consequently, many of the elements of structure discussed in the previous section are most relevant within this external narrative process.

External narrative processes are helpful because they allow the listener to understand the situation being presented *as it is understood by the speaker*. Likewise, journal entries often begin with the recounting of an event so that any forthcoming exploration can be understood in light of the details of that event. For instance, after experiencing a troubling interaction, a female client in a psychotherapy session might begin the following discourse:

> C: I went to the library yesterday. I sat down and began sorting through some of the bus scheduling information and this scragglylooking man came in and, as he walked by me, said, "Hello." To be polite, I said, "Hello," and I kept reading. He took a seat at a table facing me and kept looking at me. He was obviously not well-off and there was something strange-looking in his face. He didn't look deranged or even really rude, but he just looked very entitled. There was no question for him about staring at me all he liked. I ignored him as best as I could, not wanting to deal with him but wanting to continue on with my own activity. I read most of the information but then decided to just continue at home. But then when I got up to leave, he got up to leave also.
>
> T: Oh! What happened then?

C: Well, I meandered about in the library, hoping he would be long gone by the time I exited. But when I left he was waiting under a tree outside the main doors. I cut across the parking lot to avoid him and saw him move toward his car. So then I began walking in the opposite direction of traffic so that he couldn't come along side of me. I was walking pretty calmly, but keeping an eye peeled for his car. And then I saw him drive by, pull a U-turn, and stop his car right in front of me anyway. He offered me a lift and I declined it rather firmly and walked away in the opposite direction that his car was now facing.

It is within this narrative process that the structural qualities discussed previously can be identified. Relaying our experience within an external narrative process can help us to integrate the way situational factors may have affected our responses. The contextualization of experiences within difficult situations can allow individuals to experience a self-compassion that may be needed to help break patterns of depression and self-criticism (27). The external process of representing situational contraints and pressures can help narrators to develop an understanding of their behavior that can help them cope with their pasts and reshape their future identities.

Language clarity, concreteness, and specificity have been associated with external discourse in therapy (28, 29), and Bucci (28) suggests that these qualities of speech might best stimulate clients' associations and early memories for exploration. At this point, for instance, a therapist might ask the client to describe the entitlement in this man's demeanor and then to explore her early associations to entitlement. This quality of narrative evocativeness can be enhanced in relation to structural factors other than characterization as well, such as the description of setting or theme. Therapists who wish to enhance descriptiveness in client's speech may choose to model evocative language to induce clients into a similar level of detail or to instruct clients explicitly to paint a richly detailed scene (perhaps using Guidano's [29] moviola technique described subsequently). In journal writing, personal assignments can accomplish much the same goal.

Internal Narrative Processes   Internal narrative processes focus upon the speaker's emotional and experiential responses to a situation, event, or issue. Narrators are inwardly exploring and moving into contact with feelings, and, as a result, discourse tends to be presented in a less grammatical form than is typical of the external narrative process.

For instance, if the dialogue above continued in an internal narrative process, it might read as follows:

T: How did you feel after this episode?
C: I felt just stunned. I felt like, like—I was shocked—or was surprised that this developed from a simple "hello." I was angry too. Yeah, angry, definitely, that someone would make me feel so uncomfortable. Upset, just really upset.

In terms of coping, the process of exploring emotion may help storytellers to develop an enhanced awareness or differentiation of their feelings that, in turn, could lead to the exploration of new options or responses. Techniques in therapy that can assist in enhancing this process include Gendlin's (30) focusing, as well as process-experiential exercises (27), both of which support and guide clients to sustain states of internally focused exploration.

For instance, in the above dialogue, a therapist might decide to engage the client in an empty-chair dialogue, asking the client to imagine the presence of the stalker and to express to him, in the safety of the therapy room, the emotion that might have been unsafe to express during the incident. A corresponding journaling exercise can be envisioned in which one could decide to write exclusively in an internal narrative process for a certain period of time in order to come into contact with feelings that arise (31).

Reflexive Narrative Processes Reflexive narrative processes include analytical endeavors to make meaning of an event, thought, or emotional experience. It is within this process that narrators engage in activities such as planning, evaluating, contemplating, and interpreting the events described and their stance with reference to them. A reflexive continuation of the dialogue might read as follows:

T: Why do you think you were so upset by this incident?
C: I was upset because I didn't do anything to this person and he went out of his way to make me feel uncomfortable when it was very obvious that I was trying to avoid contact with him. I felt like it was another reminder of my being female, of my being less powerful than, and, and . . . also of my need to be defensive to be safe. And, of course, this is what I seem to be always struggling with—at home with my father, at work with my boss, and in my relationship with my husband. Always feeling that somehow I have to work to prove myself equal and worthy of respect or otherwise I won't receive it. I always need to work to defend myself. I think that this is especially affecting my relationship with my husband. I don't want to be defensive all the time.

The reflexive process allows narrators to derive meanings from their story that can assist them both in synthesizing their experiences and in identifying coping styles. The recognition of patterns of experience, feeling, and thinking often can motivate clients to begin planning new coping strategies and to examine their behavioral choices. Toward this end, most therapies incorporate the production of a macronarrative that highlights an individual's coping patterns as an important step in treatment.

In psychodynamic therapies, clients are helped to conceptualize the unconscious motivations that may have been influencing their methods of coping across situations (32, 33). In cognitive therapies, clients are taught to observe negative coping patterns in their cognition across situations (34). Similarly, in humanistic therapies, clients are encouraged to take notice of experiential or emotion-processing patterns that they repeat across situations (27). Finally, in some constructivist methods, respondents explicitly are invited to reflect on myriad micronarratives that involved their coping successfully with adversity, and then to articulate the "dependable strengths" on which they relied and on which they could draw in the future (35). The step of developing a coping macronarrative in therapy helps to frame the therapeutic endeavor in narrative terms that make sense to the client and helps to establish a "preferred story" of the client's identity anchored in the particularities of his or her life (36).

Additionally, the reflexive narrative process may have a unique role in coping. Because it is within the reflexive analysis of our experience that we interpret our behaviors as reactions to challenges, the very construal of our behavior *as* coping can be understood as a product of reflexivity. Upon reviewing our life story we can begin to see the various forms of resilience that shaped our behavior, allowing us to construct an identity for ourselves as "copers." Although we might react to hardships prior to the development of a narrative conceptualization, reflection is required for our labeling of our reaction as "coping" and our conscious consideration of our behavior as such. Reflexive processes allow us to identify ourselves as agents, who respond in characteristic styles and with varying degrees of effectiveness. Reflexively examining our micronarratives of difficult situations permits the identification of overarching macronarratives that allow for the construction of both a sense of personal continuity, as well as the possible extension or reconsideration of our identities and coping styles in response to future challenges. Having discussed the three processes within which narratives are constructed, we will now turn our attention to their basic structure, illustrating key concepts with actual psychotherapeutic examples.

Narrative Structure

Narrative psychologists have devised a number of systems for analyzing the structure of stories (37, 38), each of which has potential advantages. Our preference for focusing on the dimensions of setting, characterization, plot, theme, and fictional goal (11) derives from their correspondence with features of narratives identified by literary theorists and from their focus on features of narratives that facilitate or impede coping.

Setting The setting of a narrative refers to the "where and when" of the account; it establishes a meaningful context in which the story unfolds, in a way that makes it intelligible to both the storyteller and the audience. The "setting work" done in constructing a narrative frame for an experience can be minimal or elaborate; it can simply signal the time and place in which the story unfolds or provide rich details that make the story "come alive" for the author and audience.[1] Often, for example, problem narratives are told in such a way that their setting is implicit, taken-for-granted, or assumed, in a fashion that tends to fix the account and make it harder for the storyteller to see the experience in a new perspective. In such circumstances, it is helpful to "objectify" the narrative by anchoring it in more sensory detail, inviting the speaker to recreate the visual, auditory, tactile, or kinesthetic context in which the story took place, as a prelude to grasping a new significance in old events (39).

An example of this arose in a recent therapeutic conversation with a young woman, Annie, whose father had died four months earlier, and who was guilty and conflicted about whether to return to complete her university education in a distant city or stay with her grieving and "needy" mother in her hometown. Previous well-meaning conversations with friends about her deeply felt dilemma had focused on weighing the costs and benefits of each course of action, advising her on compromise solutions, and focusing on "her needs" rather than those of others. But none of these conversations moved her beyond an emotional impasse. Characteristically, Annie began to relate her story to her therapist in the same straightforward fashion she had in these earlier tellings, providing setting for the story in a succinctly worded sentence or two, and then moving directly into the emotional dilemma and attendant guilt with which she was wrestling. Progress was made when the therapist switched tacks and invited her to "unpack" the last vivid memory she had of her father, asking her to close her eyes and visualize the setting in all of its detail. Tears came to Annie as she reconstructed the scene: a party her father had proudly arranged for her to celebrate her academic success following her first year at college. Using a "moviola" metaphor borrowed from filmmaking (29), the therapist then asked her to gradually tighten the focus of her visualization to her father's face and eyes, envisioning in them the impish glint and proud expression she had come to prize. With gentle prompting, Annie then expressed her dilemma directly to him and waited quietly for his response. Within seconds, Annie brightened and opened her eyes, proclaiming that the problem had been resolved in a flash of "epiphany." By re-entering the story of her struggle in an experientially vivid way, she had figuratively "brought to life" her deceased father and immediately grasped the emotional truth of their relationship: that he would be equally proud of her academic achievements and of her caring so deeply for her family that she would be willing to sacrifice her educational goals for her mother's well-being. Thus, affirmed in the macronarrative of herself as both hard-working and compassionate, Annie "dissolved" the problem in an instant, resolving to return to school but maintain caring contact with her mother, and felt it entirely unnecessary to return for a second session of psychotherapy. Similar strategies of visualization for promoting an immediate "experiential shift" in a client's "symptom position" are illustrated by Ecker and Hulley (40, 41).

Characterization   The characterization of a narrative refers to the "who" of the story, its "landscape of intentionality" (3) defined in terms of the subjective worlds of the protagonist, antagonist, and supporting characters.

Difficulties can arise when the characterization of the people in the story is thin and unexamined, or when the only subjective position from which the story is viewed is that of the narrator. In such cases, it can be helpful to prompt a more empathic engagement with the intentionality of other important characters or even with different aspects of the narrator construed as autonomous "subselves" (42).

An example of the former gambit arose in the first session of marital therapy with Dan and Lisa, each of whom came primed to complain of the other's culpability in their mutual unhappiness and growing estrangement. Within minutes of beginning the session, it became clear that each partner's story was well rehearsed, having been repeated many times in an attempt to garner support from friends and family for their respective interpretations of their marital conflict. Equally clear was the very limited extent to which each incorporated the other's perspective into his or her account of their struggle, leaving the partner feeling immediately defensive and using the spouse's "talk time" to rehearse his or her counter argument. In an attempt to open the story to new possibilities, the therapist suggested a novel arrangement—that each person take turns telling the story of their difficulties *as if from the partner's perspective*. Initially surprised, Dan and Lisa then gamely started over, struggling to portray the other's point of view regarding their own role in the conflict. As a result, each began to glimpse the rather different interpretive set being brought to bear by the partner, as well as the limitations in his or her understanding of the spouse's thoughts, feelings, and motives. Just as interesting, the dynamics of listening transformed the perspective of each spouse from one of defensive preparation for a counterattack, to interested engagement with the spouse's story as a means of gauging its accuracy as a reflection of the listener's actual perspective. This experiment in "hypothetical reverse other questioning" thus set the stage for a very different account of Dan and Lisa's relationship problem, one that invited more collaboration than competition in the telling.

Plot   The plot of a story refers to the "what" of the narrative, the sequence of events that fit together into a more or less meaningful account. At a general level, coping processes are intrinsic to the plot structure of our micronarratives: our day-to-day stories hinge on how protagonists face challenges, decide how to deal with them, and then deal with the consequences of their decisions (43). As applied to self-narratives, the integration of events into a narrative plot also implies that we give shape to our sense of ourselves as unique persons by reconfiguring our moment-to-moment experiences into a life story, one made recognizable as our own through its consolidation into a coherent emotional style (44). While this ongoing effort to transform the vicissitudes of lived experience into a relatively consistent narrative identity is never fully complete, it can fail utterly in the face of events so discrepant with the perceived plot of our lives that they resist integration in any form. The experience of psychological trauma is one example (45).

An illustration of the therapeutic attempt to "emplot" a traumatic incident by relating it in a meaningful sequence arose in the course of therapy with Mark, a man in his 40's who had been violently assaulted by a gang of four young men. Pistol whipping him to the ground, two of the men had proceeded to kick Mark in the abdomen and chest, rupturing several organs and shattering his rib cage, as a third held the gun on him to discourage his desperate resistance. The fourth and most violent of the men concentrated his assault on Mark's face and head, kicking out all his teeth, breaking his jaw, and fracturing his skull in the process. Eventually, Mark lost consciousness and awoke to find himself in a hospital, where he was gradually rehabilitated and received a series of seven reconstructive surgeries to restore a semblance of his former face. No surgeries, however, could restore a semblance of his former life, as Mark lost his job, his marriage, and, in his words, his sense of "who I am" in the panicked, angry, and depressive months following his discharge.

A central focus of therapy with Mark was sifting through the horrific experience of the assault, allowing him to tell the story in all its vivid immediacy, in a way that he had been unable to do with others. As the events of that horrific experience began to consolidate into a coherent account rather than simply a jumble of emotionally charged images, Mark was able to begin considering how the attack fit into the larger pattern of who he had been, who he was now, and who he might yet become. A useful technique at this point in therapy was a "biographical grid" procedure (45, 46), which prompted Mark first to recall and then to compare and contrast critical life experiences that had shaped his sense of who he was. Beginning with preschool memories of independently riding his tricycle to the neighborhood swimming pool, Mark nominated a series of symbolically significant events, including the recent assault, and extrapolated beyond them into an imagined future. What emerged was a chronology that made better sense of the assault, which recapitulated much of the anger, uncertainty, and helplessness of his early childhood, when his father was nearly killed in an industrial accident, and Mark was functionally orphaned while his mother left town to care for her husband. Likewise, other micronarratives of his boyhood (e.g., resisting the bullying of older youths in high school by fighting back against impossible odds) echoed his vain but valiant attempts to resist his four assailants, even at the potential cost of his life. As a result of this emotionally intense life review, Mark was able to gradually assimilate the assault into the larger macronarrative of his life, whose coping themes of being a "fighter" and being resilient in the face of overwhelming loss served him well in his attempt to transcend his recent trauma.

Theme   The theme of a narrative represents its "why," providing a deeper level meaning for the emplotted events that constitute the story's surface structure. Unlike plot, which is usually explicitly represented in the story, theme is more often implicit, inferred, and brought into focal awareness only when violated. This sort of invalidation of a taken-for-granted "assumptive world" (47) frequently results in profound reverberations in the individual's meaning system, triggering a painful process of reappraisal before the viable themes of the preexisting life narrative can be reinstated or new themes established (11).

An example of this thematic invalidation occurred in the course of therapy with Brad, a trim and athletic entrepreneur who at age 40 had worked hard to build up his aging father's family business. Recently, however, he seemed beset with problems of Jobian proportions: his beloved grandmother had died two weeks before, a suit against his father by a disgruntled customer named him as a defendant, and his father's cyclic depression had returned with a vengeance. To compound Brad's turmoil, his wife Sara, herself being treated for depression, had discontinued her medication in an attempt to conceive a second child and had begun to experience wild mood swings that left Brad feeling depleted and abandoned when he needed her most. While these converging events were enough in themselves to disrupt the previously orderly and progressive narrative of his life, Brad sensed vaguely that more was at stake than simply his "stress level." Indeed, although he initially coped with these adverse events in characteristic fashion by redoubling his routine of working out and practicing yoga, these customary means of relaxing seemed less and less effective, and he found himself increasingly "paralyzed" to take action on any front.

Suspecting that Brad's life story had been disrupted at the level of theme as well as plot, his therapist prompted him to reflect on what the several stressful events had in common. Brad paused a moment, and then looked up and said, "I feel like I'm being *punished* without having done anything wrong," then fell silent for another moment and added, "I just feel *powerless*." With therapist prompting, he then rank ordered his recent misfortunes and immediately recognized that the two that were most debilitating for him—the lawsuit and Sara's moodiness—shared the additional feature of *unpredictability*. Collectively, these meanings clashed directly with the thematic underpinning of his prior macronarrative, which was based on the tacit assumptions that good efforts would be fairly rewarded, that important life events were chiefly within his control, and that a well-planned life would be predictable. Upon grasping this insight into the deeper significance of his current suffering, Brad felt much of his anxiety and anger fall away and tentatively voiced the conclusion that the recent turn of events was "God's way of telling me that bad things can happen that are out of my control." After sitting quietly for a moment with this newfound awareness, Brad and his therapist began to reformulate the disruptive plot developments in his self-narrative as promptings to undertake a "spiritual journey" whose goal would be to review and revise the thematic structure on which his life had been built.

Fictional Goal   Just as the theme of a narrative refers to the "why" behind its plot, the fictional goal of a story refers to its "wherefore," the overarching teleology that gives it a distinctive direction (11). In a constructivist view, the superordinate goal around which a self-narrative is organized is fictional, not because it is "untrue" in some objective sense, but because it is fashioned or invented by the narrator.[2] This does not imply, however, that the deepest goal structure of our personal life stories is necessarily clear to us—indeed, recognizing it beneath the welter of micronarrative interactions often requires a level of reflexivity that is rare in our day-to-day lives. Teasing out our fictional goals can be all the more daunting a task when they are tightly interwoven with those of another person who figures prominently in the plot of our self-narrative, and when we play an important role in the life story of that other person. In such cases, our lives can come to resemble a postmodern play, in which two dramatically different productions are taking place on stage at the same time, with the actors in each respective cast interactively triggering developments in the parallel story being enacted, without ever understanding their full impact.

Something of this sort developed for Brad and Sara, the couple described under the preceding section on theme. In the course of their therapy, both partners repeatedly (and heatedly) recounted micronarratives in which Brad would invite, demand, or plead for Sara to participate in some activity with his family of origin, only to be met with her lack of interest, refusal, or resentful capitulation to his request. The focus of these expectations varied from birthday parties for adult siblings to weekly brunches with his parents, but the recurrent outcome was the same: Brad ended up feeling hurt and desperate, and Sara was left feeling angry and coerced. What made the situation more perplexing was that at a surface level there was little either partner could point to to justify his or her reaction. Brad's family seemed less demanding of Sara's participation than Brad himself, and the family occasions, while perhaps a bit too predictable, were hardly "toxic" enough to account for Sara's aversion. The situation came to a head when the couple was on vacation and began discussing how to apportion their limited souvenir budget to buy gifts for their respective 12- and 13-year-old nephews. Sara immediately selected a Mickey Mouse baseball cap for her nephew, but resisted Brad's purchase of a similar gift for his nephew, justifying it on the basis of the greater economic "privilege" of Brad's family. For his part, Brad defended the purchase, citing his nephew's social ineptitude, and how wrong it would be to "leave him out." This response automatically triggered a fight about the many times Brad had attempted to invite the two nephews to do something together with them, only to have Sara's nephew tease his somewhat overweight and awkward cousin, and Sara to resist further efforts to bring the two together. The situation was never resolved, and both spouses brought the story of their stubborn standoff into their next therapy session.

Rather than debate the rational merits of each point of view—a strategy that the couple had repeatedly tried without success—the therapist pursued an experiential probe into the fictional goal implicit in each partner's account. Turning first to Brad, he asked him to close his eyes, take a moment to visualize the pudgy and tearful face of his nephew, and then say aloud, "We're sending a Mickey Mouse cap to your cousin, but not to you." Choking up, Brad was unable to complete the sentence. Gently, the therapist asked him to put words to what he was feeling. What emerged for Brad was an old and familiar "lonely pain," one he had known during his own childhood, when he himself was clumsy, overweight, and socially ostracized, prior to the development of his socially poised and athletic adult veneer. Suddenly, the deep structure of Brad's family narrative became clear to him: not only could he not "ostracize" someone whose vulnerabilities so closely resembled his own, but also he had repeatedly scripted his family interactions to maximize the sense of "inclusion" he had so desperately sought as a child. Sara's refusal to support this script represented a direct threat to the fictional goal of his self-narrative, a deep invalidation of a central premise of his life.

Turning to Sara, the therapist then pursued a similar experiential inquiry into her intransigence about limiting her involvement with Brad's relatives and discovered that being "sucked into" her husband's family felt like an abandonment of her own.[3] As each spouse tearfully reached for the other's hand, the therapist quietly suggested that the "deep sanctity" of their respective core positions—Brad's "lonely pain" and Sara's "undying loyalty"—were "almost defiled" by their squabbles about birthday parties and Mickey Mouse hats. This in turn opened a conversational space for the two partners to explore how they could support rather than unintentionally subvert the central goals of one another's life narratives.

A Healing Story

Having described and illustrated several narrative processes and structures, we will apply these briefly to a self-narrative contributed by a young woman, Jenny, who is in her early 20's. Because we believe that the concepts we have discussed apply equally well to spoken or written narratives that arise in the course of therapy and in daily life, we will expand on the psychotherapeutic storytelling embodied in the previous vignettes and focus on a written passage drawn from Jenny's personal diary.[4]

Granddaddy's Pecans

Granddaddy was such a wonderful, beautiful person; he was always so happy and nothing ever seemed to bring his spirit down. His family meant so much to him; I was his only grandchild, so he spoiled me beyond belief. Although he and my Grandma weren't rich, they made sure that I had anything that I wanted, which was usually just to go to their house and play. He had a small farm, where he lived all of his life. Granddaddy loved to be outdoors and take care of his land and his cows. He had about nine cows and always let me name them, even though I came up with ridiculous names. There was Rose, Sally,

Daisy, and Jumper, our favorite cow. Granddaddy and I used to go out into the fields together and feed them apples and pet them.

When I was a little girl, I used to spend the night with Grandma and Granddaddy every Friday night. They let me stay up late and watch television. Granddaddy would make popcorn in one of those ancient popcorn poppers that you put on the stovetop. No other popcorn has ever been as good. He would put peanuts in bottles of Coke and put them in the freezer until they were not quite frozen, but frosty. Granddaddy would let me have these treats even though Mom was scared that I would choke on the peanuts.

Several pecan trees were in Grandma and Granddaddy's front yard and Granddaddy and I used to pick pecans all of the time. Granddaddy had two or three pecans that he always kept in his pocket. I don't know how old they were, but he had had them ever since I could remember. He used to rub the pecans, so they were very smooth. All of the ridges had been rubbed out so it was difficult to even tell what they were.

One night, Grandma called my Mom in the middle of the night. Mom told me to get dressed because something had happened to Granddaddy. I put on a blue Ole Miss sweatshirt and blue pants. I remember putting on my pants backward, but I didn't care; I just wanted to get to their house as soon as I could. I wanted to get to their house and see Granddaddy sitting in his favorite chair. I knew that when I got there, everything would be all right. An eternity passed before we finally got to their house, which was actually only a few miles away. I remember walking to the door and being terrified of what I would see. I walked in and heard my Grandma crying, then saw my Granddaddy lying on the floor in front of his favorite chair. Their neighbor was performing CPR, but Granddaddy was not moving. I ran and wanted to keep going but there was nowhere to run. I ran back into the kitchen and fell to the floor screaming, "No, no, no!" My parents came into the kitchen and sat down on the floor beside me and said that Granddaddy was dead. All that I could do was scream, "No!"

I remember waking up the next morning in Granddaddy's bed. I thought for a brief moment that everything could have been a horrible nightmare, but then I realized that I had the same blue pants on backward. My Mom came into the room and just held me and we cried. The next few days were so blurry. People came and brought food; they wanted to talk to me, but I did not want to eat or talk to anyone. I just wanted everyone to go away.

I remember going to the funeral home, but being terrified to walk near the casket. Seeing Granddaddy in the casket would have made things all too final and real. Granddaddy's brother asked me if I had seen him yet and I said, "No." He told me that it would be the last time that I would be able to see him and that I might regret it if I didn't. I just cried. I remember being so scared walking up to the coffin, and there he was. My wonderful, beautiful Granddaddy was dead inside the coffin. Just a few days earlier, everything had been so perfect. I had been laughing and playing with him, and now he was gone.

All of this happened when I was in elementary school. It is still so difficult to think about, but I do think about him so much. When I go to their house, I just break down and cry. A few years ago, I was there with my Mom cleaning out the house and I opened a box where he kept his watch, glasses, medicine, and things like that. Inside the box were his pecans—his smooth, unrecognizable pecans. I picked them up and held them and just cried, remembering how he would hold them in his hands and rub them. I took one of them and put it into my pocket. I don't know why, but I did not want my Mom to see me take one. I guess that I didn't want her to see me cry and I didn't want to talk about how much that I missed Granddaddy.

The pecan is in a little box in the guest bedroom at my apartment. Every once in awhile, sometimes when I think of Granddaddy, I take the pecan out and hold it knowing that my Granddaddy's hands once held it. The same hands that used to hold the pecan and made it so unrecognizable once held and hugged me. I close my eyes and rub the pecan and imagine him. I picture him standing in a walkway in his house; he's wearing his green plaid shirt, green pants, and brown leather belt. I picture his face and see him smile at me.

Granddaddy knew how much I loved him, but I just wish that I could hug him once more. The pecan is the way that I keep him close to me. Even though I still picture him in my mind and remember the things that we did, the pecan is something that I can see and feel. Although I can't hug Granddaddy anymore, I feel close to him when I hold the pecan. I take it out from time to time and just cry; whenever I think of him I cry. I wish that I could look at the pecan or think of him and smile by remembering all of the happy and fun times, but I just think of that horrible night that I saw him lying on the floor, dead. I want to be able to think of him and smile; I don't want to cry and get so sad every time that I think about him.

It's been over ten years and I still can't talk about what happened with my family or anyone else. I'm embarrassed to cry in front of others because I want them to think that I am strong and that I have moved on with my life. This is the first time that I have tried to put this experience into words and it has been so difficult. The tears just keep flowing even though it seems that they should be all gone by now. The computer screen has gotten blurry and my tears have gotten onto Granddaddy's pecan.

Narrative Analysis

Jenny's story is characterized by strong "setting work," expressed chiefly through an external narrative process, which effectively recreates for the reader—and perhaps the writer—a series of micronarrative snapshots from the larger macronarrative of her relationship with her grandfather. The rich visual details of pet cows, an ancient popcorn popper, frosty Cokes, and above all, Granddaddy's pecans draw the reader into the account, constructing a tangible story world in which the primary narrative of her loss takes place. In contrast, "characterization work" is typically accomplished indirectly, as Jenny hints at the affective backdrop of their special relationship by portraying a few concrete interactions with her grandfather. In so doing she leaves the reader to infer the feelings and thoughts of the central figures in her story, much as one might infer the motives of characters in a play without the benefit of direct soliloquy. Into this stage setting she inserts the plot structure of her grandfather's death, related in the same psychologically suggestive, rather than explicit, narrative style. Thus, a little girl's panic, confusion, and disbelief is symbolized by her hurriedly putting on her pants backward, and waking the next morning to discover in these same uncomfortably worn trousers a cruel confirmation that her grandfather's death had not been a nightmare.

Into this externally voiced narrative Jenny sprinkles allusions to her internal state, signaled by her description of her terror, self-isolation, fear, and sadness. Her subjective view is also more subtly conveyed at various points, as when she speaks of the "eternity" that elapses driving to her grandfather's house that fateful night or the "blurry" days that followed his death. If such a story were to be presented within the context of psychotherapy, a therapist might encourage Jenny to extend this germinal internal narrative process by asking her to voice more fully the emotion she experienced at these junctures, and as her tears moistened her grandfather's pecan. If Jenny had been having difficulty functioning as a result of this mourning process, the expression of her sorrow to another person in a safe environment could be an important step. It could help her come to terms with the power of her feelings, integrating these more completely into her story of the loss, and sensitizing her to what she presently wanted from others as an audience to her account.

Jenny's "theme work" is also conveyed more by implication than by overt articulation, as themes of an idyllic youth, playful transgression of maternal restrictions, and the shattering of a sustaining attachment are presented artfully but obliquely in the text. The story concludes on a reflexive turn, as Jenny acknowledges the incompleteness of her grief journey, and speaks to her struggle as an author to put the experience into words for the first time. As she does so, the reader begins to get a sense of her fictional goal—to maintain a continuing bond with her grandfather through the telling of the story, as well as through the "linking object" provided by his pecan. Perhaps the story, in all of its concrete detail, offers Jenny "something that [she] can see and feel," much like the pecan worn smooth by the hands that once held her.

Jenny's narrative appears to enter into a reflexive narrative process just prior to its completion. Had the narrative continued in future journal entries, its thematic and goal structure might be further developed. If this story were told in the context of psychotherapy, a therapist might well question Jenny about the significance of this story in her life and about the meaning that keeping in contact with her grandfather holds for her in order to promote further reflexive investigation. It appears that Jenny's journal entry has provided her with an evocative account of an important part of her life history, further reflection on which ultimately could develop into a healing story that might be shared with supportive others.

Summary and Conclusions

The ubiquity of storytelling in its many forms suggests that it plays many roles in human life, at levels ranging from the self to social system. At the level of self-narratives—the accounts of life events that we construct for others and ourselves—narration similarly serves many functions, from the organization of inchoate experiences to the solicitation of social support. In this chapter, we have placed inflection on the way in which narration of difficult or even traumatic life experiences helps us integrate and surmount them, and have presented preliminary taxonomies of the processes and structures by which narrative activity can be understood. Equally important, we have tried to illustrate how certain guiding concepts of narrative theory can be used to focus efforts to help people explore and rewrite life stories that have been shattered, undermined, or determined by difficult life experiences. Thus, we believe that narrative ultimately serves a healing as well as a heuristic function, one that we think deserves greater attention on the part of psychotherapists and health psychologists.

Placing coping in this narrative frame shifts the emphasis from expert attempts to *instruct* others in a generic set of "coping skills," to the person's own attempt to *construct* an idiosyncratic self-narrative marked by resilience, resourcefulness, and hope. This shift toward localizing agency within the person rather than in a repertory of reified behaviors is helpful both because it acknowledges the multiple ways in which our self-narratives can be challenged by events, and because it respects the nearly inexhaustible creativity of people in responding to these challenges. In our view resilience arises—with or without professional prompting—from the double effort first to *describe* our coping responses in the micronarratives of our life story, and then to *inscribe* these as personal resources in the more or less coherent macronarratives that consolidate our sense of identity over time. "Coping" then becomes a storied construction, created and sustained within a distinctively human meaning-making process.

Notes

1. We will intentionally blur the distinction between speaker and author, and listener and reader, in discussing self-narratives, in order to emphasize their common features. Our intent here is also to emphasize that an author "speaks" through a text to an (actual or implied) audience, whose reception, interrogation, and negotiation of the meaning of the account figures prominently in its meaning (11). However, space limitations force us to focus primarily on the function of narration for the author/speaker rather than the audience in the remainder of this chapter.

2. "Fiction" derives from the Latin term *fictio*, meaning to "fashion or

mold." By linguistic extension, it refers to something invented by the imagination, especially an invented story. A secondary meaning of the term—the assumption of something as a fact irrespective of the question of its truth—is also compatible with a constructivist approach to the goal structure of self-narratives.

3. Space does not permit a full account of the exploration of Sara's fictional goal, which involved identifying a micronarrative episode in which her resistance to involvement with Brad's family was especially keenly felt. The episode involved Brad's request that Sara read some of his father's homespun philosophical writing, approximately two years after her own father's death. What she discovered in revivifying the scene was a painful stab of "disloyalty" to her father on being handed the sheaf of papers, a disloyalty that she recognized as the core of her reluctance to "get lost" in her husband's family of origin. More adequate descriptions of similar "radical inquiry" techniques have been provided by Ecker and Hulley (40, 41).

4. The entry reprinted here was written in response to the "Linking Object" exercise in *Lessons of Loss: A Guide to Coping* (48), a narratively oriented self-help book to promote the integration of grief. "Jenny" (whose name is fictionalized) generously gave permission to publish this personal account in the hope that it would be useful to others coping with loss.

References

1. Neimeyer, R. A. (1995). Client-generated narratives in psychotherapy. In Neimeyer, R. A. & Mahoney, M. J. (Eds.), *Constructivism in Psychotherapy* (pp. 231–246). Washington, DC: American Psychological Association.

2. Russell, R. L. & Lucariello, J. (1992). Narrative, yes: Narrative ad infinitum, no! *American Psychologist, 47*, 671–673.

3. Bruner, J. (1986). *Actual minds, possible worlds.* Cambridge, MA: Harvard University Press.

4. Polkinghorne, D. E. (1988). *Narrative knowing and human sciences.* Albany, NY: State University of New York.

5. Sarbin, T. R. (1986). The narrative as a root metaphor for psychology. In T. R. Sarbin (Ed.), *Narrative psychology: The storied nature of human conduct.* New York: Praeger.

6. Russell, R. L. (1991). Narrative in views of humanity, science and action: Lessons for cognitive therapy. *Journal of Cognitive Psychotherapy, 5*, 241–256.

7. Angus, L., Levitt, H. & Hardke, L. (1999). Narrative processes and psychotherapeutic change: An integrative approach to psychotherapy research and practice. *Journal of Clinical Psychology, 55*, 1255–1270.

8. Neimeyer, R. A. (1995). Constructivist psychotherapies: Features, foundations, and future directions. In Neimeyer, R. A. & Mahoney, M. J. (Eds.), *Constructivism in Psychotherapy* (pp. 11–38). Washington, DC: American Psychological Association.

9. Polkinghorne, D. E. (1992). Postmodern epistemology of practice. In Kvale, S. (Ed.), *Psychology and postmodernism* (pp. 146–165). Newbury Park, CA: Sage.

10. Neimeyer, R. A. (1998). Social constructionism in the counselling context. *Counselling Psychology Quarterly, 11*, 135–149.
11. Neimeyer, R. A. (2000). Narrative disruptions in the construction of self. In Neimeyer, R. A. & Raskin, J. (Eds.), *Constructions of disorder: Meaning making frameworks for psychotherapy* (pp. 207–241). Washington, DC: American Psychological Association.
12. Guidano, V. F. (1991). *The self in process.* New York: Guilford.
13. Howard, G. S. (1991). Culture tales: A narrative approach to thinking, cross-cultural psychology, and psychotherapy. *American Psychologist, 46*, 187–197.
14. Singer, J. A., & Salovey, P. (1993). *The remembered self.* Toronto: Free Press.
15. Spence, D. (1982). *Narrative truth and historical truth.* New York: Norton.
16. Howe, D. (1993). *On being a client.* Thousand Oaks, CA: Sage.
17. Rennie, D. L. (1984). Story telling in psychotherapy: The client's subjective experience. *Psychotherapy, 31*, 234–243.
18. Mascolo, M. F., Craig-Bray, L. & Neimeyer, R. A. (1997). The construction of meaning and action in development and psychotherapy: An epigenetic systems approach. In G. J. Neimeyer & R. A. Neimeyer (Eds.), *Advances in personal construct psychology* (Vol. 4, pp. 3–38). Greenwich, CT: JAI Press.
19. Parry, A., & Doan, R. (1994). *Story re-visions.* New York: Guilford.
20. Neimeyer, R. A. (1998). Cognitive therapy and the narrative trend: A bridge too far? *Journal of Cognitive Psychotherapy, 12*, 57–66.
21. Hermans, H. J. M. (2001). The person as a motivated storyteller. In R. A. Neimeyer & G. J. Neimeyer (Eds.), *Advances in personal construct psychology* (Vol. 5, pp. in press). New York: Praeger.
22. Atkinson, R. (1995). *The gift of stories.* Westport, CT: Bergin & Garvey.
23. Newman, F., & Holzman, L. (1999). Beyond narrative to performed conversation. *Journal of Constructivist Psychology, 12*, 23–40.
24. Angus, L., & Hardke, K. (1994). Narrative processes in psychotherapy. *Canadian Psychology, 35*, 190–203.
25. Angus, L., Hardke, K. & Levitt, H. (1996). *An expanded manual for the Narrative Process Coding System.* Toronto: York University.
26. Hardke, K. (1996). Characterizing therapy focus and exploring client process. *Psychology.* Toronto: York University.
27. Greenberg, L., Elliott, R., & Rice, L. (1993). *Facilitating emotional change.* New York: Guilford.
28. Bucci, W. (1985). Dual coding: A cognitive model for psychoanalytic research. *Journal of the American Psychoanalytic Association, 33*, 571–607.
29. Guidano, V. (1995). Self-observation in constructivist psychotherapy. In R. A. Neimeyer & M. J. Mahoney (Eds.), *Constructivism in psychotherapy* (pp. 155–168). Washington, DC: American Psychological Association.
30. Gendlin, E. T. (1996). *Focusing-oriented psychotherapy.* New York: Guilford.
31. Rainer, T. (1978). *The new diary.* Los Angeles: Tarcher.

32. Luborsky, L., & Crits-Cristoph, P. (1998). *Understanding transference.* (Second ed.). Washington, DC: American Psychological Association.
33. Spence, D. (1986). Narrative smoothing and clinical wisdom. In T. Sarbin (Ed.), *Narrative psychology.* New York: Praeger.
34. Beck, A. T. (1993). Cognitive therapy: Past, present, and future. *Journal of Consulting and Clinical Psychology, 61,* 194–198.
35. Forster, J. R. (1991). Facilitating positive changes in self-constructions. *International Journal of Personal Construct Psychology, 4,* 281–292.
36. Monk, G., Winslade, J., Crocket, K., & Epston, D. (1996). *Narrative therapy in practice.* San Francisco: Jossey Bass.
37. Mandler, J. (1984). *Scripts, stories, and scenes: Aspects of schema theory.* Hillsdale, NJ: Erlbaum.
38. McAdams, D. (1993). *The stories we live by.* New York: Morrow.
39. Goncalves, O. F. (1995). Cognitive narrative psychotherapy: The hermeneutic construction of alternative meanings. In Mahoney, M. J. (Ed.), *Cognitive and constructivist psychotherapies* (pp. 139–162). New York: Springer.
40. Ecker, B., & Hulley, L. (1996). *Depth-oriented brief therapy.* San Francisco: Jossey Bass.
41. Ecker, B., & Hulley, L. (2000). The order in clinical "disorder". Symptom coherence in depth-oriented brief therapy. In Neimeyer, R. A. & Raskin, J. (Eds.), *Constructions of disorder* (pp. 63–90). Washington, DC: American Psychological Association.
42. Sewell, K. W., Baldwin, C. L., & Moes, A. J. (1998). The multiple self-awareness group. *Journal of Constructivist Psychology, 11,* 59–78.
43. Labov, W. & Waletzky, J. (1966). Narrative analysis: Oral versions of personal experience. In Helm, J. (Ed.), *Annual Spring Meeting of the American Ethnological Society* (pp. 12–44). Seattle: University of Washington Press.
44. Arciero, G., & Guidano, V. (2000). Experience, explanation, and the quest for coherence. In Neimeyer, R. A. & Raskin, J. C. (Eds.), *Constructions of disorder* (pp. 91–117). Washington, DC: American Psychological Association.
45. Neimeyer, R. A., & Stewart, A. E. (1998). Trauma, healing, and the narrative emplotment of loss. In Franklin, C. & Nurius, P. S. (Eds.), *Constructivism in practice* (pp. 165–184). Milwaukee, WI: Families International.
46. Sewell, K. W. (1997). Posttraumatic stress: Towards a constructivist model of psychotherapy. In G. J. Neimeyer & R. A. Neimeyer (Eds.), *Advances in personal construct psychology* (Vol. 4, pp. 207–235). Greenwich, CT: JAI Press.
47. Janoff-Bulman, R., & Berg, M. (1998). Disillusionment and the creation of values. In Harvey, J. H. (Ed.), *Perspectives on loss: A sourcebook* (pp. 35–47). Philadelphia: Brunner/Mazel.
48. Neimeyer, R. A. (1998). *Lessons of loss: A guide to coping.* New York: McGraw Hill.

4

The Humor Solution

Herbert M. Lefcourt

The Impact of Stressful Experiences

Today it is common for people to associate stress with emotional upset and illness and to think of stress as anything that makes demands upon us to change or cope with challenges to the status quo. This has not always been the case, however, especially with regard to emotional disturbance and mental illness. For the greater part of the twentieth century, emotional difficulties most often were attributed to personal psychopathology with less regard given to situational events as determinants of emotional problems. Few psychologists and fewer psychiatrists examined the immediate circumstances in clients' lives as other than remote triggers precipitating latent abnormal proclivities. External stressors supposedly made visible what would have been readily apparent if the client had previously been subjected to diagnostic assessment. Rarely were "circumstances" taken to be salient causes of behavior in their own right. To be fair, some psychiatrists such as Harry Stack Sullivan and some psychologists such as Julian Rotter did consider situational variables to be, if not preeminent, at least strongly influential in determining the onset of emotional distress and mental illnesses.

Situational variables did not routinely enter into discussions about the origins of medical disease and illness until the appearance of a brief article by Thomas Holmes and Richard Rahe (1). In their article, connections were made between the occurrence of particular life events and the onset of illnesses (varying from viral infections to morbid conditions). The authors introduced a *Life Events Survey* which presented a number of situations that varied in stress potential, and that were weighted accordingly. Items ranged downward from the maximal "death of a spouse" to the relatively innocuous, "minor violations of the law." Subjects endorsed whether or not they had undergone the events in question during a given time period, and the resulting scores were the sum total of those weighted items. These scores were then used to predict the onset of illnesses and they did so reliably, with statistical significance, though the relationships never attained high magnitudes.

The life events such as death, incapacities, separations, and the like that are used as predictors of illness can be conceptualized as factors responsible for changes in relationships with valued others. What Holmes and Rahe and many other investigators found was that persons who experienced a great number of life changes in a relatively short span of time became susceptible to a variety of emotional and physical afflictions.

Life events measures of stress became familiar to the general public when they began to appear widely in popular magazines and newspapers, with encouragements for readers to predict their likelihood of becoming ill. This popularization of the stress construct resulted in scores of books about the effects of stress. It comes as no surprise, therefore, that stress has become one of the most commonly blamed causes for illness and emotional disturbance. Investigators such as Hans Selye (2) would have been amazed at the sheer volume of literature about a construct that hadn't even been named until he began his studies on the "general adaptation syndrome."

In the thirty some years that have transpired since Holmes and Rahe's seminal publication, numerous scientific books, articles, and monographs have been published attesting to the importance that life events can have upon both emotional states and physical illness. Investigators have explored the responses of people to a great variety of life experiences: the death of loved ones (3); the migration between countries and mobility within countries (4); the urban conditions that result in unpredictability and a lack of control (5); the strains involved in fulfilling difficult roles (6); the loss of work (7); and even small daily hassles (8). When it comes to strokes, coronary emergencies, or to flu and depression, current life styles and circumstances are no longer overlooked when clinicians and researchers try to understand their onset. However, at the same time that we have come to recognize the role of current life circumstances for our sense of well-being, researchers are aware that there always has been considerable variability in the responses manifested by different persons undergoing those experiences. As Johnson and Sarason (9) observed, though the effects are reliable, life events rarely account for more than 10% of the variance in the prediction of emotion-related illnesses. They, and Rabkin and Struening (10) along with Cohen and Edwards (11), suggested that the prediction of illness onset is enhanced by knowledge about individual differences that moderates the deleterious effects of stressful events. Personality predispositions, which once were the preeminent variables used to predict psychopathology, and later were ignored by those who investigated the effects of stress, now are regarded along with stress as conjoint predictors of emotional effects. They often are studied as moderator variables that minimize or maximize the impact that stress can exert upon an organism through their associations with different coping styles.

Differences in Coping Strategies in Response to Stress

Since the early 1960s, the psychological literature concerned with how humans cope with stress has become voluminous, being in the forefront of psychological writings. Flourishing in this stress research was a common model of stress posited by Richard Lazarus and Susan Folkman (8) in a volume titled *Stress, Appraisal, and Coping.*

In this Lazarus and Folkman model, stress is depicted as pressure arising from an event external to us. The situation could involve demands to achieve, to engage in some kind of frightening social interaction, or any experiences that might result in our feelings of anxiety. This "external" event, however, does not comprise stress in and of itself. Rather, *our interpretation and response* must occur before we call an event stressful, and it is in our responses to potential threats that the psychological description of coping processes originates.

In the Lazarus and Folkman model, stress comprises an event and our responses to it, the process beginning when we attend to an event and appraise it for its threat potential. This is referred to as primary appraisal. Neurotics are thought to be those persons who seem primed to believe that the worst is always about to happen; indeed, their primary appraisals often find threat in situations that would seem benign to others. As a consequence, neurotic persons often are in a state of arousal, suffering symptoms associated with their persistent hyperemotionality. Where challenging situations might elicit instrumental activity from less fearful individuals, neurotic individuals may suffer with unmitigated emotional upsets that have ramifications for the onset of illness.

When primary appraisal indicates that a situation is theatening, the subsequent "secondary appraisal" involves the person's evaluation of abilities to influence or control the given perceived stressors. If people feel capable of dealing with the particular stressors, they are more likely to engage in problem-focused coping. For example, if a person were to receive threatening information from a physician about possible coronary problems, along with the advice that it was essential to alter his life style, that patient first would appraise the physician's warning. In this primary appraisal, the patient assesses the plausibility of the physician's warnings. If the patient believes in the veracity of the threat that is inherent in the physician's diagnosis, secondary appraisal should occur. Accordingly, those who feel capable of altering their life styles would be more likely to take action, change diets, exercise, etc. As a consequence, they might allay emotional upset. In contrast, those who believed in the physician's diagnosis, but whose secondary appraisals were less hopeful with regard to altering their prognoses, would have to come to terms with their own emotional responses, either accepting them or defending themselves in some way from their erosive effects. This process is referred to as emotion-focused coping. Though many people might vary in their choice to engage in problem-or emotion-focused coping, depending on the nature of the stressful events encountered, some people probably respond to a variety of threats with a predominant coping style, always trying to alter the stressful demand, or always capitulating to the threat and working to nullify its emotional effects.

Excellent examples of how people cope with the emotional arousal accompanying uncontrollable stressful events abound in biographical writings. A remarkable case of how humor served as an emotion-focused coping response can be found in the writings of Brian Keenan (12), whose powerful book *An Evil Cradling* describes the way he and other hostages in Lebanon survived incredible ordeals during five years of captivity.

The Role of Humor as an Emotion-Focused Coping Response

To ascertain the role that humor can play as an emotion-focused coping response, we will review the literature that began with our earliest demonstration that humor can moderate the effects of stressful experiences. That humor could be a successful means for coping with emotions aroused by stress has been advanced by many notable theorists. Freud (13), for one, regarded humor to be among the best of the defensive processes. "The essence of humor is that one spares oneself the affects to which the situation would naturally give rise and overrides with a jest the possibility of such an emotional display" (p. 5). Allport (14) stated that "the neurotic who learns to laugh at himself may be on the way to self-management, perhaps to cure" (p. 280). Others have linked humor with perspective-taking. Rollo May (15), for example, suggested that humor has the function of "preserving the sense of self. . . . It is the healthy way of feeling a 'distance' between one's self and the problem, a way of standing off and looking at one's problem with perspective" (p. 54). Likewise, Viktor Frankl (16) asserted that "to detach oneself from even the worst conditions is a uniquely human capability" and that this distancing of oneself from aversive situations derives "not only through heroism . . . but also through humor" (p. 16–17). Raymond Moody (17) also alludes to the ability to detach oneself as intrinsic to humor: "A person with a 'good sense of humor' is one who can see himself and others in the world in a somewhat distant and detached way. He views life from an altered perspective in which he can laugh at, yet remain in contact with and emotionally involved with people and events in a positive way" (p. 4).

Perhaps the strongest stimulant for examining the role of humor as a coping mechanism was provided by the publication *An Anatomy of an*

Illness by Norman Cousins (18). In this book, Cousins described the therapeutic value of humor, as he laughed "himself back to health" while suffering with a serious disintegrative disease (ankylosing spondilitis). Cousin's writings have generated an enthusiasm for the use of humor in medical settings and, as well, have stimulated research efforts to assess the efficacy with which humor can moderate the emotional effects of stress. To this end, Rod Martin and I began a series of studies, described in our book *Humor and Life Stress* (19), which have become a lauching pad for many subsequent investigations.

In our first published studies (20, 21), we presented two newly created humor scales, the *Situational Humor Response Questionnaire (SHRQ)* and the *Coping Humor Scale (CHS)*. The former inquired about the likelihood that the respondent might find amusement, laughing as opposed to becoming irritated, in situations that could provoke either response. In the *CHS*, we asked our subjects if they knowingly found humor to be useful as a means of coping with difficult circumstances. After establishing the reliability and validity of these measures, we then explored whether, in fact, assertions about the efficacy of humor as a coping response could be affirmed. We did this by exploring whether our measures of humor could predict the ways in which people responded to stresses in their lives.

In our early investigations, we found reason to be encouraged about the value of humor as a means of coping with stress-derived emotional responses. Significant interactions were found between the humor scales and measures of life stress in the prediction of mood disturbance scores from the *Profile of Mood States* (POMS) (22). Subjects, whose scores on each of the humor measures indicated that they had a good sense of humor, were less likely to be predictable on the *POMS* from the stress measure than were those who had a lesser sense of humor. Those with lower humor scale scores were more apt to have become depressed, tense, confused, etc., if they had undergone stressful experiences than were those who seemed to have a better sense of humor.

In a second study, in which we substituted a measure of humor productivity (23) for our scalar measures of humor, we found similar results. The humor productivity measure consisted of subjects making up three-minute comedy routines incorporating any or all objects (old tennis shoes, a crushed beer can, toothbrush, an aspirin bottle etc.) set on a table before them, with the skits later being scored for wittiness.

As in the first study, we found a significant interaction between stress and humor in predicting mood disturbance, stress again being measured with a life event scale and mood disturbance by the *POMS*. In the analysis of that interaction, we again found that humor operated as a moderating variable. Subjects who were unable to produce humor showed a greater relationship between stress and mood disturbance than did those who were more capable of humor on this difficult and demanding task.

Finally, a subset of the subjects from our first study returned to participate in a third investigation. The same life stress and mood disturbance scores from their earlier session were used. For humor scores, however, we created another humor productivity measure, one that had more in common with humor production in a stressful situation. Subjects watched the film, *Subincision*, which Lazarus (24) had often used as a stressor in laboratory research. Subjects were asked to create a humorous monologue to accompany the film which portrays ritual genital mutilation among certain Australian aboriginal tribes. The monologues created to accompany the film were recorded and later scored for wittiness in the same way that humor productivity had been rated in the second study.

Once again, a significant interaction was obtained between stress and humor in the prediction of mood disturbance. The interaction pattern replicated our previous findings, such that those who were unable to produce humorous monologues evinced a strong relationship between stress and mood disturbance scores. Mood disturbance was more common among stressed subjects who failed to create a funny monologue than among equivalently stressed peers who succeeded at creating a funny monologue.

The results of these studies provided encouraging support for the hypothesized stress moderator role of humor. Several different measures of humor produced consistent effects: *stress had a less uniform impact upon the emotional responses of subjects who had a good sense of humor than it did for those who were with a lesser sense of humor.* In other words, while those with a good sense of humor exhibited variability in the emotional impact from stressful experiences, most of those persons with a lesser sense of humor responded to stressful experiences with negative emotions.

Shortly after the publication of these original studies (20, 21), two investigations were reported, one replicative and the other not. This naturally led investigators to question the stability of humor for moderating stress.

The disconfirming study by Porterfield (25) made use of both the CHS and SHRQ as measures of humor, and a life events scale as an index of stress. In lieu of the POMS, Porterfield used a singular measure of depression (*Center for Epidemiological Studies Scales—CES-D*) (26) as his criterion. Although there was a main effect for humor (a negative relationship between humor and depression), humor did not interact with stress in the prediction of depression. This failure to replicate our earlier significant interactive results was puzzling. Porterfield's investigation had the advantage of a rather large sample. However, it should be noted that Porterfield's subjects had very high depression scores (*Mean* = 19.42, *SD* = 10.12), more than one standard deviation higher than the normative mean (*M* = 9.25, *SD* = 8.58); accordingly, a ceiling effect may have limited the increases in depression scores. Another possible explanation for Porterfield's failure to replicate our results may have derived from the fact that the depression and humor assessments were taken very early in the students' first year on campus. Elevated depression scores could have reflected the typical freshmen sense of dislocation and loneliness before establishing friendships and a sense of belonging on campus. At such a time, heightened reports of depressive affect should not be surprising. Because humor requires a social context, having a good sense of humor may not have been as viable a tool at that early time in contrast to the students' later years in school. Being among strangers during the first weeks on campus, few students would likely feel secure enough to express humor, especially if it were typically of a self-effacing sort. Consequently, though having a good sense of humor may prove useful for alleviating the effects of stress in more normal circumstances, it may not have served as an effective moderator of stress at that early and uncertain time when the sympathetic responses of others could not be taken for granted.

In the following year, a major confirmatory study was reported (27). In this investigation, both the *CHS* and *SHRQ* were evaluated for their moderator effects upon the relationships between life stress and depression, measured by the *Beck Depression Inventory* (*BDI-*) (28) and anxiety, measured by the trait scale of the *State-Trait Anxiety Inventory* (*STAI-*) (29). The assessments of depression and anxiety were done both at the start of the study along with the other predictors, and again, two months later. At the second testing session, subjects also completed the life events measure describing stressors that had occurred since the first test administration. This investigation, then, consisted of two parallel data sets, one cross-sectional and the other prospective.

In contrast to Porterfield (25), Nezu, Nezu, and Blisseuu (27) found significant main effects *and* interactions between stress and humor in the prediction of depression at both times of testing. In the prospective analysis, where earlier measures of depression and anxiety were entered as covariates in predicting the later measures of same, the analyses were even stronger than at the first test session in predicting depression. On the other hand, anxiety was unrelated to humor. In both the cross-sectional and prospective data sets, depression scores increased, with stress occurring primarily among subjects with low scores on either measure of humor. Those who scored high on humor varied little with changing levels of stress, and they always were less depressed than their low humor counterparts.

That Nezu et al. failed to obtain parallel results with anxiety serves to remind us that the particular criterion selected can make a great difference. Anxiety, which is more often anticipatory than retrospective, may be less altered by humor than is depression; and humor may be a better tool for coming to terms with events that have already transpired (emotion-focused coping). Be that as it may, their findings with depression strongly replicated the stress-moderating effects of humor that we had found earlier.

Close on the heels of these two early follow-up investigations, three other early studies contributed to the interest in and uncertainty about the stress moderator role of humor. In one of these studies (30), humor (measured by the *CHS*) failed to moderate the effects of negative life experiences upon measures of health, illness, depression, and insomnia. However, the measurements of the criteria were questionnable, given that they were each assessed by only single questions, and the measure of depression was an abbreviated composite of the *BDI* and the *Multiple Affect Adjective Check*

List (*MAACL-*) (31). The *CHS* did produce a significant main effect upon the *MAACL* with higher humor scores being related to less depression, while the results with the *BDI* were not reported. (The authors used a very stringent criterion for significance, ignoring those results which didn't exceed the .01 level of significance). The failure to replicate may have been due to the measures used because substantial alterations and adumbrations may have compromised their reliability. Finally, because there were numerous tests of stress moderation with several variables other than humor, the authors had adopted very conservative tests of significance and therefore may have ignored trends that might have attained significance given more extensive and reliable measurements.

In a brief report that was compelling for its ecological validity, Trice and Price-Greathouse (32) found that dental patients who scored "high," and who had joked and laughed prior to treatment, became less distressed during dental surgery than did those who scored "low" on the *CHS*. Given the brevity of the description of the study, however, it was impossible to assess the veridicality of the findings, given uncertainty about whether scale scores and observed mirth were both used for subject classification, whether observers of mirth presurgery were different than raters of postsurgical behavior, and vagueness about how distress was measured. Though interesting and confirmatory, these results were obviously not free of ambiguity.

In the third of these early follow-up studies, Labott and Martin (33) examined the joint moderator effects of humor and a proclivity toward weeping during stressful circumstances as predictors of mood disturbance. These investigators had found in one study that the penchant for weeping interacted with scores from a life events scale in predicting mood disturbance. Those who are more apt to weep showed higher relationships between stress and mood disturbance than did those who were less likely to weep. With a second sample, these investigators included the *CHS* along with their other measures and found a main effect for humor, and a borderline four-way interaction between stress, humor, sex, and tendency to weep. While the tendency to weep again interacted with stress in the prediction of mood disturbance, in weepers exhibiting greater mood disturbance, humor was found to have moderated that tendency in all groups excepting males who were "high weepers." Among all nonweeping subjects, those with low humor scores manifested greater mood disturbance following stress than did those with high humor scores. Among weepers the differences between those scoring low and those scoring high on the *CHS* were less marked, and among males scores were opposite to the general findings: high humor males who also were weepers exhibited greater mood disturbance following stress than did low humor-weeping males. One limitation to the reliability of these results was a significant relationship found between humor and life event scores: high humor males had reported a lesser frequency of stressful experiences than low humor males and a lesser frequency of stress than all females regardless of their humor scores; these latter differences could have limited possible stress moderator effects.

In this study then, there were some interesting results which, like most data resulting from four-way interactions, are not entirely clear. The authors had thought that weeping would be cathartic and were expecting it to reduce the effects of stress. Their findings, however, were opposite to their hypotheses, with weepers being more dysphoric in stressful circumstances than nonweepers. Because the propensity to weep, then, might be taken as an indication of a heightened response to stress, it would seem that humor is less effective as a stress moderator among those who are the most likely to become distraught in stressful events, especially if they are male. Given that weeping is generally less frequent among males, as was indicated in the scale scores of males and females, high humor–high weeper male subjects may comprise an extreme group, being more emotionally labile and/ or more emotionally expressive than most. Nevertheless, replication for the stress-moderating role of humor was at least found among those who were less likely to weep during stressful events, indicating that humor may have more of a positive impact upon those who are somewhat less emotionally responsive in difficult circumstances.

In summarizing the findings from these early investigations, the conclusions we could draw are not dissimilar from those to be drawn in most areas of research. That is, there are tempting suggestions but no certainties. In particular circumstances, humor has been found to alter the emotional consequences of stressful events. In others, humor has been found to be a negative correlate of dysphoria, regardless of the levels of stress experienced; in essence, being similar to traits such as well-being, optimism, or cheerfulness.

More Recent Studies of Humor as a Coping Strategy

More recent studies have not completely dispeled uncertainty about the efficacy of humor as a stress moderator. For example, Overholser (34) used a life events measure of stress along with the *CHS* as moderator variables to predict depression (*BDI*), loneliness (35), and self-esteem (36). He found evidence that humor played an important role in the regression analyses, but the results were not always as expected.

Among males, the *CHS* was unrelated to depression. However, among females, *CHS* produced a strong main effect and an even stronger interaction with stress in the prediction of depression. *CHS* was negatively related to depression, but when the humor scores were used to form a low and a high group divided at the median, the relationship between stress and depression was seen only in the high humor group; and that relationship was positive. That is, among female subjects scoring in the upper half of the *CHS* distribution, the relationship between stress and depression was positive and significant. Among those in the lower half of the distribution, the relationship between stress and depression was negligible. With the other dependent variables, *CHS* produced main effects, being negatively related to loneliness among males, and positively related to self-esteem among both males and females. No interactions were found between stress and *CHS* scores in predicting these latter variables. Therefore, humor seemed to be more like a trait associated with well-being than it did a coping response in this study. However, where it did interact with stress, its results were paradoxical, seeming to be a liability among Overholser's stressed female subjects.

In three studies by a research group at Allegheny College in Pennsylvania, the effects of humor upon dysphoria have been studied experimentally with mixed results. In one study by Yovetich, Dale, and Hudak (37), humor, measured by the *SHRQ*, was used to predict self-reported anxiety, facial expressions, and heart rate while subjects sat waiting for the onset of electric shocks. During this waiting period, subjects either listened to a humorous or an interesting tape about geological events, or simply waited without external stimulation. Subjects who scored low on the *SHRQ* reported more anxiety and manifested faster pulse rates than did those who scored high on humor. However, the increased pulse rates were found only among those who had undergone the "no tape" condition. In other words, when there were no distractions (listening to a tape recording, whether humorous or merely interesting), low humor subjects evinced greater increases in heart rate than high humor subjects. In addition, they manifested increases in heart rate that were greater than all of the other subjects who had listened to either tape presentation. Other interesting findings included more smiling among high than low humor subjects while listening to the humor tapes and less reports of anxiety among those subjects who listened to the humor tape. While self-reported anxiety was more obvious among low humor subjects, especially when the time approached for the onset of electric shock, the comparisons of pulse rates at each time period varied extensively. The only reliable finding with regard to pulse rate consisted of acceleration among all subjects as the time for shock drew nearer; but this effect was most notable among the low humor subjects in the "no tape" condition. One could conclude that distractions involved in listening to the tape recordings helped to minimize the effects of anxiety while waiting for shocks and that persons with a lesser sense of humor were more apt to become anxious than were high humor subjects when there were no distractions available. However, in the final time period, before the assumed onset of shock, high humor subjects in the humor condition also exhibited increased pulse rates approaching the levels evinced by the low humor–no tape subjects. Consequently, as noted in earlier studies, the findings did not clearly support the hypothesized stress moderator role of humor.

In a second experimental study from this group of researchers (38), depression was induced by the Velten procedure (39), whereby subjects read aloud a series of progressively more depressing statements and are asked to think about them, feeling the sentiments being expressed. Danzer et al.

then examined the effect of a humorous intervention designed to undo the presumed depressive effects of the procedure. Their all female sample completed the *MAACL* before and after undergoing the Velten procedure, and again after the humor or control treatments that followed the mood induction. The humor treatment consisted of listening to 11 minutes of humorous routines by Bill Cosby and Robin Williams. The control conditions consisted of either a recorded geology lecture or an equivalent "no tape" time period. The results with the *MAACL* indicated that depression, anxiety, and hostility all increased substantially following the depression induction. After the subsequent "therapeutic" treatments, most subjects exhibited decreases in their reporting of negative affects. However, the greatest changes were found among subjects who had listened to the humor tape. These subjects' *MAACL* scores returned to baseline levels. Similar magnitude decreases were not found among control subjects for depression, anxiety, and hostility. Other data with heart rate and zygomatic muscle tension (smiles) did not produce unambiguous results, except to attest to the success of depression induction.

In a third study, Hudak, Dale, Hudak, and DeGood (40) examined the effect of humor upon responses to induced pain, an attempt at replicating an earlier investigation by Cogan, Cogan, Waltz, and McCue (41). Where the latter investigators found that tolerance for pain produced by a pressure cuff increased after subjects listened to a humorous audio tape, Hudak et al. found that responses to pain created by "transcutaneous end nerve stimulation" (*TENS*) were influenced by humorous presentation in interaction with trait-humor measured by the *SHRQ*. A humorous (*Bill Cosby Himself*) or a control video (*Annuals and Hanging Baskets*) was shown to subjects immediately after they signaled that the electrical stimulation was becoming uncomfortable in the baseline condition. Five minutes into the video presentations, pain threshold was again measured in response to *TENS*. Those subjects whose scores were in the upper half of the *SHRQ* distribution demonstrated an increase in their tolerance for pain (higher thresholds) from *TENS* compared to their baselines in both the humor and control conditions. Those in the lower half of the *SHRQ* distribution showed some increase in their thresholds for pain from their baseline levels, but only in the humor condition. However, the most marked contrast was found when subjects viewed the control video: there was a large decrease in the threshold for pain (greater intolerance) among low *SHRQ* subjects when they watched the nonhumorous tape. While zygomatic muscle tension, which indicates smiling, was most evident among high *SHRQ* subjects viewing the humorous tape, the humorous video obviously affected the pain tolerance of all subjects. On the other hand, high trait-humor subjects seemed to derive the benefit from watching either the humorous or control tape, suggesting that any distraction was effective for them, or that they may have been as amused by the *Hanging Basket* film as they were by the comedy. One way or the other, low humor subjects seemed to need the specifically comedic stimulation if they were to tolerate the induced pain.

Together, these three studies offer some support for the role of humor as a reducer of stress. In some instances, humor seemed to be more trait-like than a coping strategy for dealing with stress. In others, its effects were more notable during stressful or painful moments, suggesting that it can operate as a stress-moderator. Self-reports, facial expressions, and heart rate, indicating distress in aversive situations, have each been found to be influenced by humor. However, the inconsistent interactions among variables in these studies made the results seem conditional without providing explanations for the variability observed in the data.

To make matters even more ambiguous, Nevo, Keinan, and Teshi-movsky-Arditi (42) found only weak effects for a measure of trait-humor and humor induced by a film upon subjects in a cold pressor task. Only one subscale (Humor Productivity) of Ziv's sense of humor scales (43) was even mildly related to pain tolerance ($r = .26$, $p < .05$) and the SHRQ was unrelated to it altogether. One finding of some note in this study was that the funnier subjects thought the humorous film to be, the longer they were able to tolerate their arm being immersed in freezing water ($r = .38$, $p < .05$). In contrast to the humorous film, some subjects viewed a docu-mentary and others saw no film at all. Ironically, when subjects had been classified as low or high in humor on the basis of the Ziv measure, it was the "low humor" subjects who differentiated the most between the humor-ous and documentary film in their ratings of funniness. High humor sub-jects again may have found the documentary almost as amusing as the film that was intended to be funny.

Whether variations in the perceived funniness of the films was respon-sible for the failure of trait-humor to be a major factor in this study, or whether the procedures used in the cold-pressor task may not have been controlled (no mention was made as to whether there was a "circulating bath"), this study failed to replicate the effects of humor as a moderator of pain tolerance.

In a study with a somewhat different aim, Kuiper, Martin, and Dance (44) examined the role of humor in helping individuals maintain positive affect during their encounters with negative events. First, these investiga-tors found that positive affect increased most substantially for subjects ex-periencing positive events who had scored high on Svebak's Sense of Hu-mor Questionnaire (SHQ), (45). Two subscales within that measure, the Metamessage Sensitivity Scale (SHQ-MS), and the Liking of Humor (SHQ-LH) interacted with the Positive Life Event subscale of the Life Event Scale (LES) (46) in predicting the Positive Affect subscale of the Positive and Negative Affect Schedule (PANAS) (47). It would seem that only persons who appreciated humor seemed likely to derive positive affect from their positive experiences. It is of interest, however, that neither the CHS or SHRQ produced similar results, pointing to the specificity of certain kinds of humor measures for producing particular effects in different circum-stances. Nevertheless, when all the humor variables were used as moder-ators of the relationship between negative life events and positive affect,

the *CHS* and *SHRQ* along with the *SHQ-MS* did produce significant interactions. These interactions derived from the sharp decline in positive affect
that occurred with increasing negative life events among those who had
scored low on those humor measures. In other words, positive affect was
maintained despite negative experiences by persons who seem to have a
good sense of humor. Consequently, the authors described their focus as
being not so much upon the reduction of negative affect as upon an "enhanced quality of life." These findings add a new dimension to the work
on moderator effects of humor though their comprehension requires an
agility with English.

Carver et al. (48) have reported upon the ways in which a sample of
women coped with stresses encountered in surgery at an early stage of
breast cancer. These investigators were most interested in the effects of optimism as a moderator of the illness-distress relationship. At the same time,
they also examined the relationships of several coping mechanisms with
optimism on the one hand, and experienced distress on the other. Included
among the coping mechanisms was *use of humor*. The authors do not describe the subscale in great detail other than to say that it is composed of
three items as are each of the other subscales within the *COPE Scale* and
that it is said to have good internal consistency (49).

Among the various coping mechanisms assessed with the *COPE
Scale, use of humor* correlated significantly only with *positive reframing*.
But in each of five assessments at presurgery, postsurgery, and then at 3, 6,
and 12-month followups, *use of humor* was positively correlated with *optimism* which, in turn, was associated with less distress as measured by
subscales of the *POMS* at each point in time. As well, when coping mechanisms were examined for their direct effects upon distress at the different
time periods, *use of humor* was found to be negatively associated with
distress at all five time periods, though statistically significant at only two
of them.

Though *use of humor* was reliably related to *optimism*, its relative independence from other coping mechanisms was notable, the only other
significant correlation being with *positive reframing*, a defense similar to
"distancing." Though brief, the questions in the humor measure may have
attained their predictive power from their relevance to the stressor under
study ("I've been making jokes about it"—"it" being breast cancer). Humor,
then, seemed to be distinctive and contributed as a relatively independent
moderator of stress. Given the nature of the very real stressful circumstances explored in this study, the results are compelling.

In another study within a medical setting, the responses of patients who
had undergone orthopedic surgery were examined by Rotton and Shats
(50). They found humor to have some limited use in reducing pain. Patients
were provided either serious or humorous films to observe in the two full
days following surgery. Half of the patients in each group (humorous vs.
serious) were allowed to choose which of 20 films they could see. The other
half were shown films chosen by the experimenters. Self-reports of distress

and pain showed a marked decline from the first to the second day following surgery for all patients who were provided films. In contrast, a control group, not given the option of watching films, showed little change from day one to day two. No differences in self-reports of distress and pain were found between those who had viewed comedies and those who had viewed serious films. However, requests for "minor analgesics" (aspirins, tranquilizers) were significantly less frequent for patients who had viewed comedies in comparison with those who had viewed serious films; and having a choice of films and condition (humor vs. serious) interacted in predicting the dosage levels of "major analgesics" (Demerol, Dilaudid, and Percodan). If patients could choose the films they were to watch, then humorous film watching was associated with lower dosages of major analgesics. However, if there was no choice in the films to be watched, then humorous films resulted in greater use of such analgesics compared both to the serious film and the no-film control conditions. These findings suggest the importance of idiosyncratic preferences that people have for certain forms of humor. Watching "humorous" films that a person does not find funny may prove irritating enough to exacerbate feelings of pain. On the other hand, watching "chosen" comedies does prove beneficial with regard to muting the effects of pain.

Finally, a few recent publications have focused upon the affective responses of subjects to the stresses inherent in contemplating their own mortality. The assumption underlying this research is that many of the questions comprising life event measures of stress contain intimations about the deaths of loved ones and of the subjects themselves. In one study from our labs at the University of Waterloo (51), subjects were led to think about their own deaths during a series of tasks: subjects filled out a death certificate for themselves in which they guessed at the cause and the time of their eventual deaths; they composed a eulogy for themselves to be delivered at their funerals; and they constructed a will disposing of their worldly goods that they anticipated having at the time of their deaths. Mood disturbance, measured by the *POMS*, was assessed prior to and following these "death exercises." As had been predicted, most subjects exhibited increases in mood disturbance, reporting more depression, tension, anger, and confusion. The only exceptions to this trend were subjects who had scored high on a measure of "perspective-taking humor." These subjects showed little or no change in their moods following the completion of the death exercises. The perspective-taking humor measure consisted of an index comprising appreciation and comprehension of a set of *Far Side* cartoons (52) which had been selected for their "perspective-taking" character. Comprehension and appreciation of the cartoons required that subjects be capable of distancing themselves from the typical machinations of their own species. That is, subjects had to be able to see the nonsense in everyday human activity in order to enjoy the humor within these cartoons. We defined "perspective-taking" as "distancing" from that with which we personally are identified.

In addition to the perspective-taking humor measure, the *SHRQ* was administered and found to be negatively related to mood disturbance both before and after the death exercises. Where the *SHRQ* measure of humor produced main effects upon *POMS* scores, the perspective-taking humor measure produced an interaction. This suggests that when thinking about death, the ability to assume a humorously distant orientation from one's own group provides some protection from becoming dysphoric.

In the second study involving the contemplation of mortality as a stressor, humor was used to predict the willingness to be an organ donor represented by the signing of a form that is attached to the Ontario driver's license (53). To evaluate the signing of organ donation forms as a surrogate measure for the dread of mortality, we began by observing the correlates of form-signing. Form-signing was related to a number of other behaviors indicating fear versus acceptance of death such as the willingness to visit a mortally ill friend, to discuss death and wills with parents, etc. Organ donation form-signers seemed to be less phobic about death-related thoughts and behaviors. In turn, when organ donation signing was examined for its relationship with humor, it was found to be positively associated with humor assessed by the *SHRQ* and the cartoon measure of perspective-taking humor that we had used in the previous study. We interpreted these data to mean that humor, especially perspective-taking humor, indicated a tendency to not regard one's self too seriously; and in not being overly serious about one's self it then became possible to think about and acknowledge mortality, the end of self, without succumbing to morbid affect. Because the contemplation of mortality is regarded as a stressor in these studies, humor was said to have moderated the relationship between stressor and mood disturbance.

In another set of studies, Keltner and Bonanno have used observations of laughter, humor, enjoyment, and amusement exhibited during interviews six months after the loss of a spouse as predictive indicators of how well persons have coped with bereavement (54, 55). Though it might be questionable whether humor could determine bereavement outcomes, the readiness to laugh about characteristics of one's deceased spouse at least indicates that the surviving spouse is predisposed to respond with humor in discussions about distressing subjects. Consequently, it is reasonable to assume that humor exhibited during bereavement might be prognostic of the acceptance of mortality that we have found in our research.

In interviews with spouses whose mates had died approximately six months earlier, these investigators found differences in adjustment favoring survivors who manifested Duchenne laughter while speaking about their former partners. Duchenne laughter involves both zygomatic major muscle action that pulls the lip corners up obliquely and orbicularis oculi muscle action which pulls the skin from the cheeks and forehead toward the eyeball (56). In common parlance, Duchenne laughter could be described as laughter involving both mouth and eyes, whereas non-Duchenne laughter would involve only the mouth. The former is what we might regard as a full laugh as opposed to the latter, which appears less wholehearted or possibly overcontrolled.

Those who exhibited Duchenne laughter during their interviews reported that they felt reduced anger and were experiencing more enjoyment in their lives in contrast to the period of time immediately following their spouse's death; most important, these "full laughers" manifested dissociation from distress which was assessed by the contrast between their verbal reports and autonomic indications of distress (heart rate changes derived from electrocardiograms obtained from wrist and forearm sensor placements). Degree of Duchenne laughter was negatively correlated with the discrepancy between verbal and autonomic indications of arousal. Those who displayed more laughter exhibited more change in heart rate than they did in verbal reports of emotion. In the opposite direction, non-Duchenne laughter was positively correlated with this index, indicating that there was more verbal report than physiological indication of emotion. These findings were said to indicate a greater sensitization to distress among non-Duchenne laughers, while the former indicates a dissociation from distress among Duchenne laughers. "Full laughter," then, like humor seems to reflect a distancing from grief or dysphoria that allows people to recover and enjoy current life more fully. With regard to this latter assertion, Kelten and Bonanno did find that Duchenne laughers were less ambivalent about their "current" social involvements than were those who did not show such laughter.

Another finding with implications for the role of humor as a coping strategy concerned humor's role in facilitating the attainment of social support. Those who manifested Duchenne laughter were judged by observers to be better adjusted and happier, though nonlaughers were more likely to elicit compassion and help. While the display of laughter may arouse less nurturance, it may increase a person's attractiveness to observers in that the laughers were described as more amusing and potentially less frustrating to interact with. This emphasis upon the social responses of others to bereaved persons' displays of laughter was particularly emphasized in the study by Bonanno and Keltner (54). In that study, facial displays of enjoyment and amusement were found to be negatively related to grief-specific symptoms at 14 and 25 months following the loss, while negative emotions (anger, contempt, etc.) were positively associated with grief symptoms. In addition, facially displayed negative emotions, especially anger, were negatively correlated with perceived health outcomes at both later time periods. The authors discussed their results in functional terms about how the willingness and desire to participate with others and to obtain their social support are conveyed by emotional displays.

Overall then, the empirical literature suggests that humor does play some role in the development and maintainance of mood states. However, the role is rarely simple and straightforward. Nevertheless, the larger percentage of findings do suggest that humor can help to reduce the effects of stressors that would otherwise result in dysphoric emotions. When humorous material is provided in experimental conditions, a lessening of distress sometimes can be observed, though the effects may vary with the particular humorous presentations. On the other hand, along with the original group of studies examining the moderator effects of humor, some later findings have proven to be the opposite of hypothesized effects. Such results do little to reduce our uncertainties about the robustness and reliability of humor's stress moderator effects. However, a fairly reliable observation that may account for some of the diverse findings obtained with humor as a coping device is that men and women may differ in the ways that they use humor. As a consequence, different portents may be drawn from the assessment of mens' and womens' humor.

Sex and Humor

Recently, we have found some evidence with regard to humor as a stress moderator that may shed light upon the variability of results and conclusions that are notable in this literature (57). In one study, we engaged subjects in a series of five tasks that had all been used previously to induce stress. During each procedure, subjects' blood pressure was measured at regular intervals. As anticipated, systolic blood pressures increased above resting levels, reaching a peak toward the end of each task, and then receded toward resting levels after further five-minute lapses. When each of the humor variables, which had been assessed during a previous session, were examined opposite blood pressure scores, a similar pattern was found during the performance of each task. Women who scored high on the *CHS* measure of humor invariably exhibited lower mean blood pressures than women who scored low on the *CHS*, and lower than most male subjects regardless of their *CHS* scores. However, among males, those who scored high on the *CHS* had higher mean systolic blood pressures than those who scored low on the *CHS*, and this obtained throughout the testing sessions, even when subjects were at rest. On the other hand, though the results were not as consistent as they were with the *CHS*, males who scored high on the *SHRQ* often manifested lower systolic blood pressures than did those who had scored low on the *SHRQ*. For females, there was some similarity to this pattern found with males. However, their differences were rarely as strong. The *SHRQ* seemed particularly predictive of male blood pressures, whereas the *CHS* seemed more predictive of female blood pressures; but when the *CHS* was used with males, the results were the opposite of those found with females, high coping-humor males evincing higher systolic blood pressures than low scorers throughout the stressful tasks.

These contrasting findings suggest first that some of the variations in results that have been reported in the study of humor as a stress moderator may be attributable to the mistaken aggregation of data from males and females; second, that the particular measures of humor used may be more pertinent for males or females; and third, that the "kinds" of humor assessed by these measures may have different meanings for men and women and differing prognostic value for how effective humor will be for dealing with stressors. Though the sex of subjects often has been reported in the humor and stress moderator literature, it has not often been included as a predictor variable, usually being deleted from analyses after investigators have found minimal differences between males and females in mean humor scores. To explain the sex differences we have found, we have reexamined some of our own previous research findings and consulted the literature concerning humor and sex.

In one study (58), in which we had observed the interactions between spouses as they role played conflict situations common to many marriages (59), we came across a number of striking differences between husbands and wives with regard to their use of humor. For example, among wives, the CHS was positively associated with self-reported marital satisfaction and happiness, while the correlations among husbands were negligible. In addition, while acting out the conflicts involved in the role playing exercises, spouses were rated for "engagement" and "avoidance," the former indicating high involvement with evidence of active listening to the partner; the latter indicated attempts to withdraw, not listening or engaging in eye contact with spouses. The CHS was found to be positively related to engagement among wives, but not so among husbands. On the other hand, CHS scores were positively associated with ratings of husbands' destructiveness which, in turn, was negatively associated with marital satisfaction for husbands and wives. In contrast to scale scores, the frequency and duration of laughter during role enactments were found to be negatively related to destructiveness among husbands but not among wives. Interestingly enough, displays of laughter were unrelated to the CHS for all spouses, thereby indicating that laughter and self-reported use of humor measured by the CHS are not the same thing. Among husbands, however, laughter seems to counterindicate destructiveness, whereas self-reported use of humor suggested a tendency toward destructiveness.

In one recent investigation into the joint effects of stressful life events and interpersonal behaviors upon depression and marital stability among newlyweds, humor, anger, and sadness were found to have some paradoxical effects upon spouses. Cohan and Bradbury (60) examined the effects of negative life events and marital communication on changes in depressive symptoms and marital adjustment over an 18-month period. Spouses interacted in problem-solving tasks similar to those that we had used in our research, and the observed behaviors were coded for verbal content and expressions of affect.

When the investigators examined the impact of humor, they found that if husbands had exhibited humor during the problem-solving interactions with their wives, then there was a greater likelihood that their marriages had dissolved or gone into limbo in the ensuing 18 months if major stresses had occurred during that time. This finding appeared regardless of whether it was the husband or the wife who had undergone stressful experiences in that 18-month interim.

To make sense of these findings, the authors suggest that the husbands' humor may have reflected "disengagement from marital problem-solving" and an avoidance of problem confrontation. Given that the subjects were newlyweds, humor also may have indicated a disaffection between the spouses, with the husbands laughing *at* their wives rather than *with* them. For whatever reasons, the husband's humor held ill portents for marital stability given the advent of stressful events.

In another study focusing upon marital interaction, Gottman and Krokoff (61) found that "positive verbal expressions" including humor, which were made during marital problem-solving tasks similar to those noted above, were positively related to marital satisfaction, especially for wives. While in the same direction, the husbands' positive verbal expressions failed to reach significance in the relationship with marital satisfaction. In an interesting contrast, positive nonverbal expressions which included smiles and laughter were primarily related to their exhibitors' marital satisfaction. That is, husbands' positive nonverbal expressions were related significantly to their own marital satisfaction, but less so to their wives'; and wives' positive nonverbal expressions also were more related to their own marital satisfaction than that of their spouses.

Some of the results in the Cohan and Bradbury (60) and in the Gottman and Krokoff (61) investigations bear similarity to those in our research. A husband's humor may be associated with destructive behavior in his interaction with his wife. At the same time, humor displayed by wives can have a positive impact upon both her own and her spouses' marital satisfaction, but their husbands' humor has a less pervasive impact. That the impacts of humor can differ when the emittor and/or the recipient is male or female underlines an issue that has been discussed in the literature concerned with humor: There are various kinds of humor expressing different intentions. It is possible that males, moreso than females, may indulge in the kinds of humor that can prove to be destructive to the maintenance of relationships.

When Vaillant (62), in his longitudinal study of Harvard men entitled *Adaptation to Life*, described humor as a "mature defense mechanism," he differentiated between "self-deprecating" and wit or tendentious humor. The former was described as adaptive, allowing us to laugh at ourselves while undergoing stress, which, in turn, lessened the impact of that stressful event. Wit or hostile humor, on the other hand, was thought to be an aggressive means of controlling others and therefore, less likely to afford relief when a person is on the receiving end of stressful experiences. There is no acceptance of the inevitable, no relief from taking oneself too seriously in humor that is characterized by competition and aggression. Only in self-directed humor by which people can laugh at their own dissappointments and failings was relief to be expected.

In the literature concerning humor differences characterizing males and females there is a strong suggestion that women are more likely to engage in and appreciate self-deprecating humor, while males seem more apt to manifest wit and to enjoy jokes. Levine (63), for example, found in content analyses of the routines of stand-up comedians, that females' objects of derision were most often themselves (64% of all jokes), whereas among males self-deprecation occurred less often (7% of jokes). For jokes where the objects of derision were other persons of the same sex, male comedians exhibited a much higher frequency (26% of jokes) than females (6% of jokes). In contrast to assertions that joking is more often directed at the opposite sex, Levine found little difference in the frequency of such joking for females (3%) and males (9%). Given the changes in the relationships between men and women in the last two decades, it would be fascinating to repeat this kind of study with contemporary comedians.

In an examination of humor preferences and practices, Crawford and Gressley (64) asked subjects how likely they were to engage in different kinds of humor. While males were most apt to enjoy hostile humor (e.g., jokes making fun of racial groups), to tell jokes, and to appreciate slapstick humor, females were found to most likely engage in what the authors referred to as "anecdotal humor," the telling of funny stories about things that have happened to themselves and their acquaintances. In essence, males' humor characteristically seemed to be directed at others, whereas female humor more often focused upon herself.

In a study of "putdown humor," Zillman and Stocking (65) had subjects listen to taped renditions of disparaging humor. Subjects were asked to provide reactions to the disparager and his humor. When the narrator was a male college student disparaging either himself, a friend, or an enemy, males found disparagement of the enemy to be the funniest and the disparagement of self to be the least funny. Females showed the reverse preferences, enjoying self-disparagement over disparagement of an enemy. In a second study, the taped narration was performed by a female college student. Female subjects again enjoyed the self-disparaging version most highly, while males found it to be the least funny. In both studies, then, females were found to prefer self-disparaging humor whether it was by a male or female. Males, on the other hand, displayed a relative dislike of such humor and seemed to dislike it particularly when it was engaged in by females, though males seemed to enjoy females disparagement of other females.

If self-disparagement humor comprises what Vaillant (62) termed a mature defense mechanism which has beneficial properties, then it would seem that females are more apt to be the possessors of this mature strategy with its attendant benefits; and if, when females respond to the questions in the *CHS* they are alluding to their use of self-directed humor, then our positive findings for high *CHS* females in our study of systolic blood pressure responses during stressful tasks (57) may become explainable. If elevated *CHS* scores reflected womens' tendency to laugh at themselves as they fumbled through our stressful tasks, they may have been better able to accept their failures, inabilities, and frustrations in those tasks more easily than men. Conceivably, female subjects, with a propensity to use humor as a coping strategy, may have begun to think of the experiment as something to share and laugh at with their friends, anticipating social support in the process. If males, on the other hand, mean that they engage in wit and joking aimed at others when they score highly on the *CHS*, then we might not expect to find the surcease of distress that was found among women, indicated by their lowered systolic blood pressure. That is, humor which is associated with competition and attempts at control should be of less help for minimizing distress, when one is engaged in circumstances where wit or other-directed humor is inappropriate.

Conclusions

In this brief review, I have presented evidence suggesting that humor can be an effective means of coping with stressful experiences, lessening their impact upon moods and emotions. However, men and women may differ in their preferences for certain kinds of humor, and that these differences may have ramifications for well-being indicates that humor, per se, is not a singular, universal panacea for managing stress. Additionally, that there are diverse kinds of humor that express different intents which result in different emotional outcomes indicates that there is need for more research to help elucidate the complexities in this literature.

In looking ahead to what future research may uncover, based upon what our research with perspective-taking humor has revealed, I would like to offer a prognosis for humor as a coping strategy. In his play, *Death of a Salesman*, Arthur Miller revealed to his audiences the agony that haunts people who feel that they are failures, an agony so great that the protagonist Willy Loman commits suicide rather than accept his failures. It was Freud who argued that humor is the antidote to taking oneself so seriously, a gift that comes from the internalization of parental acceptance of our failures. This gift, which Erik Fromm described as "mother love," provides us the feeling that we are loved and worthy even if we do not achieve or succeed. If I were to guess which form of humor will be found to have the greatest importance for us as a means of coping with stressors, it would be perspective-taking humor, the kind of humor that allows us to have distance from our own experiences so that ultimately we enjoy this "gift" of not having to take either our failures or successes too seriously.

References

1. Holmes, T. H., & Rahe, R. H. (1967). The social readjustment rating scale. *Journal of Psychosomatic Research, 11*, 213–218.
2. Selye, H. (1956). *The stress of life*. New York: McGraw-Hill.
3. Stroebe, M. S., & Stroebe, W. (1983). Who suffers more? Sex differences in health risks of the widowed. *Psychological Bulletin, 93*, 279–301.

4. Coelho, G. V., & Ahmed, P. I. (1980). *Uprooting and development: Dilemmas of coping with modernization.* New York: Plenum.
5. Glass, D. G., & Singer, J. E. (1972). *Urban stress: Experiments on noise and social stressors.* New York: Academic Press.
6. Pearlin, L. I. (1983). Role strains and personal stress. In H. B. Kaplan (Ed.), *Psychosocial stress* (pp. 1–30). New York: Academic Press.
7. Kasl, S. (1995). Theory of stress and health. In C. Cooper (Ed.), *Handbook of stress, medicine, and health* (pp. 13–26). New York: CRC Press.
8. Lazarus, R. S., & Folkman, S. (1984). *Stress, appraisal, and coping.* New York: Springer.
9. Johnson, J. H., & Sarason, I. G. (1979). Moderator variables in life stress research. In I. G. Sarason & C. D. Spielberger (Eds.), *Stress and anxiety, Vol. 6* (pp. 151–167). Washington, D.C.: Hemisphere.
10. Rabkin, J. G., & Struening, E. L. (1976). Life events, stress, and illness. *Science, 194,* 1013–1020.
11. Cohen, S., & Edwards, J. R. (1988). Personality characteristics as moderators of the relationship between stress and disorder. In R. W. J. Neufeld (Ed.), *Advances in the investigation of psychological stress* (pp. 235–283). New York: John Wiley.
12. Keenan, B. (1992). *An evil cradling.* New York: Viking Penguin.
13. Freud, S. (1928). Humour. *International Journal of Psychoanalysis, 9,* 1–6.
14. Allport, G. W. (1950). *The individual and his religion.* New York: Macmillan.
15. May, R. (1953). *Man's search for himself.* New York: Random House.
16. Frankl, V. (1969). *The will to meaning.* New York: World Publishing.
17. Moody, R. (1978). *Laugh after laugh: The healing power of humor.* Jacksonville, FL: Headwaters Press.
18. Cousins, N. (1979). *Anatomy of an illness.* New York: Norton.
19. Lefcourt, H. M., & Martin, R. A. (1986). *Humor and life stress.* New York: Springer-Verlag.
20. Martin, R. A., & Lefcourt, H. M. (1983). Sense of humor as a moderator of the relationship between stressors and moods. *Journal of Personality and Social Psychology, 45* (6), 1313–1324.
21. Martin, R. A., & Lefcourt, H. M. (1984). The Situational Humour Response Questionnaire: A quantitative measure of sense of humor. *Journal of Personality and Social Psychology, 47* (1), 145–155.
22. McNair, D. M., Lorr, M., & Droppleman, L. F. (1971). *The profile of mood states.* San Diego, CA: EDITS.
23. Turner, R. G. (1980). Self-monitoring and humor production. *Journal of Personality, 48,* 163–172.
24. Lazarus, R. S. (1966). *Psychological stress and the coping process.* New York: McGraw-Hill.
25. Porterfield, A. L. (1987). Does sense of humor moderate the impact of life stress on psychological and physical well-being? *Journal of Research in Personality, 21,* 306–317.
26. Radloff, L. S. (1977). The CES-D scale: A self-report depression scale for research in the general population. *Applied Psychological Measurement, 1,* 385–401.
27. Nezu, A. M., Nezu, C. M., & Blissett, S. E. (1988). Sense of humor as a

moderator of the relation between stressful events and psychological distress: A prospective analysis. *Journal of Personality and Social Psychology, 54* (3), 520–525.

28. Beck, A. T., Ward, C. H., Mendelson, M., Mock, J., & Erbaugh, J. (1961). An inventory for measuring depression. *Archives of General Psychiatry, 4,* 561–571.

29. Spielberger, C. D., Gorsuch, R. L., & Lushene, R. E. (1970). *The state-trait anxiety inventory.* Palo Alto: Consulting Psychologists Press.

30. Anderson, C. A., & Arnoult, L. H. (1989). An examination of perceived control, humor, irrational beliefs, and positive stress as moderators of the relation between negative stress and health. *Basic and Applied Social Psychology, 10* (2), 101–117.

31. Zuckerman, M. (1960). The development of an Affect Adjective Check List for the measurement of anxiety. *Journal of Consulting Psychology, 24,* 457–462.

32. Trice, A. D., & Price-Greathouse, J. (1986). Joking under the drill: A validity study of the CHS. *Journal of Social Behavior and Personality, 1,* 265–266.

33. Labott, S. M., & Martin, R. B. (1987). Stress-moderating effects of weeping and humor. *Journal of Human Stress, 3* (4), 159–164.

34. Overholser, J. C. (1992). Sense of humor when coping with life stress. *Personality and Individual Differences, 13* (7), 799–804.

35. Russell, D., Peplau, L., & Cutrona, C. (1980). The revised UCLA Loneliness Scale: Concurrent and discriminant validity evidence. *Journal of Personality and Social Psychology, 39,* 472–480.

36. Rosenberg, M. (1965). *Society and the adolescent self-image.* Princeton, NJ: Princeton University Press.

37. Yovetich, N. A., Dale, J. A., & Hudak, M. A. (1990). Benefits of humor in reduction of threat-induced anxiety. *Psychological Reports, 66* (1), 51–58.

38. Danzer, A., Dale, J. A., & Klions, H. L. (1990). Effect of exposure to humorous stimuli on induced depression. *Psychological Reports, 66* (3), 1027–1036.

39. Velten, E. J. (1968). A laboratory task for the induction of mood states. *Behavior Research & Therapy, 6,* 473–482.

40. Hudak, D. A., Dale, J. A., Hudak, M. A. & DeGood, D. E. (1991). Effects of humorous stimuli and sense of humor on discomfort. *Psychological Reports, 69* (3 Pt.1), 779–786.

41. Cogan, B., Cogan, D., Waltz, W., & McCue, M. (1987). Effects of laughter and relaxation on discomfort thresholds. *Journal of Behavioural Medicine, 10* (2), 139–144.

42. Nevo, O., Keinan, G., & Teshimovsky-Arditi, M. (1993). Humor and pain tolerance. *Humor—International Journal of Humor Research, 6* (1), 71–88.

43. Ziv, A. (1984). *Personality and sense of humor.* New York: Springer.

44. Kuiper, N. A., Martin, R. A., & Dance, K. A. (1992). Sense of humor and enhanced quality of life. *Personality and Individual Differences, 13*(12), 1273–1283.

45. Svebak, S. (1974). Revised questionnaire on the sense of humor. *Scandinavian Journal of Psychology, 15,* 328–331.

46. Sarason, I. G., Johnson, J. H., & Siegel, J. M. (1978). Assessing the impact of life changes: Development of the life experiences survey. *Journal of Consulting and Clinical Psychology, 46,* 932–946.
47. Watson, D., Clark, L. A., & Tellegren, A. (1988). Development and validation of brief measures of positive and negative affect: The PANAS scales. *Journal of Personality and Social Psychology, 54,* 1063–1070.
48. Carver, C. S., Pozo, C., Harris, S. D., Noriega, V., Scheier, M. F., Robinson, D. S., Ketcham, A. S., Moffat, F. L., & Clark, K. C. (1993). How coping mediates the effect of optimism on distress—A study of women with early stage breast cancer. *Journal of Personality and Social Psychology, 65* (2), 375–390.
49. Carver, C. S., Scheier, M. F., & Weintraub, J. K. (1989). Assessing coping strategies: A theoretically based approach. *Journal of Personality and Social Psychology, 56,* 267–283.
50. Rotton, J., & Shats, M. (1996). Effects of state humor, expectancies, and choice on post-surgical mood and self-medication: A field experiment. *Journal of Applied Social Psychology, 26,* 1775–1794.
51. Lefcourt, H. M., Davidson, K., Shepherd, R. S., Phillips, M., Prkachin, K., & Mills, D. (1995). Perspective-taking humor: Accounting for stress moderation. *Journal of Social and Clinical Psychology, 14*(4), 373–391.
52. Larson, G. (1988). *The Far Side Gallery 3.* Kansas City, MO: Andrews and McMeel.
53. Lefcourt, H. M., & Shepherd, R. S. (1995). Organ donation, authoritarianism, and perspective-taking humor. *Journal of Research in Personality, 29,* 121–138.
54. Bonanno, G. A., & Keltner, D. (1997). Facial expressions of emotion and the course of conjugal bereavement. *Journal of Abnormal Psychology, 106,* 126–138.
55. Keltner, D., & Bonanno, G. A. (1997). A study of laughter and dissociation: Distinct correlates of laughter and smiling during bereavement. *Journal of Personality and Social Psychology, 73,* 687–702.
56. Keltner, D., & Ekman, P. (1994). Facial expressions of emotion: Old questions and new findings. *Encyclopedia of Human Behavior (Vol. 2)* (pp. 361–369). New York: Academic Press.
57. Lefcourt, H. M., Davidson, K., Prkachin, K. M., & Mills, D. E. (1997). Humor as a stress moderator in the prediction of blood pressure obtained during five stressful tasks. *Journal of Research in Personality, 31,* 523–542.
58. Miller, P. C., Lefcourt, H. M., Holmes, J. G., Ware, E. E., & Saleh, W. E. (1986). Marital locus of control and marital problem solving. *Journal of Personality and Social Psychology, 51,* 161–169.
59. Gottman, J. M. (1979). *Marital interaction: Experimental investigations.* New York: Academic Press.
60. Cohan, C. L., & Bradbury, T. N. (1997). Negative life events, marital interaction, and the longitudinal course of newlywed marriage. *Journal of Personality and Social Psychology, 73* (1), 114–128.
61. Gottman, J. M., & Krokoff, L. J. (1989). Marital interaction and satisfaction: A longitudinal view. *Journal of Consulting and Clinical Psychology, 57,* 47–52.
62. Vaillant, G. E. (1977). *Adaptation to life.* Toronto: Little, Brown & Co.

63. Levine, J. B. (1976). The feminine routine. *Journal of Communication, 26* (3), 173–175.
64. Crawford, M., & Gressley, D. (1991). Creativity, caring, and context: Women's and men's accounts of humor preferences and practices. *Psychology of Women Quarterly, 15,* 217–231.
65. Zillman, D., & Stocking, S. H. (1976). Putdown humor. *Journal of Communication, 26,* 154–163.

5

Forgiving

Michael E. McCullough

Although forgiveness has a long and rich history in religious views of optimal human functioning (1), the capacity to forgive has been largely unexplored during the first century of scientific psychology (2). In the past decade, however, the concept of interpersonal forgiving has begun to receive sustained research attention from researchers in developmental psychology (e.g., 3, 4), social psychology (e.g., 5, 6, 7), and clinical/counseling psychology (e.g., 8, 9, 10). This emerging body of work has provided some initial clues about: (a) the nature of forgiveness; (b) the relevance of forgiveness to health, well-being, and relationships; and (c) the effectiveness of educational and clinical interventions for encouraging forgiveness. In the present chapter, I review this body of research.

What Is Forgiveness?

Before embarking on a discussion of the existing research on forgiving, it is useful to outline the psychological context in which forgiveness takes place, and also to define what I mean by the term "forgiving." What I will delineate here should not be mistaken for a consensual definition of forgiveness. Indeed, developing a definition of forgiveness upon which all researchers can agree has been one of the more difficult tasks in the field of forgiveness research in the last decade (2, 11). Nevertheless, the theorizing and research I have been conducting generally has followed the conceptual and definitional principles that I lay out in the present chapter.

The Social Context of Forgiveness

First, forgiving occurs in the context of an individual's perception that the action or actions of another person were noxious, harmful, immoral, or unjust. These perceptions typically elicit emotional responses (e.g., anger or fear), motivational responses (e.g., desires to avoid the transgressor or harm the transgressor in kind), cognitive responses (e.g., hostility toward or loss of respect for the transgressor), or behavioral responses (e.g., avoidance or aggression) that would deteriorate good will toward the offender and social harmony.

To understand this psychological context, I believe we must look into humans' ancient past. I posit that it has been adaptive over the history of human development for humans to acquire two basic motivational responses to psychological and/or physical threat. The first of these motivational responses is the motivation to avoid the source of the threat. When attacked or otherwise threatened by another organism, animals are frequently motivated to avoid further contact with the offending organism. Behaviors that are apparently energized by the avoidance system include temporary behavioral withdrawal, ignoring, and the long-term disruption of prosocial interactions. The second of these motivational responses is the motivation to attack defensively or seek retribution against the source of the threat. Indeed, primatologists have documented that certain species of old world primates (including chimpanzees and perhaps macaques, as well as humans) coordinate retaliatory responses after having been victimized by another animal—sometimes even after considerable time has passed (e.g., 12).

As humans have grown cognitively more complex over many thousands of years, these two basic motivational systems have become increasingly sophisticated. The emergence and refinement of the sense of self and refinements in the use of language have widened the range of transgressors' actions that "victims" can perceive to be threatening or offensive. Whereas competing for sexual mates, food, or positions in social hierarchies might have been the primary social events that motivated our ancestors to avoid or seek revenge against aggressors, modern humans are capable of perceiving threat in a variety of more subtle social actions. In the context of ongoing relationships, for example, the subtlest glances or apparently innocent references can be interpreted as slights or forms of ridicule that challenge a person's self-worth or sense of acceptance from other persons, thereby eliciting motivations to avoid or seek revenge. Indeed, even words themselves (and their implications) can be perceived as threatening, whereas overt behaviors were probably the main threats that our ancestors recognized.

In response to these threats, then, people fundamentally are motivated to (a) avoid the source of threat; (b) retaliate against the source of threat; or (c) both. These distinct motivations, along with a motivation toward benevolence or positive interpersonal relations (which typically decreases when someone hurts, insults, or otherwise offends us), work in concert to create the psychological state that people refer to as "forgiveness."

Defining Forgiveness

Put succinctly, when a person forgives, he or she counteracts or modulates his or her motivations to avoid or seek revenge so that the probability of restoring prosocial and harmonious interpersonal relations is increased. When an offended relationship partner reports that he or she has *not* forgiven a relationship partner for a hurtful action, the offended partner's perception of the offense is posited to stimulate relationship-destructive levels of the two negative motivational states, that is, high motivation to avoid contact with the offending partner, and high motivation to seek revenge or see harm come to the offending partner. Conversely, when an offended relationship partner indicates that he or she *has* forgiven, his or her perceptions of the offense and offender no longer create motivations to avoid the offender and seek revenge. Rather, the victim experiences relationship-constructive transformations in these motivations and the return of constructive, positive motivations. Thus, forgiveness is not a motivation *per se*, but rather a complex of prosocial *changes* in one's basic interpersonal motivations following a serious interpersonal offense.

The idea that forgiveness can be understood exclusively in terms of something as simplistic as "motivational change" is not accepted unanimously by forgiveness researchers (e.g., 2,11). Nevertheless, the motivations to avoid and to seek revenge against an aggressor are both common and apparently basic to human functioning, so I believe that a motivational definition is both theoretically and empirically useful. Moreover, locating forgiveness at the motivational level, rather than at the level of overt behaviors, accommodates the fact that many people who would claim to have forgiven someone who has harmed them might not behave in any particularly prosocial way toward the transgressor. Rather, by invoking a motivational definition, I simply am suggesting that someone who forgives has experienced a reduced *potential* for avoidant and vengeful behavior (and an increased potential for benevolent behavior), which might or might not be expressed overtly.

One implication of this conceptualization is that forgiving can be viewed as a prosocial phenomenon with similarities to other prosocial psychological changes. Social and developmental psychology are full of examples of such prosocial changes. The well-established link between empathy and helping is a prime example. Because of empathy, we can come to care for a stranger's welfare and then intervene to promote his or her welfare (e.g., 13). In the psychology of close relationships, such prosocial psychological phenomena include accommodation (14), which is the inhibition of destructive responses and the enacting of constructive responses following a partner's destructive interpersonal behavior. Another prosocial process is willingness to sacrifice (15), which is "the propensity to forego immediate self-interest to promote the well-being of a partner or relationship" (15, p. 1374). What forgiving, empathy-motivated helping, accommodation, and willingness to sacrifice have in common is that a person acts in a manner that often has a personal cost (e.g., psychological effort, relinquishment of one's righteous indignation and, potentially, a loss of face) *to produce a benefit for another person or a relationship.* In the case of forgiving, one's negative interpersonal motivations are being transformed so that prosocial motivations toward the transgressor can emerge or reemerge.

Understanding Avoidance and Revenge Motivations

Understanding the avoidance system and the revenge system—as well as the factors that interfere with and enhance them—are crucial for learning how forgiveness operates.

The Avoidance System Individual differences in the functioning of the avoidance system are related to individual differences in the disposition to experience negative affect (i.e., neuroticism) and perhaps also in the disposition to be agreeable in social interactions (i.e., agreeableness). Negative affectivity or neuroticism involves emotional instability and a broad range of negative affects, including anxiety, sadness, irritability, and nervous tension (16). Neuroticism also involves a tendency to view ambiguous stimuli in a negative and threatening light. Some scholars have suggested that people high in neuroticism direct their attention differentially to negative stimuli (see 17 for review). Agreeableness is a prosocial orientation toward others that includes such qualities as altruism, kindness, and trust. People low in agreeableness have greater amounts of conflict with peers, assert more power during conflict, and have difficulties in relational closeness and commitment (18, 19), as well as empathy deficits (see, e.g., 20). It also is worth noting that adjectives such as "forgiving" (and "vengeful") often are used as prototypical descriptions of the agreeable (or disagreeable) person (e.g., 21, 22).

Aside from the contribution of personality factors to people's motivations to avoid individuals who have offended or harmed them, avoidance motivations appear to be sensitive to the relational and situational context in which an offense occurs. In a recent study (17), we presented participants with a series of eight real-life and fictional scenarios in which they had been (or were to imagine that they had been) offended by a relationship partner (i.e., a same-sex friend or an opposite-sex friend). For example, one real-life scenario instructed participants to think about the worst thing that a close friend had ever done to them. One fictional scenario asked participants to imagine that a close friend of the opposite sex had betrayed a confidence in a way that had humiliating consequences for the participant.

In response to each of the eight scenarios, participants completed the Avoidance and Revenge scales of the Transgression-Related Interpersonal Motivations Inventory (TRIM; 6). These scales are self-report measures that assess people's motivations to avoid and seek revenge against specific persons who have transgressed against them. We used variance components analyses to examine the extent to which responses to the offenses could be attributed to stable individual differences, the additive effects of various aspects of the scenarios; and error or other factors not modeled. These analyses were similar to standard analyses of variance (ANOVA), but the goal in variance components analyses is to estimate the amount of variance that can be attributed to each term in the model rather than to determine the statistical significance of the model's terms. Individual differences accounted for a considerable amount of the variability in people's avoidance scores (i.e., 18–37% in historical scenarios and 14–15% in fictional scenarios), but by no means did individual differences explain the lion's share of the variance in people's responses.

The remainder of the variance was distributed among effects due to (a) offense severity; (b) relationships in which the offense occurred; (c) the two-way interactions involving individual differences, offense severity, and type of relationship in which the offense occurred; and (d) error and other factors not modeled. With the exception of the main effect of offense severity among the fictional offense scenarios (which accounted for 54% of the variance in people's avoidance motivations), each of these additional terms accounted for less than 10% of the variance in people's avoidance responses. Nevertheless, the main finding of interest from these analyses is that although people demonstrated individual differences in their motivations to avoid their offenders, these differences among persons are probably not the most important factor driving people's avoidance motivations in any given offense situation. In other words, to lump people into those who are "avoidant" and those who are not "avoidant" would be a highly error-laden enterprise with limited value for predicting who would be avoidant in the context of a novel interpersonal offense. Thus, avoidance motivations also are strongly influenced by offense severity, characteristics of the relationships in which the offenses occur, and other factors that we have not yet isolated.

The Revenge System   The second motivational system intrinsic to forgiveness is the revenge system. Among the personality dimensions in the Big Five taxonomy, agreeableness appears to be the trait with the most relevance to the operation of the revenge system (23, 24). Specifically, people who are highly agreeable tend to be considerably less motivated to seek revenge against transgressors (17).

In contrast to the avoidance system, which appears to be mostly under the control of social and relational factors, individual differences are apparently the primary determinant of whether an individual will be motivated to seek revenge in response to a specific interpersonal offense. In the previously described McCullough and Hoyt study (17), in which we conducted variance components analyses, stable differences among persons explained the largest proportion of the variance in people's revenge responses across a variety of offense scenarios. For historical offenses, individual differences among persons explained 32–60% of the variability; for fictional scenarios, individual differences among persons explained 32–48% of the variability. Smaller amounts of additional variance were explained by other factors. In other words, it does seem meaningful to conclude that some people are simply more vengeful than others (see also 25). However, the revenge system, like the avoidance system, also appears to be highly sensitive to contextual aspects of the offense and the relationship in which the offense occurs.

Longitudinal Course of Avoidance and Revenge

As discussed previously, I believe that the avoidance and the revenge systems are two very old motivations that underlie much of primates' responses to threats and transgressions that they have received. Even so, it appears that many primates have a need to reconcile following conflict (12, 26). Because of the innately social nature of primates' lives, the motivations to avoid and seek revenge are frequently juxtaposed against a strong motivation to maintain a positive set of relations with others. Indeed, Baumeister and Leary (27) reviewed a massive amount of evidence suggesting that humans also have a foundational need for at least a few positive, supportive interpersonal relationships (27).

Either via the motivation to maintain positive human relationships or processes such as habituation or extinction, people's motivations to avoid or seek revenge from transgressors should subside over time for many (if not most) interpersonal transgressions. However, in analyses we conducted as part of a study of people who had been offended by another person in the previous several weeks, we did not find any evidence of a general trend toward reductions in avoidance and revenge motivations during an eight-week longitudinal follow-up (25).

It is hard to know what to make of this counterintuitive null result. The measurement of avoidance and revenge was adequate (i.e., internal consistency reliabilities were approximately $alpha$ = .90 for both administrations and people's avoidance and revenge scores were correlated at r = .50 and .47 across administrations, as we have found in other research). Inadequate statistical power could have been a problem (indeed, people's mean scores *did* decrease over time, although not significantly so). Also, failure to measure individuals during the time periods during which their motivations were changing could have been an issue (a common dilemma in longitudinal research; see 28). What we *did* find, however, was that individual differences in how people's motivations changed over time—particularly their motivations to seek revenge—were related to individual differences in vengefulness. People high in dispositional vengefulness were not only more motivated to seek revenge against specific offenders cross-sectionally, but also slower to reduce those revenge motivations over time.

Determinants of Forgiveness

Aside from individual differences, such as a disposition toward revenge, that might explain why some people seem to experience reductions in their avoidance and/or revenge motivations over time, researchers have isolated a number of psychological variables that seem to be associated with people's capabilities of forgiving. These include (a) cognitive and emotional processes such as empathy, perspective-taking, rumination, and suppression; (b) relationship qualities such as closeness, adjustment, and commitment; and (c) apology.

Empathy and Perspective-Taking Empathy and perspective-taking are important facilitators of many prosocial human activities, including willingness to help others (e.g., 13), and apparently, forgiving. Cross-sectionally, the extent to which someone feels empathic affect toward an offender and understands the cognitive perspective of the offender are highly correlated with measures of forgiving (7, 29) and measures of avoidance and revenge motivations, in particular (6).

In addition, empathy appears to mediate the well-established effect of apologies on people's willingness to forgive their offenders. That is, people appear to forgive apologetic offenders, in large part, because the apology itself helps people feel more empathic toward the offenders (6, 7). Also, the link between attributional processes and intentions to retaliate against someone appear to be mediated partially by empathy (30). Moreover, interventions for encouraging forgiveness appear to work, in part, through enhancing the offended person's empathy for the offender, as well as his or her ability to adopt the cognitive perspective of the offender (6). Indeed, empathy is, as far as I am aware, the only psychological construct that researchers have shown to facilitate forgiveness for specific real-life transgressions when manipulated experimentally (6, 31).

Rumination and Suppression The more that people ruminate about an offense they have incurred, the more difficult forgiving the offense appears to be. Intrusive rumination about the offense (i.e., being troubled by thoughts, affects, and images about the offense) and attempts to suppress those ruminations are related (in cross-sectional designs) to higher levels of avoidance and revenge motivations (6, 25). Longitudinal changes in rumination and suppression also are correlated with longitudinal changes in forgiveness, so that people who become less ruminative and suppressive also appear to become more forgiving (6, 25). Thus, rumination might play an important role in perpetuating *interpersonal* distress following interpersonal events, just as it appears to perpetuate psychological distress in general (32, 33). This conclusion is consistent with conclusions of other researchers who have examined rumination as a dispositional variable (e.g., 34): People who have trouble extinguishing ruminative thoughts in general also have a more difficult time forgiving.

Relational Closeness, Commitment, and Satisfaction   In discussing the variables that influence the avoidance and revenge systems earlier in this chapter, I noted the importance of relational factors. One of the most important
relational factors is relational quality. Specifically, people are most likely
to forgive in relationships that are characterized by closeness, commitment,
and satisfaction. Based on their results, several researchers (35, 36, 37, 38)
have noted that relationship partners more readily forgive one another for
interpersonal offenses in relationships that are characterized by closeness,
commitment, and satisfaction (but see also 37 for evidence that people are
actually *less* likely to forgive in intimate relationships if the offense is the
refusal of a relatively low-cost favor).

The link between relationship closeness/commitment/satisfaction and
forgiveness is probably quite robust. We recently studied over 100 couples
who reported on the extent to which they had forgiven their partner for two
different offenses (the worst thing their partner had ever done to them, and
the most recent serious thing that their partner had done to them). Both
the forgivers' and their partners' self-reported degree of closeness/commit-
ment/satisfaction were related to forgivers' degree of forgiveness in the context of both offenses. Moreover, in a follow-up study, we found that the
closeness-forgiveness relationship was mediated, in part, by a greater
willingness of offending relationship partners to apologize, and a greater
capacity for offended relationship partners to empathize with their offenders (6). Therefore, empathy and apology may serve as psychological bridges
between relationship closeness and forgiving.

Apology   A final variable that seems to have great import for forgiveness is
the extent to which the offender makes sincere apologies or expressions of
remorse (6, 7, 34, 39, 40). This robust link, of course, would probably be
predicted by many general theories, including theories of reality negotiation (e.g., 41) and attributional theories (e.g., 30). Sincere apologies and
expressions of remorse might be the most potent factors under the offender's control for influencing the likelihood that an offended relationship
partner will forgive the offender. The effects of apologies on forgiving appear largely to be mediated by empathy (6, 7). In other words, people are
willing to forgive apologetic offenders because such apologies and expressions of contrition appear to produce empathy for the offender.

Is Forgiving *Really* That Good? Is Revenge *Really* That Bad?

Thus far in this chapter I have addressed only theoretical issues related to
the basic nature of forgiveness and its personality and social determinants.
However, a major impetus for research on interpersonal forgiving has been
the prospect that forgiving might contribute to beneficial personal and interpersonal outcomes. To date, several researchers have examined the as-

sociation of forgiving with measures of psychological well-being, health, and relational well-being. Their preliminary results appear to be consistent with the generally held assumption that forgiving is, in general, linked with better adjustment and well-being, whereas seeking revenge is, in general, associated with worse adjustment and well-being.

Links with Psychological Well-Being

Dispositional Evidence   Based on initial evidence, it appears that people who are more forgiving and less vengeful tend to have slightly higher degrees of well-being. Using a nationally representative sample, for instance, Poloma and Gallup (42) found that people who reported higher use of forgiveness as a strategy for coping with interpersonal offenses (along with other constructive coping strategies such as praying for the offender, trying to discuss the matter with the person, or attempting to do something nice for the offender) had higher scores on a single-item measure of life satisfaction ($r = .16$). Similarly, Mauger et al. (43) found that people's scores on a multiitem self-report measure of their tendency to forgive others was correlated at $r = .16$ with scores on the MMPI depression subscale (with positive scores indicating a negative association of forgiving and depressive symptoms).

The disposition toward vengeance manifests an opposite pattern. Caprara and his colleagues (e.g., 44, 45) have found that people's scores on a measure of tendencies to retaliate after aggression are positively related to negative affect and neuroticism. Similarly, we (25) found that highly vengeful people (measured with a subset of items from Mauger et al.'s (43) Forgiveness of Others Scale) had significantly lower life satisfaction and higher negative affect. Also, Poloma and Gallup (42) reported that those who "try to get even" or "hold a resentment" are slightly lower in life satisfaction ($r = -.14$).

I infer from these results that people who are dispositionally more forgiving (or less vengeful) appear to have slightly less negative affect and slightly higher satisfaction with life. However, we should not mistake these observations for causal data; rather, these initial findings provide only modest initial evidence that a substantive, causal relationship between the disposition to forgive and psychological well-being might exist.

Offense-Specific Evidence   In addition to the dispositional evidence cited already in the present chapter, researchers also have begun to examine the relationship between forgiving individual offenders and various measures of psychological well-being (e.g., 25, 46, 47, 48, 49). For example, Aschleman (46) conducted a cross-sectional survey of 30 divorced or permanently separated mothers with children aged 10 to 13. Each mother completed the Enright Forgiveness Inventory (48) to indicate the extent to which she had forgiven the child's father for any offenses that the father had committed against her. In addition, mothers completed self-report measures of well-being, depressive symptoms, and anxiety symptoms. The extent to which mothers had forgiven the fathers was positively related to several measures of well-being, including self-acceptance and purpose in life. Also, forgiving was inversely related to self-reported anxiety and depressive symptoms.

Weinberg (50) examined how various strategies for coping with the unnatural death of a loved one influenced survivors' overall adjustment to the death. Weinberg surveyed a group of adults who had experienced the death of a loved one. A subset of these respondents blamed a third person for the unnatural death. Among respondents who blamed a third person for the death, those who reported that they "thought about or sought revenge" reported significantly lower scores on a single-item measure of adjustment than did respondents who blamed a third person for the death but did not report seeking revenge.

These cross-sectional relationships between forgiving a specific offender and adjustment, of course, do not provide persuasive evidence that causal processes are at work. Indeed, the only longitudinal research on the subject casts some doubt on whether forgiving has a causal influence on subsequent adjustment. As discussed earlier in this chapter, we (25) conducted an eight-week longitudinal study involving approximately sixty undergraduate students who had been injured by another person in the previous two months. At the baseline assessment, participants completed the TRIM Inventory (6), as well as a measure of the extent to which they ruminated about the offense and attempted to suppress their ruminative cognitions about the offense. They also completed a measure of life satisfaction. Eight weeks later, participants completed the same instruments again.

We did not find strong evidence for causal association between forgiving and well-being in either cross-sectional or longitudinal analyses. In cross-sectional analyses, we found that people who had high motivations to avoid and seek revenge against their offenders had lower satisfaction with life (although the relationships were not significant; $rs = -.20$ and $-.11$). In longitudinal analyses, however, we found little evidence that people who became more forgiving over the eight-week time period became any more satisfied with their lives (rs of residualized change scores $= -.04$ and $-.13$). Because subjective well-being (like other measures of mental health or psychological distress) is probably influenced by a host of psychosocial factors, people's responses to individual offenses that they have incurred might not have very robust effects on their subjective well-being. Thus, whether forgiving actually *promotes* psychological well-being remains very much in question at the time of this writing.

Other explanations exist for why some researchers find links between measures of forgiving and measures of psychological well-being and adjustment. The vagaries of sampling error might be responsible in part for the inconsistencies (51). Substantive explanations include the possibility that the forgiving-adjustment association might occur only among people who have encountered specific types of offenses. For example, forgiveness might be relevant for psychological well-being only when forgiveness is being used to buffer people against particularly stressful interpersonal of-

fenses (48). The respondents in the McCullough et al. (25) study were forgiving interpersonal offenses that, although perhaps more severe than normal, certainly represented the types of offenses that one might expect to
incur in the course of an average year of college life (e.g., a relationship
break-up, sexual infidelity in a romantic relationship, a racial slur). Conversely, Aschleman's (46) and Trainer's (49) participants had experienced
separation and/or divorce—exceptionally severe life events. Perhaps the
links of forgiving and adjustment are apparent only in the context of such
serious life events. Subkoviak, Enright, Wu, Gassin, Freedman, Olson, and
Sarinopoulos (48) suggested the related possibility that forgiveness might
be most relevant for psychological well-being when it is used to buffer people against interpersonal offenses that have occurred in the context of certain types of relationships (e.g., spousal, romantic, and family relationships), but not in others. From such explanations we can infer that
forgiveness may not exert a "main effect" on mental health, but rather might
interact with relationship type, perceived stressfulness of the offense, or
some other property of offenses to influence mental health and well-being.
To date, researchers have emphasized the "main effects" of forgiveness, so
in the future researchers need to examine interactions with relationship
type or offense severity to shed more light on how forgiveness might influence mental health and well-being.

Links with Physiological Measures

Forgiving appears to be associated with several physiological parameters.
Witvliet, Ludwig, Chamberlain, Thompson, and Ahmad (52), for example,
examined the physiological effects of four types of mental strategies for
coping with interpersonal offenses: (a) focusing on the hurt; (b) nursing a
grudge; (c) empathizing with the offender's human qualities; and (d) forgiving. Participants completed laboratory trials during which they were
instructed to recall a specific offense as they engaged in each of these four
types of imagery. During the trials, Witvliet and her colleagues measured
participants' heart rates, diastolic blood pressure, arterial pressure, and skin
conductance. Although all four imagery conditions led to increases in heart
rate and blood pressure, there were significant differences such that participants in the forgiving imagery conditions (i.e., empathizing and forgiving)
manifested lower heart rate, diastolic blood pressure, and mean arterial
blood pressure than did participants in the unforgiving imagery conditions
(i.e., focusing on the hurt and nursing a grudge). The physiological data
were consistent with respondents' self-reported affects during the imagery
sessions. During the trials in which participants were instructed to focus
on the hurt or nurse a grudge, they reported that their imagery was more
negative than when they were empathizing or forgiving. Whether the physiological effects associated with forgiveness imagery actually lead to clinically significant changes in physical health remains to be investigated.
However, several teams of investigators are examining currently the links

of forgiving to physiological indicators of emotion and health, so hopefully we will see answers to these questions in the coming years.

Links with Relational Well-Being

People who can forgive their transgressors also are more likely to restore positive relations with their transgressors. Conversely, it is probably true that people who cannot forgive exhaust and then abandon their relationships at a quicker rate than do forgiving relationship partners. Because the lack of positive, supportive relationships has been linked to nearly every psychological and physical malaise from suicide to immunosuppression (27), forgiveness might be associated with mental and physical well-being by helping people maintain stable, supportive relationships.

Indeed, researchers have reported a variety of associations between forgiving and relational well-being. As mentioned earlier, researchers have found positive correlations between forgiveness and self-reported relational closeness and adjustment (35, 36, 38). We (6) also found that forgiving not only occurs more frequently in the context of satisfactory, committed, close relationships, but also that forgiving appears to help people restore relational closeness following interpersonal transgressions.

In another study, Holeman and Myers (53) reported an important link between forgiving and relational well-being. Using a sample of 63 married women who were survivors of childhood sexual abuse, Holeman and Myers found that women who reported high scores on the Enright Forgiveness Inventory (i.e., who had forgiven the people who had sexually abused them) had higher marital adjustment than did respondents who reported low scores on the Enright Forgiveness Inventory (i.e., who had not forgiven the people who had sexually abused them). Holeman and Myers' (53) results are important because they are consistent with the view that people who can forgive in one relationship (in this case, a perpetrator of sexual abuse) also might reap social benefits in other relationships (in this case, their marriages).

In another study, Kelln and Ellard (5) instructed participants to complete a laboratory task in which they were working with a piece of seemingly fragile electronic equipment. In reality, however, the task was a bogus one, as was the "fragile apparatus." Participants later were led to believe that they had severely damaged the equipment. The independent variable was the experimenter's (actually a confederate's) response to the damaged equipment. The experimenter either (a) did nothing in response to the breakage; (b) sought retribution by reneging on a previous arrangement to pay the participant $4 for participating; (c) both reneged on the arrangement to pay and offered a verbal gesture of forgiveness to the participant; or (d) only made a verbal expression of forgiveness. In a fifth (control) condition, the participants were not led to believe that they had broken the equipment.

The dependent variable was the number of envelopes that respondents offered to distribute around campus for the experimenter as part of an unrelated task. Kelln and Ellard found significant differences among experimental groups, with participants in the "forgiveness only" condition indicating a willingness to deliver twice as many envelopes ($M = 18.08$ envelopes, $SD = 4.35$) as did participants who received (a) no intervention ($M = 9.13$ envelopes, $SD = 5.89$), (b) retribution and forgiveness ($M = 9.27$ envelopes, $SD = 5.38$), or (c) retribution only ($M = 7.29$ envelopes, $SD = 6.33$). The "forgiveness only" participants also volunteered to deliver considerably more envelopes than did participants who completed the bogus laboratory task without being led to believe that they had broken the equipment. Thus, participants who were forgiven were willing to do considerably more work on behalf of the completely forgiving experimenter than they were for the experimenter in any of the other conditions.

Kelln and Ellard interpreted this finding in the context of equity theory, arguing that the gift-like quality of forgiveness increased respondents' feelings of inequity, prompting them to restore equity by doing something kind for the experimenter. These findings also may be interpreted as evidence that people who are inclined to forgive their transgressors might engender greater social support from the forgiven transgressor than they might from any other response to the offense. Thus, forgiving appears to stimulate positive social interactions—even among people who hardly know each other.

If we can conclude that forgiving is "good" for relationships, then we also can surmise that revenge is "bad" for relationships. For example, people who use revenge as a problem-solving style encounter difficulty in maintaining friendships. To examine this possibility empirically, Rose and Asher (54) presented over 600 elementary schoolchildren with 30 conflict scenarios, in which they were instructed to place themselves in the shoes of the protagonist who had been insulted, injured, or frustrated by another child. Participants then were instructed to indicate what their goals would be in responding to the conflict. Among the six possible goals that respondents could choose was the goal of "trying to get back" at their friend. Rose and Asher used peer ratings to determine how many best friends each respondent had, how well each respondent was accepted by peers, and how hostile and positive each respondent was perceived to be by close friends. Endorsing revenge as a conflict resolution goal was negatively related to the quality of respondents' social relationships. The more frequently respondents reported that they would attempt to "get back" at their friends in the 30 conflict scenarios, the fewer best friends they had ($r = -.18$), the more hostile ($r = .25$) and less positive ($r = -.13$) their friends rated them to be, and the less they were accepted by their peers ($r = -.08$).

Can Forgiving Be a Maladaptive Coping Response?

Forgiveness might not be a good thing for all people in all circumstances. It is possible that in certain interpersonal situations, people who cope by forgiving might put themselves at risk for serious psychosocial problems (55). Also, some researchers suggest that forgiveness might be a marker for relational disturbance in some relationships, including those characterized by physical abuse (56). In Katz et al.'s study, 145 undergraduate women in dating relationships completed a survey in which they indicated the extent to which they would blame themselves if their romantic partner physically abused them. Participants also indicated the likelihood that they would forgive their partners and the likelihood that they would terminate the abusive relationship. Katz et al. found that women who reported that they would blame themselves for the physical abuse would be more likely to stay in the relationship. They also found evidence that the association between self-blame and staying in the abusive relationship was mediated by the women's willingness to forgive the violent partners.

Therefore, it appeared that women who would blame themselves would be more likely to stay in the relationship precisely because they were more willing to forgive the partner for the physical abuse. It is not clear whether forgiving actually *causes* such perilous situations, but the possibility that forgiving too easily is a potential marker for relational peril should be investigated seriously. Conducting such investigations and acknowledging that forgiving could be a red flag for psychosocial distress also would help to bridge ideological gaps between therapists and researchers who advocate for the positive effects of forgiveness and those who warn against its potential dangers.

Helping People Cope by Helping Them Forgive: Educational and Therapeutic Interventions

Research on the use of forgiveness in clinical applications is growing. In recent years, a variety of group and individual interventions for encouraging people to forgive have been developed and tested. In many of these studies people have been encouraged to forgive based on the intervention program outlined by Enright (see, e.g., 11). Other clinical researchers have based their intervention studies on the theoretical work of McCullough and colleagues (e.g., 7, 31). Other researchers presently are launching evaluations of intervention programs.

In general, participants in such intervention programs appear to make strides in forgiving their transgressors as a result. Worthington, Sandage, and Berry (57) conducted a meta-analysis of data from 12 group intervention studies. They reported that these group interventions were generally effective, improving group members' forgiveness scores by 43% of a standard deviation (Cohen's $d = .43$). Among the eight intervention studies that involved six hours of client contact or more, group members' forgiveness scores were 76% of a standard deviation higher than were those of members of control groups (Cohen's $d = .76$). Thus, it appears that participation in short-term interventions (particularly those involving at least six hours of client contact) are at least moderately effective in helping people to forgive specific individuals who have harmed them.

Individual psychotherapy that includes forgiveness as a treatment goal also appears to be more efficacious than no-treatment control conditions. In two published studies (8, 9), researchers have investigated whether individual psychotherapy protocols based on forgiveness are effective in helping people forgive specific offenders, and whether these interventions yield improvements in psychological well-being. In these two studies, researchers randomly assigned participants to either a psychotherapy intervention designed to help them forgive a specific relationship partner or to a no-treatment control group. In both studies, participants in the forgiveness interventions forgave to a greater extent than did participants in the control conditions. Moreover, participants in the forgiveness interventions also experienced reductions in anxious and depressive symptoms relative to people in the control conditions.

Other researchers have found that psychoeducational interventions can be effective in reducing vengefulness—even among people for whom vengefulness has been a chronic and serious problem. For example, Holbrook (58) examined the efficacy of a cognitive-behavioral training group in reducing vengeful thoughts and attitudes among 26 male prison inmates who had a history of reactive aggression (i.e., violence motivated by the desire to retaliate). Holbrook found that inmates' scores on a measure of beliefs and attitudes about revenge significantly decreased from the beginning to the end of the training sessions. These results provide a basis for hope that even individuals who have entrenched, serious problems with vengefulness might benefit from interventions designed to reduce their vengefulness.

Forgiveness at the Societal Level

In this chapter, I have focused almost exclusively on the nature and consequences of forgiving for individuals and relationships. Another aspect that has not received the attention that it merits is how forgiveness might exert influences at the societal level. This is unfortunate because—as I am sure that nearly everyone who reads this chapter would agree—it would be more pleasant to live in a society where people were quick to forgive and slow to retaliate.

Indeed, the problems associated with the lack of forgiveness at a societal level eventually will hit almost everyone. Nearly one-half of all interpersonal delinquency in student samples (e.g., a serious fight at work or school, hurting someone badly enough to require medical attention, etc.) is motivated by anger and revenge (59). Also, people who endorse vengeance have higher levels of retaliatory behavior in the laboratory, on the highways, and in their personal lives (60, 61, 62). The desire for vengeance is frequently cited as a motive for many destructive interpersonal behaviors, including homicide, suicide, rape, arson, shoplifting, and adultery. Put simply, a substantial amount of human misery can be attributed to people's difficulties in modulating their revenge motivations. As researchers continue to address the nature and consequences of forgiveness at the level of the individual and relationships, we also would be well advised to direct effort at developing strategies for helping society to become a more forgiving place.

Conclusions

After more than nearly a century of scientific psychology, researchers finally have begun to give sustained attention to the concept of forgiveness, how it operates, and how it affects people's lives. In this chapter, I have discussed these initial empirical and theoretical contributions in the context of my own theorizing about the nature of forgiveness. I have proposed that the capacity to forgive is best understood as a motivational phenomenon: When people forgive, they reduce their motivations to seek revenge against (and to maintain relational breaches with) people who have damaged them, thereby allowing prosocial motivations to emerge or reemerge.

The capacity for the motivational transformations that I call "forgiving" appears to be related to a variety of psychological factors, including (a) individual differences; (b) aspects of the situation in which the interpersonal offense takes place; (c) qualities of the offended person's relationship to the offender; and (d) apology. The disposition to avoid one's offenders appears to be stronger in people who are high in neuroticism and low in agreeableness, and the disposition to seek revenge against one's offenders appears stronger in people who are low in agreeableness. Empathy for one's offender, and the related cognitive perspective-taking, appear to reduce both avoidance and revenge motivations. Cognitive rumination about the offense and, ironically, attempts to suppress those ruminations, appear to inhibit forgiving. People are more forgiving in close and committed relationships than they are in distant and less committed ones. Finally, providing believable accounts, excuses, and apologies, as well as expressions of genuine remorse, are reliable means by which transgressors can increase their likelihoods of being forgiven.

Forgiving appears to be related positively, albeit weakly, to many measures of mental health and well-being. To date, however, there is not compelling evidence that these associations are robust or causal. Based on initial evidence, it appears that forgiving is related to lower levels of physiological arousal. Additionally, people who readily forgive individuals who have harmed them appear to experience more positive relationships. Individual and group interventions for promoting forgiveness and reducing revenge appear to be moderately effective and might even help people to make improvements in their mental health and well-being. In light of the concern that forgiveness might not be salutary in all relationships, and that it might even be a risk factor in some relationships, future clinical researchers should devote attention to determining the types of clients, relationships, and transgressions that can be treated effectively by forgiveness interventions, and those for which forgiveness interventions would be ineffective or harmful for one or more of the parties involved.

Over the last decade, many investigators have entered the field of forgiveness research. I would surmise that at least fifty different research groups worldwide currently are conducting empirical research on forgiveness. If each of these research teams publishes only one study on forgiveness, this practically will double the fund of scientific information that we have about forgiveness currently—a situation that will render this chapter's findings obsolete. I will gladly welcome such obsolescence because it will signal that science is truly making progress in understanding forgiveness. Indeed, there is ample reason for hope that the next decade will be a golden era for forgiveness research.

References

1. McCullough, M. E., & Worthington, E. L., Jr. (1999). Religion and the forgiving personality. *Journal of Personality, 67*, 1141–1164.
2. McCullough, M. E., Pargament, K. I., & Thoresen, C. E. (2000). The psychology of forgiveness: History, conceptual issues, and overview. In M. E. McCullough, K. I. Pargament, and C. E. Thoresen (Eds.), *Forgiveness: Theory, research, and practice* (pp. 1–14). New York: Guilford.
3. Enright, R. D., Santos, M. J., & Al-Mabuk, R. (1989). The adolescent as forgiver. *Journal of Adolescence, 12*, 95–100.
4. Girard, M., & Mullet, E. (1997). Forgiveness in adolescents, young, middle-aged, and older adults. *Journal of Adult Development, 4*, 209–220.
5. Kelln, B. R. C., & Ellard, J. H. (1999). An equity theory analysis of the impact of forgiveness and retribution on transgressor compliance. *Personality and Social Psychology Bulletin, 25*, 864–872.
6. McCullough, M. E., Rachal, K. C., Sandage, S. J., Worthington, E. L., Jr., Brown, S. W., & Hight, T. L. (1998). Interpersonal forgiving in close relationships II: Theoretical elaboration and measurement. *Journal of Personality and Social Psychology, 75*, 1586–1603.
7. McCullough, M. E., Worthington, E. L., Jr., & Rachal, K. C. (1997). Interpersonal forgiving in close relationships. *Journal of Personality and Social Psychology, 73* (2), 321–336.
8. Coyle, C. T., & Enright, R. D. (1997). Forgiveness intervention with post-abortion men. *Journal of Consulting and Clinical Psychology, 65*(6), 1042–1046.
9. Freedman, S. R., & Enright, R. D. (1996). Forgiveness as an intervention goal with incest survivors. *Journal of Consulting and Clinical Psychology, 64*, 510–517.
10. McCullough, M. E., & Worthington, E. L., Jr. (1995). Promoting forgiveness: A comparison of two brief psycho-educational interventions with a waiting-list control. *Counseling and Values, 40*, 55–68.
11. Enright, R. D., & Coyle, C. T. (1998). Researching the process model of forgiveness within psychological interventions. In E. L. Worthington, Jr. (Ed.), *Dimensions of forgiveness: Psychological research and theo-

logical perspectives (pp. 139–161). Radnor, PA: Templeton Foundation Press.

12. de Waal, F. (1996). *Good natured: The origins of right and wrong in humans and other animals.* Cambridge, MA: Harvard University Press.
13. Batson, C. D. (1991). *The altruism question.* Hillsdale, NJ: Erlbaum.
14. Rusbult, C. E., Verette, J., Whitney, G. A., Slovik, L. F., & Lipkus, I. (1991). Accommodation processes in close relationships: Theory and preliminary empirical evidence. *Journal of Personality and Social Psychology, 60,* 53–78.
15. Van Lange, P. A. M., Rusbult, C. E., Drigotas, S. M., Arriaga, X. B., Witcher, B. S., & Cox, C. L. (1997). Willingness to sacrifice in close relationships. *Journal of Personality and Social Psychology, 72,* 1373–1395.
16. Benet-Martinez, V., & John, O. P. (1998). Los Cinco Grandes across cultures and ethnic groups: Multitrait multimethod analyses of the Big Five in Spanish and English. *Journal of Personality and Social Psychology, 75,* 729–750.
17. McCullough, M. E., & Hoyt, W. T. (1999 August). *Recovering the person from interpersonal forgiving.* Paper presented at the annual meeting of the American Psychological Association, Boston, MA.
18. Asendorpf, J. B., & Wilpers, S. (1998). Personality effects on social relationships. *Journal of Personality and Social Psychology, 74,* 1531–1544.
19. Graziano, W. G., Jensen-Campbell, L. A., & Hair, E. C. (1996). Perceiving interpersonal conflict and reacting to it: The case for agreeableness. *Journal of Personality and Social Psychology, 70,* 820–835.
20. Ashton, M. C., Paunonen, S. V., Helmes, E., & Jackson, D. N. (1998). Kin altruism, reciprocal altruism, and the Big Five personality factors. *Evolution and Human Behavior, 19,* 243–255.
21. John, O. P. (1990). The "Big Five" factor taxonomy: Dimensions of personality in the natural language and in questionnaires. In L. A. Pervin (Ed.), *Handbook of personality: Theory and research* (pp. 66–100). New York: Guilford.
22. McCrae, R. R., & Costa, P. T., Jr. (1987). Validation of the five-factor model of personality across instruments and observers. *Journal of Personality and Social Psychology, 52,* 81–90.
23. McCrae, R. R. (1999). A mainstream perspective on personality and religion. *Journal of Personality, 67,* 1209–1218.
24. McCullough, M. E. (2000). Forgiveness as human strength: Theory, measurement, and links to well-being. *Journal of Social and Clinical Psychology, 19,* 43–55.
25. McCullough, M. E., Bellah, C. G., Kilpatrick, S. D., & Johnson, J. L. (in press). Vengefulness: Relationships with forgiveness, rumination, well-being, and the Big Five. *Personality and Social Psychology Bulletin.*
26. de Waal, F. (1989). *Peacemaking among primates.* Cambridge, MA: Harvard University Press.
27. Baumeister, R. F., & Leary, M. R. (1995). The need to belong: Desire for interpersonal attachments as a fundamental human motivation. *Psychological Bulletin, 117,* 497–529.

28. Cohen, P. (1991). A source of bias in longitudinal investigations of change. In L. M. Collins and J. L. Horn (Eds.), *Best methods for the analysis of change* (pp. 18–30). Washington, D.C.: American Psychological Association.

29. McCullough, M. E. (1995). *Forgiveness as altruism: A social-psychological theory of interpersonal forgiveness and tests of its validity*. Unpublished doctoral dissertation, Virginia Commonwealth University, Richmond, VA.

30. Weiner, B. (1995). *Judgments of responsibility*. New York: Guilford.

31. Sandage, S. J., & Worthington, E. L., Jr. (1999 August). *An ego-humility model of forgiveness: An empirical test of group interventions*. Poster presented at the 107th annual meeting of the American Psychological Association, Boston, MA.

32. Greenberg, M. A. (1995). Cognitive processing of traumas: The role of intrusive thoughts and reappraisals. *Journal of Applied Social Psychology, 25*, 1262–1296.

33. Holman, E. A., & Silver, R. C. (1996). Is it the abuse or the aftermath? A stress and coping approach to understanding responses to incest. *Journal of Social and Clinical Psychology, 15*, 318–339.

34. Metts, S., & Cupach, W. R. (1998 June). *Predictors of forgiveness following a relational transgression*. Paper presented at the Ninth International Conference on Personal Relationships, Saratoga Springs, NY.

35. Nelson, M. K. (1993). *A new theory of forgiveness*. Unpublished doctoral dissertation, Purdue University, West Lafayette, IN.

36. Rackley, J. V. (1993). *The relationships of marital satisfaction, forgiveness, and religiosity*. Unpublished Dissertation, Virginia Polytechnic Institute and State University, Blacksburg, VA.

37. Roloff, M. E., & Janiszewski, C. A. (1989). Overcoming obstacles to interpersonal compliance: A principle of message construction. *Human Communication Research, 16*, 33–61.

38. Woodman, T. (1991). *The role of forgiveness in marital adjustment*. Unpublished doctoral dissertation, Fuller Graduate School of Psychology, Pasadena, CA.

39. Darby, B. W., & Schlenker, B. R. (1982). Children's reactions to apologies. *Journal of Personality and Social Psychology, 43*, 742–753.

40. Ohbuchi, K., Kameda, M., & Agarie, N. (1989). Apology as aggression control: Its role in mediating appraisal of and response to harm. *Journal of Personality and Social Psychology, 56*, 219–227.

41. Snyder, C. R., & Higgins, R. L. (1988). Excuses: Their effective role in the negotiation of reality. *Psychological Bulletin, 104*(1), 23–35.

42. Poloma, M. M., & Gallup, G. H. (1991). *Varieties of prayer*. Philadelphia: Trinity Press International.

43. Mauger, P. A., Perry, J. E., Freeman, T., Grove, D. C., McBride, A. G., & McKinney, K. E. (1992). The measurement of forgiveness: Preliminary research. *Journal of Psychology and Christianity, 11*(2), 170–180.

44. Caprara, G. V., Barbaranelli, C., & Comrey, A. L. (1992). A personological approach to the study of aggression. *Personality and Individual Differences, 13*, 77–84.

45. Caprara, G. V., Manzi, J., & Perugini, M. (1992). Investigating guilt in relation to emotionality and aggression. *Personality and Individual Differences, 13*, 519–532.
46. Aschleman, K. A. (1996). *Forgiveness as a resiliency factor in divorced or permanently separated families.* Unpublished master's thesis, University of Wisconsin at Madison.
47. Strasser, J. A. (1984). *The relation of general forgiveness and forgiveness type to reported health in the elderly.* Unpublished doctoral dissertation, Catholic University of America, Washington, D.C.
48. Subkoviak, M. J., Enright, R. D., Wu, C., Gassin, E. A., Freedman, S., Olson, L. M., & Sarinopoulos, I. (1995). Measuring interpersonal forgiveness in late adolescence and middle adulthood. *Journal of Adolescence, 18*, 641–655.
49. Trainer, M. F. (1981). *Forgiveness: Intrinsic, role-expected, expedient, in the context of divorce.* Unpublished Dissertation, Boston University, Boston, MA.
50. Weinberg, N. (1994). Self-blame, other blame, and desire for revenge: Factors in recovery from bereavement. *Death Studies, 18*, 583–593.
51. Hunter, J. E., & Schmidt, F. L. (1990). *Methods of meta-analysis.* Newbury Park, CA: Sage.
52. Witvliet, C. V., Ludwig, T., Chamberlain, K., Thompson, E., & Ahmad, D. (1999 August). *Forgiveness and unforgiveness: Responses to interpersonal offenses influence health.* Paper presented at the Annual Meeting of the American Psychological Association, Boston, MA.
53. Holeman, V. T., & Myers, R. W. (1998). Effects of forgiveness of perpetrators on marital adjustment for survivors of sexual abuse. *The Family Journal: Counseling and Therapy for Couples and Families, 6*, 182–188.
54. Rose, A. J., & Asher, S. R. (1999). Children's goals and strategies in response to conflicts within a friendship. *Developmental Psychology, 35*, 69–79.
55. McCullough, M. E., Rachal, K. C., Sandage, S. J., & Worthington, E. L., Jr. (1997, August). *A sustainable future for the psychology of forgiveness.* Paper presented at the meeting of the American Psychological Association, Chicago, IL.
56. Katz, J., Street, A., & Arias, I. (1997). Individual differences in self-appraisals and responses to dating violence scenarios. *Violence and Victims, 12*(3), 265–276.
57. Worthington, E. L., Jr., Sandage, S. J., & Berry, J. W. (2000). Group interventions to promote forgiveness: What researchers and clinicians ought to know. In M. E. McCullough, K. I. Pargament, & C. E. Thoresen (Eds.), *Forgiveness: Theory, research, and practice* (pp. 228–253). New York: Guilford Press.
58. Holbrook, M. I. (1997). Anger management training in prison inmates. *Psychological Reports, 81*, 623–626.
59. Pfefferbaum, B., & Wood, P. B. (1994). Self-report study of impulsive and delinquent behavior in college students. *Journal of Adolescent Health, 15*, 295–302.
60. Caprara, G. V. (1986). Indicators of aggression: The dissipation-rumination scale. *Personality and Individual Differences, 7*, 763–769.

61. Collins, K., & Bell, R. (1997). Personality and aggression: The dissipation-rumination scale. *Personality and Individual Differences, 22*, 751–755.

62. Stuckless, N., & Goranson, R. (1992). The vengeance scale: Development of a measure of attitudes toward revenge. *Journal of Social Behavior and Personality, 7*(1), 25–42.

6

Coping with the Inevitability of Death: Terror Management and Mismanagement

Eric Strachan

Tom Pyszczynski

Jeff Greenberg

Sheldon Solomon

> . . . *To die: to sleep.*
> *No more; and by a sleep to say we end*
> *The heart-ache and the thousand natural shocks*
> *That flesh is heir to: 'tis a consummation*
> *Devoutly to be wish'd. To die: to sleep.*
> *To sleep? perchance to dream. Ay, there's the rub;*
> *For in that sleep of death what dreams may come,*
> *When we have shuffled off this mortal coil,*
> *Must give us pause. There's the respect*
> *That makes calamity of so long life.*
> —*Hamlet*, act III, scene i

Shakespeare understood the problem of death anxiety. His prose brilliantly captures a singularly human theme: *the anticipation of death is terrifying.* And what is particularly remarkable about the power of death in Hamlet's case is that the young prince *wants* to die. He has lost the instinct for self-preservation that is characteristic of most living things—for him death is "a consummation devoutly to be wish'd" and still it gives him pause. It seems, then, that the anticipation of death for a typical, content person might be powerful indeed. Does awareness of death have the power in "real life" that it does on the stage? If so, how do people cope with death anxiety? How do we muster the strength to "bear the slings and arrows of outrageous fortune," knowing that in the end the effort is futile and life is finite? The uncertainty that we all share concerning the actual hour of our death leaves us with a lurking fear that we might die before we have "finished." In other words, we might die without completing that which we have defined as meaningful—that which makes our life worth living. Does this lurking (implicit) knowledge of the inevitability of death, juxtaposed with our instinct for survival, affect our daily lives? The purpose of this chapter is to examine these questions.

We will be discussing the problem of coping with death anxiety from the perspective of Terror Management Theory (1, 2, 3). This theory provides an explanation for two fundamental human characteristics—the desire to maintain a favorable self-image (i.e., self-esteem) and the need to promote the truth of particular cultural worldviews—by recognizing the power that death anxiety holds over every human being. Thus, in the majority of the chapter we discuss Terror Management Theory and its explanations for coping with death anxiety in everyday life. The latter part of the chapter is dedicated to one of the more recent ideas to emerge from Terror Management theory; namely, the hypothesis that anxiety disorders (such as specific phobias and obsessive-compulsive disorder) are maladaptive attempts to focalize this core human fear. As the point of transition between these two sections, we will consider the role of the personality trait known as neuroticism. We believe this trait is a reflection of how well (or poorly) people are able to buffer death anxiety via the mechanisms of self-esteem and belief in cultural standards of value. But more on that later.

As a final note before we begin, it is probably wise to clarify what this chapter is not about. Some readers may have turned to these pages hoping for an understanding of how people cope with the death of a loved one. Others may be seeking a discussion of how the terminally ill cope with the impending end of their lives. Although Terror Management Theory may have useful implications for these important issues, the central focus of Terror Management Theory is on how people cope with knowing that death is inevitable, when death is not pending in the immediate future. The concerns of the terminally ill, for example, reflect what we would term *fear* of death, rather than death *anxiety*. As McKinney (4) writes, "fear is an emotion produced by present or impending danger. The cause is apparent. Anxiety, on the other hand, is the emotion when the cause is vague or less understandable" (p. 177). Terror Management Theory deals with the impact of awareness of death when that awareness is not the focus of attention and when death is ostensibly unrelated to whatever behavior is occurring. We will describe how people deal rationally with their conscious thoughts of death and provide a more extended examination of how death anxiety affects us in ways of which we are unaware.

Terror Management Theory

Imagine this. You are a municipal court judge in your hometown. You have a full docket of cases for the day, including the arraignment of a woman accused of prostitution. Cases like this are not uncommon in your daily work and you don't think much about it. In the back of your mind as you drive to work is the phone call you received before you left from someone trying to convince you of the need for advanced planning of your own funeral. The salesperson was polite and reasonably effective; you spent some time considering the prospect of your own death (which hopefully will occur in the distant future) and what that would mean for your family. When you arrive at the courthouse, you put these thoughts aside and begin the day's work. First up, the alleged prostitute. You set bond for her at $455 and move on to the next case. At the lunch break, your clerk jokes that either you are having a hard day or you did not like something about that woman accused of prostitution. She tells you that in similar previous cases you usually have assessed a bond closer to $50. As an arbiter of justice, this discrepancy is worrisome, especially given your realization that you have no good explanation for it. What happened?

This fictional scenario is derived from an actual empirical study conducted by Rosenblatt, Greenberg, Solomon, Pyszczynski, and Lyon (5) to test one of the major hypotheses derived from Terror Management Theory, the *mortality salience hypothesis*. The hypothesis can be stated thusly: If a psychological structure (e.g., a coping strategy) provides protection against death anxiety, then reminders of death should increase the need to maintain that structure. In other words, reminders of death should make people cling more tenaciously to anything that protects them from their fear of death. Note that implicit in the hypothesis is that anticipation of death is something from which people need protection and that such mechanisms do, in fact, exist. In the Rosenblatt et al. study, municipal court judges were randomly assigned to conditions in which half were reminded of their own death and half were not. Reminders of death came in the form of two open-ended questions about one's thoughts, feelings, and expectations about death. Each of these judges was then asked to set bond for a hypothetical alleged prostitute. Rosenblatt et al. hypothesized that judges reminded of death (known as *mortality salient*) would assess higher bond than control judges (the basis of this prediction will be discussed in greater detail below). The results? Average bond set by mortality salient judges was $455 compared to only $50 for those in the control condition. Thus, the actual data matched the prediction exactly (and strongly)—thinking about death had a powerful impact on a behavior that had seemingly little to do with death. Since that initial finding, more than 90 separate studies conducted in different laboratories located in seven countries have provided empirical support for Terror Management Theory. Death anxiety affects our everyday behavior in ways of which we are only now becoming aware.

Discussing empirical results before we have clarified the general nature of Terror Management Theory might seem like putting the cart before the horse. But unfolding the theory in this way may enable the reader to maintain an idea of the potential "real life" effects of death anxiety as we discuss theoretical origins. We turn, now, to that task.

Background

Perhaps the best place to begin an overview of the theory is with the proposition that major differences exist between the cognitive abilities of humans and those of other animals. Humans have the capacity to delay behavior in order to consider alternatives (to act rather than just react), to deliberate over past, present, and future, to imagine that which does not exist and, perhaps even more remarkably, to then turn the products of that imagination into reality. In other words, humans can conceive of a situation (problem, solution, opportunity, predicament, etc.) as something that exists over time. We can imagine what the next and hopefully best step should be to address the situation, and we can implement that step using knowledge (including tools, things) we already have, and knowledge that we do not yet have but can acquire. We can use our hands (in cooperation with our brains) to change the world into that which we desire (i.e., the future we want to produce). There is an important exception, of course—we cannot change the world into a place where we never die. Some things cannot be manipulated.

Consider, too, that these abilities imply a capacity for interpreting the world in multiple ways. People live their lives in a subjective world of humanly created concepts rather than one of "objective" reality. Our ability to manipulate objects and situations and to reassess their meanings and values implies that radically different interpretations and implementations of the same object or situation are not only possible, but likely. To paraphrase Hamlet, nothing is good or bad or useful or useless, except thinking and manipulating make it so. And it is not even necessary that we undertake actual exploration of the situation or object. We are capable of imagining exploration and making decisions about meaning and value based on that alone. This is a powerful and dangerous ability. Powerful, for example, because we can determine the utility of something before we actually need it (e.g., knowing the utility of a rope and harness before starting to climb a sheer rock face rather than trying to figure it out while falling). Dangerous, for example, because it is but a short step from imagining frightening outcomes in actually benign situations to avoiding those situations, without ever discovering that there was really nothing to fear in the first place.

It is worth noting that other species—primarily humankind's closest cousins (genotypically speaking) the gorillas and chimpanzees—have been observed making and using simple tools and perhaps even passing the techniques on in a kind of "cultural" transmission (6). Although this may hint at some moderately active level of the abilities just discussed, the noted sociobiologist E. O. Wilson (7) forcefully argues that "the human intellect is vastly more powerful than that of the chimpanzee" (p. 26). This statement is not, of course, particularly surprising, but it is relevant in the current context—there is an *important* difference between humans and other animals, even those animals closest in genotype and ability. That difference, according to Terror Management Theory, rests in the ability to think ahead and manipulate (in vivo or abstractly), to conceive of things as meaningful, and to act based on systems of meaning. This is in contrast to the experience of, say, chimpanzees who (as far as scientists can determine) act and react concretely, without the benefit of "abstract exploration" or consideration of meaning. As Jordan Peterson (8) recently put it:

> Simple animals perform simple operations and inhabit a world whose properties are equally constrained (a world where most "information" remains "latent"). Human beings can manipulate—take apart and put together—with far more facility than any other creature. Furthermore, our capacity for communication, both verbal and nonverbal, has meant almost unbelievable facilitation of exploration, and subsequent diversity of adaptation. (p. 66)

The "latent information" that Peterson addresses is the symbolic meaning of things in the world—the fine detail that separates the meaning of a Porsche from a Plymouth. As the capacity for abstraction and manipulation increases, so does possible meaning. Again, the same object can have vastly different symbolic meaning for different people.

Another unique cognitive capacity that all humans share is equally remarkable, though often taken for granted: *awareness of oneself as a unique entity, separate from all other living (and nonliving) things.* To put it formally, humans are self-conscious—aware of *individual* existence and distinction from other objects in the world. This capacity for self-awareness plays a central role in the ongoing regulation of behavior and provides freedom from rigid control by innate fixed response patterns. Remarkable as it may be, though, self-consciousness is a double-edged sword (as perhaps are all these capacities)—it creates the potential for both promise and terror in the face of life's seemingly unlimited possibilities. Promise because knowledge of the vastness of the universe, combined with awareness of a distinct place in that universe, allows for consideration of myriad alternatives to construct a life that is generally rewarding (if one is sufficiently productive, clever, and lucky). Terror because knowledge of life, combined with an understanding and anticipation of the future, leads to the inevitable conclusion that no matter how life is constructed, it will ultimately end in death, perhaps in a death that is excruciatingly painful, that could come at any time.

Again, our primate cousins have evidenced some behavioral manifestations of a primitive form of self-consciousness. For example, chimpanzees and orangutans are apparently able to recognize themselves in a mirror (6). Gallup's (9) method of testing self-consciousness (self-awareness at the very least) included painting small dots on the bodies of chimpanzees in places that would not be visible except in a mirror (e.g., above the eyebrow). After a certain age, the chimpanzees would explore their own bodies, their "selves," rather than the image, to determine the nature of the change. Other than humans (over the age of 18 months) no other species has demonstrated such self-awareness. But there is no evidence that the level of self-consciousness or awareness demonstrated in chimpanzees has the affective and motivational consequences that it has for humanity. Specifically, there is no evidence that apes give their own death a moment's consideration. E. O. Wilson (7) takes up this very point:

> If [for nonhuman primates] consciousness of self and the ability to communicate ideas with other intelligent beings exist, can other qualities of the human mind be far away? [Primatologist David] Premack has pondered the implications of transmitting the concept of personal death to chimpanzees, but he is hesitant. "What if like man," he asks, "the ape dreads death and will deal with this knowledge as bizarrely as we have? . . . The desired objective would be not only to communicate the knowledge of death but, more important, to find a way of making sure the apes' response would not be that of dread, which, in the human case, has led to the invention of ritual, myth, and religion [abstract meaning]. Until I can suggest concrete steps in teaching the concept of death without fear, I have no intention of imparting the knowledge of mortality to the ape." (p. 27, brackets added)

It would be interesting to discover if nonhuman primates could, in fact, grasp the concept of their own death, and if that knowledge would produce dread as it does in humans. If other beings had the capacity to understand death, it seems probable that the only reaction possible (initially at least) would be one of dread. How do you live a satisfying life when the final outcome is always death?

Ernest Becker (10,11), a cultural anthropologist whose integrative, multidisciplinary work forms the base for a substantial part of Terror Management Theory, proposed, like Premack, that knowledge of death (and not, it seems, merely self-conscious knowledge of life) in a creature instinctively programmed for survival creates the potential for abject terror. He writes, "the irony of man's condition is that the deepest need is to be free of the anxiety of death and annihilation; but it is life itself which awakens it" (11, p. 66)—"life itself," and an intellect capable of a great deal of abstraction and thought. Humankind is smart enough to grasp the inevitability of death (and the threat posed by unfamiliar things that may be dangerous and cause death). Fortunately, the same cognitive capacities that put humans into this paradox also provide a solution. That solution is culture, broadly speaking, and particularly culture that purports to grant its adherents immortality.

This is where the discussion of capacity for thought, manipulation, and abstraction has been leading. Humanity, in its effort to be free of the paralyzing terror inherent in intelligent self-consciousness, creates for itself a world of meaning, in which humans are the prime players, in which the meaning of the many things (including people) in the world are (more or less) clearly defined, and in which adherence to cultural standards guarantees immortality. The meaning of objects in the world comes from the tenets of shared experience. For example, in most of the United States, a Porsche is *more desirable* (of greater intrapsychic, and not just material, value) than a Plymouth and reflective of a greater amount of success in the meaningful activity of pursing the American Dream. Immortality can come in many forms, but the two basic groupings are literal immortality (e.g., belief in heaven) and symbolic immortality (e.g., belief that one will live on by becoming part of something larger and longer lasting than oneself, such as one's family, one's nation, one's accomplishments, etc.). Thus, the problem of death is solved by imbuing life with eternal meaning and value; as a result, life can be lived fully on that bedrock of stability. If one lives up to the values of one's culture, the reward is eternal life (or, at least, eternal meaning).

Thus, we now have the beginnings of a Terror Management Theory of coping with death anxiety. Humans are self-conscious and capable of infinite abstraction. Because of those abilities, we are aware of the inevitability of death, which is terrifying for an animal born with an innate desire for continued life. Protection from death comes in the form of culture which grants us immortality if we live up to its standards and expectations. But culture has to be up to the task. It not only needs to provide critical information about how to live (e.g., which foods to eat, which are dangerous, and how society should be organized) but also needs to present a compelling picture of how death can be transcended. In other words, culture needs to be both practical (i.e., it needs to contain information about how to stay alive and prosper) and transcendent (i.e., it needs to contain standards that define the path to immortality). Often, the two are intertwined: pursing the American Dream not only helps one make decisions about how to live day-to-day, but also how to live forever through one's accomplishments. Culture must elevate humanity to a special and unique place in the world and provide the opportunity for each person to be an object of primary value in a meaningful universe.

Difficulties arise, however, when someone else has a different perspective on the meaning or value of an important aspect of life; or, more seriously, has a different perspective on the meaning or value of almost every aspect of life, such as is the case when two people adhere to different cultural worldviews (e.g., Fundamentalist Iraqi Muslims and Capitalist American Christians). The very existence of someone who does not understand and value the world in the same way as another throws the ultimate truth of that valuation into question. That is, the truth of the person's view of the world, which assured death transcendence, is now in doubt, thereby arousing the threat of existential terror.

Death is the ultimate unknown and thus it holds a unique place for Homo sapiens (literally "Man, the Wise"). It is unknown, which is terrifying, but more than that it is *unknowable*. Peterson's (8) contention that the unknown is initially terrifying is followed by the notion that the unknown is also promising. The unknown object or phenomenon might be turned to one's advantage if one is able to adequately explore and successfully control it. Death, however, cannot be adequately explored. Its meaning cannot be determined because the experience of it removes the explorer from the playing field. Humans can experience the death of another and place the meaning of that into the cultural canon, but personal death remains elusive. Death must be transcended because it cannot be manipulated. We must achieve the security of (expected) immortality because the intrapsychic consequences (i.e., paralyzing terror) of facing death without a secure worldview are too great. It is something to be avoided at all costs.

That is why Rosenblatt et al.'s (5) mortality salient municipal court judges were so harsh on the hypothetical alleged prostitute. All of the judges presumably adhere to the tenets of the American legal system. Those tenets are rooted in American culture, English common law, and other traditions. They form the basis of a coherent system of meaning that is part of an overall immortality-granting cultural worldview. In other words, the law these judges practice helps shield them (abstractly, symbolically) from death. There is an unconscious supposition that if the law (cultural meaning) is upheld, immortality will be the result. Thus, when reminded of death (when re exposed to the ultimate source of terror), there is a need to cling more tenaciously to the shield, the law. Hence, the greatly increased penalty imposed by mortality salient judges on the alleged prostitute—on someone who rejects the cultural standards of value and thus calls their ultimate truth (and eternal security) into question.

Two Hypotheses

The Mortality Salience Hypothesis Research designed to test terror management theory has been focused on two major hypotheses: the *mortality salience hypothesis* and the *anxiety buffer hypothesis*. We already have discussed the mortality salience hypothesis at some length and have provided Study 1 of Rosenblatt et al. (5) as an example of this line of research. As a reminder, in the mortality salience hypothesis, we state that: If a psychological structure (e.g., a coping mechanism) provides protection against the fear of death, then reminding people of death should increase their need for that structure. The Rosenblatt et al. study is exemplary of the notion that mortality salience leads to harsher evaluations of moral transgressors because those transgressors threaten the security (immortality) granted by culture (12, 13). The mortality salience hypothesis also has been tested in other ways. To cite just a few examples, mortality salience has been shown to lead to (a) enhanced positive evaluations of those who support the cultural worldview and strengthened negative evaluations of those who challenge it (14, 15); (b) increased preference for ingroup members over outgroup members (14); (c) increased estimates of social consensus for culturally valued attitudes (16); (d) increased stereotyping and a preference for those who conform to stereotypes over those who violate them (17); (e) decreased aggression toward those who support the worldview and increased aggression toward those who threaten it (18); (f) increased propensities to behave in accord with the standards of the cultural worldview (19, 20); (g) increased identification with the standards of the cultural worldview among those who are successfully meeting them (21); and (h) greater stress and difficulty behaving in ways that violate such standards (22). For a comprehensive review of the effects of mortality salience on diverse forms of human behavior, see Greenberg, Solomon, and Pyszczynski (1).

The bottom line message, then, is that the cultural worldview—defined in many ways in these studies but generally following the theme of standards of value and behavior—does appear to provide the protection against death anxiety that we have proposed. Culture teaches people how to be secure in a world where the only certainty is death, and reminders of death make people cling to culture with renewed vigor. Culture defines the world (the good, the bad, and the unimportant) so as to allow us to make decisions about how to proceed in our daily lives. The things that are valued most highly by the culture are the things that provide the greatest potential for protection against anxiety, and vice versa. And make no mistake, people are capable of enough abstraction that just about anything can sit on the throne of the transcendental. That is why people die trying to distinguish themselves as the greatest daredevil or the first person to climb Mt. Everest without any boots on. That kind of behavior might seem silly to the average reader, but to adherents of the daredevil culture (or the climbing-Mt.-Everest-without-boots-on culture) it is the ultimate in heroic and meaningful behavior.

The Anxiety Buffer Hypothesis   On the other side of the terror management theory coin sits the anxiety buffer hypothesis, in which we state that: If a psychological structure provides protection against anxiety, then augmenting that structure should reduce anxiety in response to subsequent threats. Central to this hypothesis is that self-esteem serves an anxiety-buffering function similar to that of culture. Specifically, one's self-esteem can be thought of as an internal estimation of how well one is living up to the standards of value salient in one's culture generally and also in one's life—that is, the specific salient standards for a college professor are different than those for a ballet dancer, even if both are guided by their American nationality. This provides a compelling explanation as to why self-esteem is so important: *the greater one's self-esteem, the more secure, protected, and immortal one feels.* That is a very important point. To address our question from the opening of the chapter, it is high self-esteem that allows people to "bear the slings and arrows of outrageous fortune." Without self-esteem, the world would be a threatening place indeed. And even if the threats to self-esteem are not consciously perceived as threats to eternal life (and we contend that they are not), the anxiety implicit in intelligent self-consciousness still takes its toll.

Evidence for this hypothesis is provided by studies in which participants with either dispositionally high levels of self-esteem or self-esteem that has been experimentally bolstered show less anxiety and anxiety-related behavior in response to threats. For example, increasing participants' self-esteem by means of bogus feedback on a personality or intelligence test has been shown to lead to lower self-reports of anxiety in response to a graphic death-related video and lower levels of physiological arousal in response to threat of painful electric shock (23). Other research has shown that both experimentally increased and dispositionally high levels of self-esteem lead to an elimination of the otherwise robust tendency for subjects to distort their self-reports of emotionality in whatever direction they were led to believe is associated with a long life expectancy (24). These latter studies were derived from previous evidence that people distort their perceptions and judgments so as to deny their vulnerability to serious illness and premature death (25; 26). In other words, if people are told that laughing a lot leads to a longer, healthier life, they are more likely to report that they laugh a lot in comparison to people who were told that laughing has no impact on life expectancy. Bolstering self-esteem reduces that tendency towards distortion—we do not need to pretend that our physical health is better than it is if we view ourselves as valuable contributors to a meaningful universe.

Two Modes of Defense

Proximal Defenses   The research just mentioned brings to light an important point in terror management theory: that people have at their disposal two modes of dealing with death (2). The first deals with immediate, rational threats to life—threats that bring to light what we referred to above as *fear* of death. *Proximal defenses* are the mechanisms that, according to the theory, are brought to bear against such threats. These are relatively rational cognitive maneuvers that push conscious death-related thoughts out of consciousness, often by simply seeking distractions, but sometimes, as above, by distorting our perceptions of reality. A person might, for example, quickly flip past the pages of a weekly news magazine with gruesome photos of ethnic slaughter in Kosovo and focus on the more mundane coverage of the Dow Jones reaching 11,000 points. Or that same person might study the gruesome photos and accompanying story and thank his or her lucky stars that nothing like that ever happens in America (thus distorting this nation's violent past and present).

Proximal defenses are (quasi-)rational responses to the rational fear of death. They address the problem of death in immediate, conscious, and concrete terms. And even here the effects of culture can be felt. Culture in this case influences perceptions of what constitutes healthy, acceptable, and sustainable living (hopefully based on some reasonably "factual" criteria). The practical aspects of culture need to provide adherents the information necessary to live a long life or else the people within the culture itself are likely to die out.

Distal Defenses   Distal defenses make up much of we have addressed so far in this chapter. They are the main tools that humans use to cope with the death anxiety that is inherent in being human. They are defenses against the ever-present knowledge that death is our inevitable fate. Just as we know our names, regardless of what happens to occupy our currently conscious thoughts, so too do we know that someday we must die. This knowledge has an ongoing effect on our thoughts and behavior by motivating us to find meaning in the cultural worldview and to live up to the standards of value that it prescribes. Research has shown that the impact of this knowledge on our ongoing thoughts and behavior increases as it becomes more accessible, that is, as it comes closer to current consciousness. Once such thoughts enter consciousness, they must be dealt with in a more rational way. Thus, proximal defenses are activated.

What is perhaps most intriguing about the distal defenses is that they bear no obvious semantic or logical connection to the problem of death. As we have argued throughout this chapter, humankind copes with its knowledge of the inevitability of death by imbuing life with abstract cultural meaning and value. By being a good Christian, a proud American, a caring parent, or a productive scholar, we establish ourselves as valued contributors to the meaningful universe specified by our culture. If our culture promises some form of literal immortality, such as heaven, reincarnation, or nirvana, living a meaningful and valuable life qualifies us (in our eyes and the eyes of other members of the culture, if not in actual fact) for eternal life. Even if we do not subscribe to such beliefs, being a valued contributor to a meaningful culture gives us symbolic immortality—we become part of something larger and more significant than our individual selves which goes on forever.

The distal defenses of finding meaning in life and value in self acquire their anxiety-buffering properties by virtue of our early interactions with our parents, caretakers, and other agents of the culture. This process begins long before the child is capable of understanding death or engaging in abstract thought. It develops out of a primitive aversive reaction to hunger, thirst, discomfort, and other harbingers of threat to continued existence. This precognitive aversive reaction to threats to continued existence is the "primal terror" from which a fear of the abstract concept of death later emerges. The protection from this fear provided by self-esteem, faith in the cultural worldview, and consensual validation of these structures is rooted in similarly primitive preverbal experiences, in which the child associates safety with the parental affection that results from accepting their beliefs and living up to their standards.

From the first days of life, the helpless infant's fears are assuaged by the love, approval, and protection provided by the parents or primary caregivers. Although this approval and affection is initially given unconditionally, as the child matures and his or her capacities develop, the parents begin to provide more of these entities when the child behaves in accord with their own beliefs and standards (which are derived from the cultural worldview). Once the child acquires language, the parents provide verbal rules that correspond to the culture's standards and use the cultural worldview to answer the child's emerging questions about how the world works. All the while, the approval and protection that the parents provide is increasingly tied to the child's acceptance of the cultural worldview and behaving in accord with its dictates.

Gradually, children come to realize that their parents are mortal creatures with flaws and that there are things from which even their parents cannot protect them. At this point, the child requires protection from something larger and more powerful than the parents, which is provided by the culture at large in the form of deities, group identifications, and social roles and institutions. Very gradually, the child's own perceptions, evaluations, and beliefs, strengthened by the consensual validation provided by significant others and society at large, take on the ability to provide the protection formerly provided by the parents. People are confident that their beliefs are correct and that they are indeed living up to the culture's standards when others agree with their beliefs and self-evaluations; as a consequence, they feel relatively free from anxiety. This confidence is threatened, however, when others disagree with us or criticize our behavior, thus leaving us susceptible to anxiety.

Of course, we adults realize that death is inevitable, even if our conception of the world is absolutely correct and we perfectly live up to all the standards of that worldview. We nonetheless continue to feel comforted when our self-esteem and faith in the cultural worldview is intact because the protection that these structures provide has little to do with rationality or logic. As Vandenberg (27) writes:

> Death anxiety is rarely experienced directly because it is too disruptive and overwhelming. . . . These existential uncertainties are not necessarily eliminated or diminished through the use of logical-mathematical thought. Indeed, these uncertainties may give rise to other ways of considering the world, ways that may be non-logical in nature. (p. 1279)

It is the early experiential connection between these structures and security that underlies the feeling of safety that self-esteem and one's cultural worldview provides. Distal defenses address the problem of death indirectly and symbolically, by providing a sense that one is a permanent part of a meaningful, eternal universe.

The Mismanagement of Terror: Anxiety Disorders

Overview

So far we have attempted to outline the Terror Management Theory of coping with death anxiety as it has developed over the past 15 years. We have given consideration to both proximal and distal defenses against death anxiety and underscored which kind of defense is used for which kind of death-related threat. Critical to understanding our perspective is understanding that the basic, default state for all living things (at least those with some sort of central nervous system) is a readiness to experience fear or anxiety. This is a simple consequence of being instinctively programmed for survival. What we learn through the processes of enculturation and individual exploration (i.e., manipulation and abstraction) is how to be secure in a world where the only certainty is death. In other words, we learn how to shape or interpret the world such that we are immortal beings of primary importance in a meaningful, eternal universe.

We have proposed that death holds a special place in the thinking of humans (i.e., it is the ultimate terror) because, despite the fact that we desperately want to live, we know we must die. Intrapsychic stability requires that we transcend death—make it a nonissue by living forever. Culture provides us the roadmap to immortality by delineating the practical, day-to-day steps for successful living and, more important, by showing us the path to immortality. That is why culture is focused on the heroic, the eternally meaningful (8, 11). One might imagine that if another fear, say, the fear of mountains were the ultimate terror, then our human cultures would likely be structured around staying at sea level and would grant us symbolic protection against the threat of increased elevation. Our reformulated theory would, of course, be called terra management theory, and experimental manipulations would involve reminding people of Mt. Everest and assessing the impact on moral transgression. But mountains can be explored and even manipulated and do not undermine our basic needs and desires; thus, they could never hold the threat that death does. The underlying structure of culture sends an implicit message about what it is that fundamentally motivates us.

Whence, then, comes the discussion of anxiety disorders? Is there any reason to expect that there is some connection between fundamental existential anxiety and the development of diagnosable anxiety disorders? And by the way, what exactly are the anxiety disorders? The answer to the latter question is that anxiety disorders, as the name suggests, are the group of psychological disorders whose main characteristic is the excessive experience of anxiety. In other words, they are the disorders in which extreme, unreasonable, and disruptive anxiety *is* the pathology. The focus of the anxiety varies from diagnosis to diagnosis and can be limited to specific objects or situations (namely, phobias such as spider phobia, snake phobia, and claustrophobia) or can be extremely broad with nearly every stimulus being anxiety provoking (i.e., generalized anxiety disorder).

There are numerous theories of etiology (i.e., cause) for each of the anxiety diagnoses and a complete review of any one of them (let alone all of them) would go well beyond the constraints of this chapter (for reviews see 28, 29). Suffice it to say that, like most diagnoses in clinical psychology, there are several etiological models for each of the anxiety disorders that delineate accounts of onset, course, and treatment. Given that numerous models already exist, one might question why a terror management model is needed at all. The answer to that question is threefold and we will consider each below. First, research in our laboratories has begun to implicate the degree of individual neuroticism—that is, consistent, high, but not necessarily pathological levels of anxiety—in terror management processes. Second, we do not believe that any of the models provide a compelling account of the *severity* of the anxiety characteristic of anxiety disorders or an explanation for why afflicted individuals often realize that their fears are indeed unreasonable. Third, there may be important (and empirically testable) clinical implications of a model of anxiety disorders based on Terror Management Theory.

Neuroticism

To begin, neuroticism, as a scientific construct, is many things to many people. For the purposes of this discussion, we define neuroticism as trait anxiety—that is, the amount of anxiety one feels on a regular basis, independent of situational factors (in the lab, terror management researchers use the Neuroticism subscale of the Eysenck Personality Inventory [30] as the operational definition of neuroticism). However, we have also indicated our belief that neuroticism is a dimension of personality that reflects how well one is able to use the mechanisms of culture and self-esteem to buffer the threat inherent in self-conscious knowledge of death. Recall, too, our proposal that anxiety is the default state of being for humans which suggests that all humans are "neurotic" when stripped of anxiety-buffering defenses. Thus, it is the combination of these factors that make up our first reason for proposing a Terror Management Theory of anxiety pathology: we suggest that highly neurotic people have difficulty finding meaning and transcendence in daily living and thus experience the anxiety inherent in intelligent self-consciousness to a greater extent (and on a more regular basis) than those low in neuroticism. This ties several points from the chapter together: neuroticism, or trait anxiety, exists because anxiety is the basic state of being for humans. Differences in degree or level of neuroticism exist based on how successfully anxiety is buffered by culture. And failure to successfully buffer death anxiety affects behavior in ways ostensibly unrelated to death (e.g., distal defenses or neuroticism).

Although we have only recently begun exploring the role of neuroticism in terror management processes, several studies have shown that individuals high in neuroticism show especially strong reactions to reminders of their mortality. For example, Goldenberg, Pyszczynski, McCoy, Greenberg, and Solomon (31) have shown that neurotic individuals are especially threatened by the physical aspects of the human sexual experience and that this threat results from the reminder of one's creaturely animal nature that sex has the potential to provide. In an initial study, Goldenberg et al. found that reminding neurotic individuals of their mortality led them to view the physical but not romantic aspects of sex as less appealing. Mortality salience tended to have the opposite effect on individuals low in neuroticism. A second study showed that inducing neurotics to think about the physical aspects of sex increased the accessibility of death-related thoughts, as measured by a word-stem completion measure (e.g., COFF_ _; which could be completed as either COFFIN or COFFEE; more death-related completions indicate greater accessibility of death-related thoughts). Neurotics induced to think about the romantic aspects of sex or nonneurotic individuals showed no such effect on the accessibility of death-related thoughts. A third study replicated this finding and showed that inducing neurotics to think about romantic love but not another pleasant topic eliminated the increased death-thought accessibility produced by thoughts of physical sex. Taken together, these studies suggest that the anxiety and distress that many individuals experience concerning the topic of sex may be rooted in the existential problem of being a physical creature with a sophisticated mind that is struggling to elevate itself above the rest of the natural world in order to deny its ultimate mortality. Sex is a problem and is regulated, restricted, and imbued with abstract meaning by cultures worldwide because it has the potential to remind us of our underlying physical animal nature.

Although our initial studies showed a connection between sex and existential concerns only for neurotics, more recent research has shown similar effects for a general population when the problem of creatureliness is especially salient. By so doing, these newer studies shed light on what may lie at the core of neurotic tendencies. Goldenberg, Pyszczynski, Greenberg, Solomon, and Cox (32) have shown that making the problem of creatureliness salient by having participants read a short essay arguing that humans are biological animals no different from other living things leads individuals regardless of level of neuroticism to show increased death thought accessibility after thinking about physical sex and to find physical sex less appealing after being reminded of their mortality. This, of course, is exactly what one would expect if the connection between anxiety concerning death and sex results from the creaturely aspects of the sexual experience. It also suggests that neurotics are particularly troubled by these issues because they have difficulty maintaining abstract cultural meaning in human activities when our creaturely nature is salient, as is the case with many activities involving the human body. Recall, too, that when sex was explicitly associated with love—a unique, meaningful, and transcendent human experience—neurotics were far less troubled by thoughts of physical sex.

The upshot of this research is that difficulty maintaining abstract cultural meaning in the face of the animalistic creaturely side of human existence may be at least partly responsible for the neurotic individual's proneness to experience high levels of anxiety. Of course, neuroticism is no doubt a complex phenomena with multiple determinants, and a great deal of additional research will be needed to fully evaluate our proposition that difficulties maintaining meaning play a central role in this phenomenon. Nonetheless, these initial findings pave the way for a terror management analysis of anxiety and anxiety-related problems.

Excessive Fear

If the empirical relationship between neuroticism and terror management processes does not directly implicate death anxiety in anxiety disorders, it at least serves as a reasonable basis for hypothesizing about such a relationship. What happens when an individual's cultural anxiety buffer is insufficient or nonexistent? What happens when one believes firmly in a worldview (i.e., the buffer is intact) but constantly feels that one is failing to live up to the standards of value (i.e., self-esteem is low)? Our hypothesis is that one possible result might be the development of a specific anxiety disorder. Perhaps a quote from Irvin Yalom (33) will drive the point home. In a chapter from his classic *Existential Psychotherapy*, Yalom writes:

> The paradigm that I shall describe in this chapter rests, as do most paradigms of psychopathology, on the assumption that psychopathology is a graceless, inefficient mode of coping with anxiety. An existential paradigm assumes that anxiety emanates from the individual's confrontation with the ultimate concerns in existence. . . . All individuals are confronted with death anxiety, must develop adaptive coping modes—modes that consist of denial-based strategies such as suppression, repression, displacement, belief in personal omnipotence [think proximal defenses], acceptance of socially sanctioned religious beliefs that "detoxify" death, or personal efforts to overcome death through a wide variety of strategies that aim at achieving symbolic immortality [think distal defenses]. Either because of extraordinary stress or because of an inadequacy of available defensive strategies, the individual who enters the realm called "patienthood" has found insufficient the universal modes of dealing with death fear and has been driven to extreme modes of defense. (pp. 110–111, brackets added)

This leads nicely into a discussion of our second reason for a terror management model of anxiety disorders. Our initial empirical work on the connection between death anxiety and anxiety disorders has focused on spider phobia (34) and obsessive compulsive disorder. Although an extensive literature exists on these types of disorders, there is little research that actually addresses the excessive nature of the fear. Instead, that excessive fear is merely taken for granted—a phobia is, by definition, an excessive, irrational fear. A terror management model, however, can account for the excessive nature of the fear. More precisely, the terror management model proposes that the fear is not actually excessive. Rather, it is an accurate reflection of the threat posed by that which is actually feared—death.

Consider a study by Thorpe and Salkovskis (35) which demonstrated that phobics report higher levels of belief in harm cognitions (related to exposure to the phobic stimulus) than control subjects. Without going into great detail, the relevant point is that the harm cognitions endorsed by the phobic participants—for example "I would go mad"—were not specific to the phobic stimulus (to avoid confounding symptoms with negative cognitions). In fact, the phobic participants tended to endorse items relating to the dangerousness of the phobic object, such as "I would come to physical harm" relatively less frequently. Thus, the picture the authors created is one of confusion felt by phobics who "know" they will not really be harmed but fear some "nameless and dreadful" consequence of contact nonetheless. As the authors write, "this would suggest that spider phobics endow spiders with *more meaning* than do non-spider phobics" (p. 814; emphasis added). In other words, the fear felt by spider phobics is much greater than the threat posed by spiders. It is not, however, greater than the threat posed by death, the ultimate terror.

Empirical Support

All of this, of course, is merely speculation without experimental results. Fortunately, initial data exist in the form of a study by Strachan (34). In that study, spider phobic and nonspider phobic participants were reminded either of death or a neutral topic. They were then asked to complete a series of tasks relevant to spider fear. It was hypothesized that (similar to the mortality salience hypothesis), if death anxiety is the root of spider phobia, then reminding phobic participants of death should increase their fear reactions to spider stimuli and that no such effect should be found for nonphobics. The study supported the hypothesis. Specifically, significant effects for reminders of death were found among the phobics, but not the nonphobics, in terms of behavioral avoidance of, and perception of threat from, spider stimuli. That is, death salient spider phobics spent less time voluntarily viewing pictures of spiders than non-death salient spider phobics. Also, those same death salient spider phobics perceived the spiders in the pictures to be more threatening than the control spider phobics. No differences were found for the nonphobics. Thus, reminders of death (the actual, underlying, distal fear) increased fear reactions to the proximal stimulus as should be the case if the death anxiety hypothesis is correct.

In another study, we investigated the effects of mortality salience on the hand-washing behavior of individuals scoring high on a measure of obsessive-compulsive tendencies. One common manifestation of obsessive-compulsive disorder is a fear of contamination, often manifested as excessive hand-washing. Some individuals afflicted with this disorder wash their hands so frequently and with such vigor that they literally become raw and blistered. Participants first filled out a series of questionnaires that contained a pair of open-ended questions about either the prospect of their own death or the prospect of dental pain. Under the guise of getting them ready for physiological recording, some sticky, gooey electrode paste was smeared on their hands. In fact, this provided the context for assessing how vigorously they washed their hands afterward. The data showed that when washing off the paste, high obsessive-compulsive participants ran the water for a significantly longer time in the mortality salient condition than in the dental pain control condition. Thus, as in the spider phobia study, reminders of mortality led to increased anxiety-related symptoms among those who typically have problems with those symptoms.

To reiterate the terror management model, then, we propose that anxiety disorders, such as spider phobia, are "graceless, inefficient modes" of coping with death anxiety. In other words, what is ultimately feared in spider phobia and obsessive-compulsive disorder is death rather than spiders, contamination, or other specific stimuli from daily life. We suspect that the association between the phobic stimulus and death arises when there is an excess of death-related anxiety—due to a breakdown in the cultural anxiety buffer or confrontation with a reminder of one's mortality—which prompts a search of the environment for a source worthy of the anxiety. Thus, the fear of death becomes focalized on something less threatening and more manageable. To paraphrase Yalom (33), it is better to be afraid of "some thing" than of "no thing," presumably because fear of "no thing" means that nothing can be done about it. That is to say, fear motivates most animals that experience it to act in some way that reduces the experience of it. If there is no obvious cause for these feelings—which is the defining feature of anxiety—there is no obvious course of action to eliminate it. Once the anxiety has a name and a shape, however, it has boundaries that allow one to work around it—an advantage not offered by death. Phobic fear is extreme fear, but in as much as it is associated with a particular stimulus, it is also a circumscribed fear.

Implicit in this hypothesis, of course, is that the anxiety is not recognized as death anxiety per se (else there would be no need to find an alternative source of fear), an idea amply supported in the terror management literature (1). That is, conscious thoughts of death are quickly and automatically pushed out of consciousness, although they remain highly accessible in the sense described by Wegner and Smart (36). Thus, these accessible but non-conscious thoughts "continue to pose problems for the individual" (2), and such existentially anxious individuals search out a source, from the environment, for their problem (i.e., anxiety).

Clinical Implications

This section will be somewhat shorter than we would like, in large part because we have not yet conducted any type of treatment outcome research on the terror management model of anxiety disorders. That being said, however, there are several major clinical implications that can be drawn from the model. If research continues to confirm a connection between anxiety disorders, neuroticism, and death anxiety, special care should be taken to include self-esteem and worldview components in treatment plans for anxious people. Our reasoning for this is based on the idea that self-esteem is a reflection of how "immortal" a person feels based on the anxiety-buffering properties inherent in adherence to a specific cultural worldview. Thus, bolstering self-esteem and faith in a meaningful worldview should increase the efficacy of treatment of anxiety disorders and may serve to reduce the severity of symptoms. To the extent that anxiety pathology is a reflection of the inadequacies of the individual's standard means of buffering anxiety, bolstering those standard means should decrease the "need" for alternative sources of security (or at least anxiety displacement).

Some indirect evidence for this notion can be drawn from another set of findings from the Strachan (34) study. In that study, there was a significant negative correlation between participants' neuroticism and self-esteem ($r = -.65$, $p < .0005$) scores, and also between spider fear (as measured by a self-report questionnaire) and self-esteem ($r = -.32$, $p = .01$) scores. These data are correlational and thus we do not claim that low self-esteem *causes* high neuroticism and spider fear. We do, however, emphasize that low self-esteem is strongly related to high neuroticism and (to a lesser degree) spider fear, which is consistent with the notion that problems with self-esteem may be contributing to these anxiety-related problems. We also emphasize that this is an empirical question that is amenable to laboratory experimentation.

Additionally, based on previous results, one can infer that worldview affirmation can be of value. Following mortality salience, worldview defense has been shown in two studies to reduce the accessibility of death-related thoughts, presumably because it quells the individual's death anxiety (37). Worldview defense also has been found to be beneficial in depressed individuals. Based on Pyszczynski and Greenberg's (38) analysis of depression, Simon et al. (39) proposed that depressed individuals suffer from inadequate terror management because of both low self-esteem and a lack of faith in life as being meaningful. They hypothesized that mortality salience would therefore provoke a particularly strong reaction in mildly depressed individuals, resulting in particularly strong worldview defense. In support of this hypothesis, they found that mildly depressed individuals (with elevated scores on the Beck Depression Inventory) displayed even stronger worldview defense in the form of pro-American bias after mortality salience than did nondepressed individuals. Simon et al. (40) further proposed that because mortality salience motivated depressed individuals to bolster their worldviews, this would enhance their sense that life was meaningful. In a study to assess this idea, they found that mildly depressed individuals in general perceive life as less meaningful than do the nondepressed, but that this deficit was eliminated if the depressed participants were allowed to defend their worldview following mortality salience. This research thereby provides at least preliminary support for the idea that treatments for psychological disorders such as depression and anxiety disorders that encourage bolstering the individual's worldview may help alleviate psychological distress.

Conclusion

Although a great deal more research is needed, the existing evidence supports the idea that a number of psychological disorders may indeed reflect maladaptive efforts to cope with the knowledge of inevitable death. A useful next step may be to assess treatment approaches that acknowledge the problems of existential meaning and promote healthier modes of coping with this most unique human problem. To end where we began (with an understanding that by *conscience* Shakespeare means "the ability to think").

> *For who would bear the whips and scorns of time, . . .*
> *When he himself might his quietus make*
> *With a bare bodkin? Who would fardels bear,*
> *To grunt and sweat under a weary life,*
> *But that the dread of something after death,*
> *The undiscover'd country from whose bourn*
> *No traveller returns, puzzles the will,*
> *And makes us rather bear those ills we have*
> *Than fly to others that we know not of?*
> *Thus conscience does make cowards of us all.*

References

1. Greenberg, J., Solomon S., & Pyszczynski, T. (1997). Terror management theory of self-esteem and cultural worldviews: Empirical assessments and conceptual refinements. In M. Zanna (Ed.), *Advances in experimental social psychology* (vol. 30, pp. 61–139). San Diego: Academic Press.
2. Pyszczynski, T., Greenberg, J., & Solomon, S. (1999). A dual process model of defense against conscious and unconscious death-related thoughts: An extension of terror management theory. *Psychological Review, 106*, 332–336.
3. Solomon, S., Greenberg, J., & Pyszczynski, T. (1991). Terror management theory of self-esteem. In C. R. Snyder & D. Forsyth (Eds.), *Handbook of social and clinical psychology: The health perspective* (pp. 21–40). New York: Pergamon.
4. McKinney, W. T. (1988). Animal models. In C. G. Last & M. Hersen (Eds.), *Handbook of anxiety disorders* (pp. 171–180). Oxford: Pergamon Press.
5. Rosenblatt, A., Greenberg, J., Solomon, S., Pyszczynski, T., & Lyon, D. (1989). Evidence for terror management theory I: The effects of mortality salience on reactions to those who violate or uphold cultural values. *Journal of Personality and Social Psychology, 57*, 681–690.
6. DeWaal, F. (1996). *Good natured: The origins of right and wrong in humans and other animals.* Cambridge, MA: Harvard University Press.
7. Wilson, E. O. (1978). *On human nature.* Cambridge, MA: Harvard University Press.

8. Peterson, J. B. (1999). *Maps of meaning: The architecture of belief.* London, Routledge.
9. Gallup, G. (1982). Self awareness and the emergence of mind in primates. *American Journal of Primatology, 2,* 237–248.
10. Becker, E. (1971). *The birth and death of meaning* (2nd ed.). New York: Free Press.
11. Becker, E. (1973). *The denial of death.* New York: Free Press.
12. Florian, V., & Mikulincer, M. (1997). Fear of death and the judgement of social transgressions: A multidimensional test of terror management theory. *Journal of Personality and Social Psychology, 73,* 369–380.
13. Ochsmann, R., & Reichelt, K. (1994). Evaluation of moral and immoral behavior: Evidence for terror management theory. Unpublished manuscript, Universitat Mainz, Mainz, Germany.
14. Greenberg, J., Pyszczynski, T., Solomon, S., Rosenblatt, A., Veeder, M., Kirkland, S., & Lyon, D. (1990). Evidence for Terror Management Theory II: The effects of mortality salience on reactions to those who threaten or bolster the cultural worldview. *Journal of Personality and Social Psychology, 58,* 308–318.
15. Greenberg, J., Pyszczynski, T., Solomon, S., Simon, L., & Breus, M. (1994). The role of consciousness and accessibility of death-related thoughts in mortality salience effects. *Journal of Personality and Social Psychology, 67,* 627–637.
16. Pyszczynski, T., Wicklund, R. A., Floresku, S., Koch, H., Gauch, G., Solomon, S., & Greenberg, J., (1996). Whistling in the dark: Exaggerated estimates of social consensus in response to incidental reminders of mortality. *Psychological Science, 7,* 332–336.
17. Schimel, J., Simon, L., Greenberg, J., Pyszczynski, T., Solomon, S., Waxmonsky, J., & Arndt, J. (1999). Stereotypes and terror management: Evidence that mortality salience enhances stereotypic thinking and preferences. *Journal of Personality and Social Psychology, 5,* 905–926.
18. McGregor, H., Lieberman, J. D., Solomon, S., Greenberg, T., Arndt, J., Simon, L., & Pyszczynski, T. (1998). Terror management and aggression: Evidence that mortality salience motivates aggression against worldview threatening others. *Journal of Personality and Social Psychology, 74,* 590–605.
19. Greenberg, J., Simon, L., Pyszczynski, T., Solomon, S., & Chatel, D. (1992). Terror management and tolerance: Does mortality salience always intensify negative reactions to others who threaten one's worldview? *Journal of Personality and Social Psychology, 63,* 212–220.
20. Taubman Ben-Ari, O. T., Florian, V., & Mikulincer, M. (1999). The impact of mortality salience on reckless driving: A test of terror management mechanisms. *Journal of Personality and Social Psychology, 76,* 35–45.
21. Goldenberg, J. L., McCoy, S., Pyszczynski, T., Greenberg, J., & Solomon, S. (2000). The body as a source of self-esteem: The effect of mortality salience on identification with one's body, interest in sex, and appearance monitoring. *Journal of Personality and Social Psychology, 79,* 116–130.
22. Greenberg, J., Porteus, J., Simon, L., Solomon, S., & Pyszczynski, T. (1995). Evidence of a terror management function of cultural icons: The

effects of mortality salience on the inappropriate use of cultural symbols. *Personality and Social Psychology Bulletin, 21,* 1221–1228.

23. Greenberg, J., Solomon, S., Pyszczynski, T., Rosenblatt, A., Burling, J., Lyon, D., Simon, L., & Pinel, E. (1992). Assessing the terror management analysis of self-esteem: Converging evidence of an anxiety-buffering function. *Journal of Personality and Social Psychology, 63,* 913–922.

24. Greenberg, J., Pyszczynski, T., Solomon, S., Pinel, E., Simon, L., & Jordan, K. (1993). Effects of self-esteem on vulnerability-denying defensive distortions: Further evidence of an anxiety-buffering function of self-esteem. *Journal of Experimental Social Psychology, 29,* 229–251.

25. Jemmott, J. B., Ditto, P. H., & Croyle, R. T. (1986). Judging health status: Effects of perceived prevalence and personal relevance. *Journal of Personality and Social Psychology, 50,* 899–905.

26. Quattrone, G. A., & Tversky, A. (1984). Causal versus diagnostic contingencies: On self-deception and on the voter's illusion. *Journal of Personality and Social Psychology, 46,* 237–248.

27. Vandenberg, B. (1991). Is epistemology enough? An existential consideration of development. *American Psychologist, 46,* 1278–1286.

28. Last, C. G., & Hersen, M. (Eds.) (1988). *Handbook of anxiety disorders.* Oxford: Pergamon Press.

29. Tuma, A. H., & Maser, J. D. (Eds.) (1985). *Anxiety and the anxiety disorders.* Hillsdale, NJ: Erlbaum.

30. Eysenck, H. J., & Eysenck, S. B. G. (1967). *Personality structure and measurement.* London: Routledge & Kegan Paul.

31. Goldenberg, J. L., Pyszczynski, T., McCoy, S. K., Greenberg, J., & Solomon, S. (1999). Death, sex, and neuroticism: Why is sex such a problem? *Journal of Personality and Social Psychology, 77,* 1173–1187.

32. Goldenberg, J. L., Pyszczynski, T., Greenberg, J., Solomon, S., & Cox, C. (1999). *Stripping sex of its meaning: Understanding human sexual ambivalence.* Manuscript submitted for publication, University of Colorado, Colorado Springs, CO.

33. Yalom, I. D. (1980). *Existential psychotherapy.* New York: Basic Books.

34. Strachan, E. (1999). *The effects of mortality salience on fear reactions in spider phobia: Terror mismanagement?* Manuscript in preparation, University of Colorado, Colorado Springs, CO.

35. Thorpe, S., & Salkovskis, P. (1995). Phobic beliefs: Do cognitive factors play a role in specific phobias? *Behavior Research and Therapy, 33,* 805–816.

36. Wegner, D. M., & Smart, L. (1997). Deep cognitive activation: A new approach to the unconscious. *Journal of Consulting and Clinical Psychology, 65,* 984–995.

37. Arndt, J., Greenberg, J., Solomon, S., Pyszczynski, T., & Lyon, D. (1997). Suppression, accessibility of death-related thoughts, and worldview defense: Exploring the psychodynamics of terror management. *Journal of Personality and Social Psychology, 73,* 5–18.

38. Pyszczynski, T., & Greenberg, J. (1992). *Hanging on and letting go: Understanding the onset, progression, and remission of depression.* New York: Springer-Verlag.

39. Simon, L. Harmon-Jones, E., Greenberg, J., Solomon, S., & Pyszczynski, T. (1996). Mild depression, mortality salience and defense of the world-view: Evidence of intensified terror management in the mildly depressed individual. *Personality and Social Psychology Bulletin, 22,* 81–90.
40. Simon, L., Greenberg, J., Harmon-Jones, E., Solomon, S., Pyszczynski, T., Arndt, J., & Abend, T. (1997). Terror management and meaning: Evidence that the opportunity to defend the worldview following MS increases the meaningfulness of life in the depressed. *Journal of Personality, 66,* 359–382.

7

Managing Hostile Thoughts, Feelings, and Actions: The LifeSkills Approach

Redford B. Williams
Virginia P. Williams

Persons with a hostile personality type—characterized by tendencies toward cynical thoughts, angry feelings, and aggressive actions—are more likely than their less hostile counterparts to develop major, life-threatening illnesses over the course of their lives. They are also more likely to experience anxiety, depression, and social isolation—all of which add further to their risk of illness, as well as reducing their levels of happiness and well-being. As a result, it is especially important for persons with this personality type to acquire coping skills that will enable them to adapt better to their environments and thereby avoid the physical and emotional consequences likely to ensue if the thought, feeling, and action tendencies growing out of their personality are given free rein.

In this chapter, we shall first review: (1) the epidemiological evidence documenting the health-damaging effects of hostility and associated psychosocial characteristics; (2) the biobehavioral mechanisms whereby these characteristics lead to poor health; and (3) clinical trials documenting the benefits of behavioral interventions aimed at ameliorating the impact of psychosocial risk factors on health and disease. In the remainder of this chapter, we shall describe one particular approach—the LifeSkills Workshop—that we have developed to train persons with a hostile personality, as well as other psychosocial risk factors, in the use of coping skills that will enable them to adapt in a healthier way to the situations they encounter in daily life.

Hostility and Associated Psychosocial Risk Factors

Epidemiological Evidence

Following the initial report of an association between high scores on a hostility (Ho) scale from the Minnesota Multiphasic Personality Inventory and increased severity of angiographically documented coronary atherosclerosis (1) and two subsequent reports (2, 3) of a prospective association between increased Ho scores and increased risk of coronary heart disease (CHD) and all-cause mortality, a large body of research has evaluated the role of hostility as a psychosocial risk factor. A recent comprehensive review (4) of this research concluded that the psychological trait of hostility, characterized by a cynical mistrust of others, a low threshold for anger, and the aggressive expression of this anger (5), increases risk not only for CHD but also virtually any physical illness.

It has become increasingly clear in recent years that hostility is not the only psychosocial characteristic that is "coronary-prone" or health-damaging generally. Thus, depression, whether viewed as a subclinical psychological predisposition or a clinical disorder, has been shown predisposed to increased risk of CHD (6) or all-cause mortality (7) in healthy people, as well as increased risk of dying in CHD patients (8). Another negative emotion, anxiety, also has been found to predict increased CHD risk (9). Similarly, social isolation (the lack of emotionally supportive relationships) predicts increased CHD and all-cause mortality (10), as well as a poor prognosis in CHD patients (11). Job stress, whether defined as demand/control or effort/reward imbalance, also has been shown to increase CHD risk in healthy people (12), though an impact on prognosis in CHD patients has not been confirmed (13). And finally, lower socioeconomic status (SES) also predisposes to increased CHD risk and all-cause mortality in healthy people (14) and poorer prognoses in CHD patients (11).

These psychosocial risk factors do not occur in isolation from one another, but tend to cluster in the same individuals and groups. For example, working women who report high job strain are characterized also by increased levels of hostility, anger, depression, anxiety, and social isolation (15). Furthermore, when psychosocial risk factors do cooccur, especially in lower SES groups, their impact on mortality is compounded (16).

In addition to the effects of hostility and other psychosocial risk factors that contribute over a period of years to the *gradual* development of atherosclerosis and other health problems, the emotion of anger has an *acute* impact on angina and risk of myocardial infarction (MI). When CHD patients keep a diary of physical and mental activities during ambulatory ECG monitoring, high-intensity physical and mental activities leading to anger or other negative emotions are of equal potency in triggering ischemic episodes, whether silent or accompanied by angina—with strenuous physical activity and intense anger together being the most potent triggers (17, 18). Among patients undergoing exercise testing, angina also develops sooner and lasts longer among those who are depressed (19). Acute episodes of intense anger are associated with a twofold increased risk of MI during the two hours following the anger episode (20). Among persons with lower educational levels, this risk increases to over threefold. (21) It has been estimated that such episodes of intense anger are responsible for at least 36,000 (2.4% of 1.5 million) heart attacks in the United States each year (22).

Biobehavioral Mechanisms

Both hostility and depression are associated with alterations in autonomic balance and hypothalamic-pituitary-adrenal (HPA) axis function that could account for at least some of their health-damaging effects. When anger is induced in laboratory studies (23–25), for example, persons who score high on the same hostility scale that predicts increased risk of CHD and all-cause mortality exhibit larger sympathetic nervous system (SNS)-mediated cardiovascular responses than do low scorers. Hostile persons also show increased SNS activation during everyday life, as documented by larger increases in daytime urinary epinephrine excretion (26) and down regulation of lymphocyte beta adrenergic receptors (27). Increased SNS outflow has been documented in patients with major depression (28).

There is also evidence that parasympathetic (PNS) function is reduced in both hostile and depressed persons. In laboratory research (29), hostile participants show decreased PNS antagonism of SNS effects on myocardial function. Also, both hostility (30) and depression (31) are associated with decreased PNS function during ambulatory ECG monitoring.

Increased and dysregulated hypothalamic-pituitary-adrenal (HPA) axis function has long been a known accompaniment of depression (32). Persons with hostile personality also have been found in recent research to exhibit increased HPA activation, both in ambulatory (33) and laboratory (25) conditions.

Biologic changes similar to those documented in depressed and hostile persons are also present in persons who are socially isolated and/or exposed to high demand/low control jobs or life situations. Increased urinary catecholamine excretion has been found (34), for example, in persons reporting low social support. Persons in high-strain jobs exhibit (35) increased ambulatory blood pressure and increased left ventricular mass index—both likely the result of chronically increased SNS function. Working women with young children living in the home—clearly a high demand/ low control situation!—show greater 24-hour urinary cortisol excretions than do working women without children at home (36).

Psychosocial risk factors are also associated with increased behavioral/ physical risk factor levels. In two large-scale prospective (37) and cross-sectional (38) studies, each involving over 5,000 subjects, researchers found that hostility associated with statistically significant increases in cigarette smoking, alcohol consumption, body mass index, 24-hour caloric intake, and cholesterol/HDL ratio. Yet other researchers find that hostility predicts increased incidence of hypertension (2). Increased smoking (39) and alcohol consumption (40) are also well-documented in depression. Persons with low social support are less likely to succeed in smoking cessation programs (41) or to adhere to prescribed medical regimens (42).

These biobehavioral characteristics have been postulated to increase risk via a variety of biologically plausible pathogenic mechanisms—including excessive cardiovascular arousals that promote atherogenesis via mechanical injury of arterial endothelium (43), or alterations in immune functions that reduce ability to kill cancer cells. Related to these issues, Adams (44) proposed that effects of biobehavioral factors on the cellular and molecular biology of the monocyte/macrophage system deserve increased attention in research aimed at identifying possible mediators in the final common pathway at the cellular/molecular level.

In addition to these long-term biobehavioral mechanisms, based on evidence from laboratory studies, we can see more immediate physiological effects of anger that are biologically plausible triggers of acute CHD events. When CHD patients are engaged in a personally relevant, emotionally arousing speaking task during radionuclide ventriculography, for example, the frequency and size of their regional myocardial wall-motion abnormalities are similar to those induced by exercise and more severe than those caused by a more neutral mental challenge like mental arithmetic (45). Moreover, CHD patients who exhibit mental stress-induced decreases in left-ventricular ejection fraction (LVEF) are 2.8 times more likely to suffer a cardiac event over a five-year follow-up than patients without falls in LVEF (46). In another study, when CHD patients recalled a recent event that made them angry, they exhibited a significant fall of greater than 5% in LVEF (47).

Based on the foregoing review, we offer the following synthesis: *psychosocial risk factors do not themselves lead directly to increased risk of disease and death. Rather, their health-damaging effects probably are mediated by the behavioral/physical and biological characteristics that cooccur with the psychosocial risk factors.* Related to this point, Williams has proposed (48, 49) that reduced function of the neurotransmitter serotonin in the central nervous system could be responsible for this clustering of psychosocial risk factors and health-damaging biobehavioral characteristics in the same individuals and groups (e.g., lower SES). Further support for such a role of brain serotonin systems comes from research showing that a functional polymorphism of the promoter region of the gene that encodes for the serotonin transporter is associated with a tendency to experience increased levels of negative emotions (50).

Behavioral Interventions

It should be clear from the foregoing discussion that, over the past 20 years, behavioral medicine researchers have made remarkable progress in identifying psychosocial risk factors for CHD and other major illnesses, as well as characterizing the biobehavioral mechanisms that are likely to account for the role of psychosocial risk factors in the development and course of disease. While this progress is extremely gratifying, the ultimate goal of these researchers has always been to identify targets for interventions that would ameliorate the impact of psychosocial risk factors on the development and course of disease. With respect to this goal, there already is encouraging evidence that behavioral interventions can improve prognosis in CHD, cancer, and other chronic medical conditions.

CHD, Cancer, and Other Chronic Diseases

In a number of randomized clinical trials to improve prognosis in both CHD (51, 52) and cancer (53, 54), researchers using group-based behavioral interventions targeting psychosocial factors have observed favorable outcomes in those receiving the interventions. Based on these encouraging results, we can make a strong case (55) for large-scale clinical trials of behavioral interventions, in which the aim is to improve patients' ability to cope with the stresses accompanying psychosocial risk factors. The National Heart, Lung, and Blood Institute is currently supporting just such a trial—the ENRICHD study, the first large-scale, multicenter, randomized clinical trial of a psychosocial intervention, in this case targeting depression and social isolation with the goal of reducing morbidity and mortality in CHD patients (56).

Another application for behavioral interventions is in patients with chronic medical conditions that, while not necessarily life-threatening, are associated with much suffering and costly use of medical diagnostic and treatment services. In the Hawaii Medicaid study (57), patients with chronic medical conditions who were high utilizers of medical services were randomly assigned to one of three groups: no mental health treatment; traditional one-on-one psychotherapy for up to 50 sessions over a year; or, a highly structured group-based intervention consisting of no more than eight sessions of training in various coping skills. Compared to the other two groups, both of which showed *increases* of 17–26% in medical costs during the year following randomization, the patients in the structured group intervention showed a *decrease* of 20% in costs for medical-surgical services.

Several inferences can be derived from the results of the Hawaii Medicaid study, as well as the other behavioral intervention studies we covered in the foregoing review. Those references include the following:

- *Group settings* are more efficient than one-on-one approaches and enable patients to learn from one another, thereby serving as a powerful source of social support.
- Applying principles of *cognitive behavior therapy* and *behavior therapy*, along with *social skills training,* enables patients to gain "hands-on" practice in the development of coping skills they can use to handle the stressful situations and resulting negative emotions they need to face in the here and now, as well as increasing the likelihood that their contacts with other people will result in emotionally supportive social relationships.
- Some technique or method for reducing autonomic arousal—meditation, progressive muscle relaxation, and the like—appears helpful to enable patients to decrease troubling thoughts and emotions and blunt potentially dangerous physiologic hyperarousal.
- Treatment can be effective even when limited to a fixed number of sessions, often no more than six to eight, during which each skill to be mastered is presented in a manualized, protocol-driven format that enables each patient to learn to practice and apply the skill to actual problems he or she is currently encountering at work, home, or play.

The LifeSkills Workshop

Over the past decade, the authors have been developing and refining what is now a highly structured, manualized, and protocol-driven workshop aimed at reducing levels of psychosocial risk factors and improving coping skills. Originally aimed at reducing the cynical mistrust, anger, and aggression that are characteristic of persons with a hostile personality type (58), this workshop now focuses on a more general set of eight skills that will help participants to manage a broader range of negative emotions (not just anger), use action skills to cope better with the stresses of everyday life, and build more supportive and positive interpersonal relationships (59). Thus, in addition to our earlier focus on reducing the levels of negative, health-damaging psychosocial risk factors, using the "LifeSkills Workshop" in its current embodiment, we aim to increase levels of positive, health-promoting characteristics—example, social support, self-efficacy (60), sense of coherence (61), and optimism (62). In addition to the elements common to the successful behavioral interventions outlined above, elements from the Recurrent Coronary Prevention Project (51) and cognitive behavior therapy (63) also are incorporated into the LifeSkills Workshop.

The Workshop teaches participants to use eight "LifeSkills" that are grouped into two sets.

Set I. Skills to help you understand yourself and others, including:

- *Identification of thoughts and feelings*
- *Evaluation (and management) of negative thoughts and feelings*
- *Communication using effective speaking and listening skills*
- *Empathy*

Set II. Skills to help you act effectively, when called for by evaluation of thoughts and feelings. These include:

- *Problem solving*
- *Assertion*
- *Acceptance (only when no harm will ensue to yourself or others)*
- *Enhancing the positives in your interpersonal relationships*

Typically, the length of the Workshop is 12 hours, conducted over six sessions of two-plus hours, with a 10-minute break in the middle. Alternative schedules are possible—example, two sessions per week over three weeks, one session per day over six days, or three sessions per day massed over two consecutive days. The latter format is less desirable, because it allows for little practice of "homework" assignments designed (see following) to facilitate use of the skills in the real world. The six sessions are organized to teach the eight LifeSkills as follows:

Session 1—Introduction; scientific evidence; becoming aware of thoughts and feelings.
Session 2—Evaluating negative thoughts and feelings; use of deflection strategies, including meditation/relaxation, when action is not required.
Session 3—Problem solving; speaking up; assertion.
Session 4—Saying "No," listening.
Session 5—Empathy; evidence regarding higher levels of stress in the modern world; the option of acceptance.
Session 6—Increasing the positives; deciding what really matters.

Central to the LifeSkills Workshop is the use of a common format for teaching each skill:

- Facilitator explains the skill and rationale for its use.
- Facilitator models use of the skill, using a personal example.
- Facilitator models use of the skill, using an example from the life of one participant.
- "Hands-on" exercises for each participant to practice the skill during the Workshop, with the facilitator as coach.
- Homework assignment to use the skill in real life.
- Checking in at the next session to report how the homework went.

A number of study aids have been developed to facilitate participants' mastery of the skills being taught:

- The book *LifeSkills* by Williams and Williams (59) as a text providing background reading, both during the Workshop and to maintain skills afterward.
- The *LifeSkills Workbook*, which is used as each skill is covered during the Workshop.
- A small notebook that fits in a shirt pocket, used to keep the "Thoughts and Feelings Log."

- A laminated pocketcard containing the "I AM WORTH IT!" roadmap tool that participants use to evaluate negative thoughts and feelings as recorded in their Log and in real life.
- A set of over 75 overheads to present the material relevant to each skill, including cartoons that provide a humorous perspective.
- A video with dramatizations of the right and wrong ways to practice assertion (additional video modules are currently being developed for the other skills).

The Workshop guidelines make it clear to participants that the LifeSkills Workshop is not designed as psychotherapy for some psychological or physical disorder, but rather as *training* in coping skills that will help participants enhance wellness by more effective management of the stresses that we all face in today's world and by building more positive and supportive relationships with others.

Experience over the past decade, during which over 2,000 persons have taken the LifeSkills Workshop, indicates that participants enjoy taking the Workshop and doing the in-session exercises. Analogous to an "open label" trial undertaken to show that a new version of an older drug with well-documented efficacy does indeed have the expected beneficial effects, pre- and post-Workshop assessments have been done with participants in several workplace settings. As shown in Figures 7.1 and 7.2, in both government agency and university settings, employees taking the LifeSkills Workshop show decreases in measures of hostility and depression and increases in a measure of social support.

Of course, in the absence of a control group, we cannot rule out regression to the mean or response bias (participants wanting to give a good report after the Workshop) in accounting for these favorable outcomes. Suggesting these confounds were not at work is the finding that participants rated their home and work environments as equally stressful before and after the

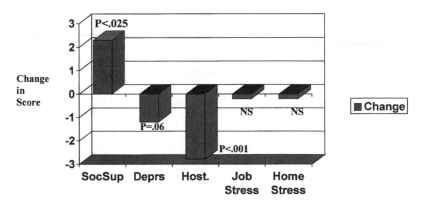

Figure 7.1. Changes in psychosocial risk characteristics among workers at a government agency who took the LifeSkills Workshop.

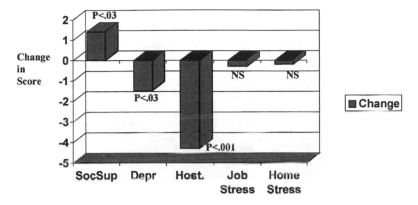

Figure 7.2. Changes in psychosocial risk characteristics among personnel in a university human resources department who took the LifeSkills Workshop.

Workshop. This pattern of results suggests that, although participants' environments were no less stressful following the Workshop, their ability to cope with environmental stress—as indexed by increased social support and decreased hostility and depression—was improved following the Workshop. Before such a conclusion can be accepted, it will be necessary to conduct larger-scale randomized trials of the LifeSkills Workshop, and these are currently being planned.

There has been one small-scale randomized clinical trial that evaluated the impact of a hostility reduction workshop, adapted from an earlier, version (59) of the LifeSkills Workshop, on a number of outcomes in patients who had suffered a myocardial infarction (64). Since the focus was on hostility reduction, this intervention included about 40% of the eight Life-Skills, including the following: (a) Identification of thoughts and feelings; (b) Evaluation (and management) of negative thoughts and feelings; and (c) Assertion. As shown in Figures 7.3 and 7.4, both hostility and diastolic blood pressure levels were unchanged or higher, both after the workshop and at two-month follow-up, in patients randomized to usual care. In contrast, patients randomized to hostility reduction training showed decreases in both hostility and blood pressure that were sustained and enhanced following training. A subsequent six-month follow-up of the patients in this study revealed that the average number of days in hospital was reduced from 2.5 days in usual care patients to 0.6 days in patients who received hostility reduction training.

When considered along with the encouraging results from the behavioral intervention trials described above for patients with heart disease, cancer, and other chronic medical conditions, these findings are encouraging that behavioral interventions like the one embodied in the LifeSkills Workshop not only have considerable promise to reduce psychosocial risk factors and

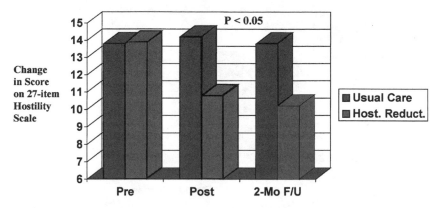

Figure 7.3. Changes in hostility levels following completion of a hostility reduction workshop and at two months follow-up in a clinical trial of persons randomized to hostility reduction or usual care. (Adapted from Gidron et al., 1999)

improve coping skills, but also to improve medical outcomes in patients with major medical disorders. Since the full LifeSkills Workshop has not yet had a rigorous evaluation in a randomized clinical trial, we emphasize here the term "encouraging" to describe our current stance regarding the potential utility of the LifeSkills Workshop. We have carried out a limited but rigorously designed and conducted randomized trial to evaluate a video module presenting one of the LifeSkills—assertion—and the results clearly show that, at least for this component of the full Workshop, instruction in the skills is superior to a control condition.

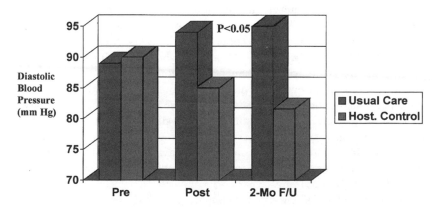

Figure 7.4. Changes in diastolic blood pressure levels following completion of a hostility reduction workshop and at two months follow-up in a clinical trial of persons randomized to hostility reduction or usual care. (Adapted from Gidron et al., 1999)

In this study, evaluating a prototype video module that was developed to teach assertion skills in the context of the Workshop, we randomly assigned subjects to view either the assertion video (using dramatizations of the right and wrong ways to practice assertion in a domestic conflict situation) or a control video (demonstrating Cherokee blowgun construction techniques). Subjects wrote what they would say and do in response to conflict situations, presented in written scenarios, before and after viewing the videos. The quality of subjects' use of assertion skills and the amount of aggression expressed in their responses to the scenarios were scored by raters unaware of both the condition (assertion vs. control) and timing (pre vs. post) of the responses. Subjects randomized to the control video showed no changes in either assertion practice or aggression after viewing the video. In contrast, those who viewed the assertion video show highly significant increases in assertion scores and decreases in aggression scores.

Based on these findings, it appears that video modules can be a useful adjunct to the Workshop exercises in teaching coping skills. They also support the interesting corollary that persons trained to use assertion skills will become less aggressive. Video modules for the other seven LifeSkills are currently being developed. We shall be testing the impact of these videos—both as an adjunct to the Workshop and as a stand-alone product—on psychosocial risk factors and biomarkers of stress in a randomized trial currently in the planning stage.

Final Thoughts

In behavioral medicine research, investigators have identified psychosocial characteristics that increase the risk of developing a major, life-threatening medical illness and having a poor prognosis once disease is present. Considerable progress also has been made toward identifying the biobehavioral mechanisms responsible for the health-damaging effects, as well as developing behavioral interventions for ameliorating the potential harm.

As we look toward the future, in addition to the ongoing research on psychosocial risk factors and biobehavioral mechanisms, it will be important to expand the research effort aimed at developing and refining behavioral interventions. This latter effort should include not only randomized clinical trials, but also development of manualized and protocol-driven behavioral treatment packages that can be delivered with the expectation of relatively comparable benefits in differing settings.

We also should begin to think of these behavioral intervention packages as products that can be bought and sold. It was not until someone thought of standardizing the preparation of the foxglove leaves that were used in the eighteenth and nineteenth centuries to treat patients with "dropsy" (congestive heart failure), and packaging them into standardized preparations of "digitalis leaf" tablets, that the modern pharmaceutical industry really began. Perhaps those of us interested in developing the most effective behavioral interventions and seeing them used as widely as possible toward the betterment of human health should begin to think about ways to launch the modern "behavio-tech" industry.

Acknowledgments
Preparation of this chapter was supported in part by grants P01-HL36587 from the National Heart, Lung and Blood Institute; K05-MH79482 from the National Institute of Mental Health; Clinical Research Unit Grant M01-RR-30; and the Fetzer Institute, Kalamazoo, Michigan. Portions are adapted from an earlier review by one of the authors (Williams, R. B. [1999]. Clinical Crossroads: A 69-year-old man with anger and angina. *JAMA, 282*, 763–770).

References

1. Williams, R. B., Haney, T. L., Lee, K. L. Blumenthal, J. A., & Kong, Y. (1980). Type A behavior, hostility, and coronary atherosclerosis. *Psychosomatic Medicine, 42* (6), 539–549.
2. Barefoot, J. C., Dahlstrom, W. G., & Williams, R. B. (1983). Hostility, CHD incidence, and total mortality: A 25-year follow-up study of 255 physicians. *Psychosomatic Medicine, 45*, 59–63.
3. Shekelle, R. B., Gale, M., Ostfeld, A. M., & Paul, O. (1983). Hostility, risk of coronary disease, and mortality. *Psychosomatic Medicine, 45*, 219–228.
4. Miller, T. Q., Smith, T. W., Turner, C. W., Guijarro, M. L., & Hallet, A. J. (1996). A meta-analytic review of research on hostility and physical health. *Psychological Bulletin, 119*, 322–348.
5. Barefoot, J. C., Peterson, B. L., Dahlstrom, W. G., Siegler, I. C., Anderson, N. B., & Williams, Jr., R. B. (1991). Hostility patterns and health implications: Correlates of Cook-Medley Hostility scale scores in a national survey. *Health Psychology, 10*, 18–24.
6. Anda, R., Williamson, D., Jones, D., Macera, C., Eaker, E., Glassman, A., & Marks, J. (1993). Depressed affect, hopelessness, and the risk of ischemic heart disease in a cohort of U.S. adults. *Epidemiology, 4*, 285–294.
7. Barefoot, J. C., & Schroll, M. (1996). Symptoms of depression, acute myocardial infarction and total mortality in a community sample. *Circulation, 93*, 1976–1980.
8. Frasure-Smith, N., Lesperance, F., & Talajic, M. (1994). Post-myocardial infarction depression and 18-month prognosis. *Circulation, 90*, 1614–1620.
9. Kawachi, I., Sparrow, D., Vokonas, P. S., & Weiss, S. T. (1994). Symptoms of anxiety and risk of coronary heart disease. The normative aging study. *Circulation, 90*, 2225–2229.
10. House, J. S., Landis, K. R., & Umberson, D. (1988). Social relationships and health. *Science, 241*, 540–545.
11. Williams, R. B., Barefoot, J. C., Califf, R. M., Haney, T. L., Saunders,

W. B., Pryor, D. B., Hlatky, M. A, Siegler, I. C., & Mark, D. B. (1992). Prognostic importance of social and economic resources among medically treated patients with angiographically documented coronary artery disease. *Journal of the American Medical Association, 267,* 520–524.

12. Bosma, H., Peter, R., Siegris, J., & Marmot, M. (1998). Two alternative job stress models and the risk of coronary heart disease. *American Journal of Public Health, 88,* 68–74.

13. Hlatky, M. A., Lam, L. C., Lee, K. L., Clapp-Channing, N. E., Williams, R. B., Pryor, D. B., Califf, R. M., & Mark, D. B. (1995). Job strain and the prevalence and outcome of coronary artery disease. *Circulation, 92,* 327–333.

14. Adler, N. E., Boyce, T., Chosncy, M. A., Folkman, S., & Syme, S. L. (1993). Socioeconomic inequalities in health: No easy solution. *Journal of the American Medical Association, 26,* 3140–3145.

15. Williams, R. B., Barefoot, J. C., Blumenthal, J. A., Holms, M. J., Luecken, L., Pieper, C. F., Siegler, I. C., & Suarez, E. C. (1997). Psycho social correlates of job strain in a sample of working women. *Archives of General Psychiatry, 54,* 543–548.

16. Kaplan, G. A. (1995). Where do shared pathways lead? Some reflections on a research agenda. *Psychosomatic Medicine, 57,* 208–212.

17. Gabbay, F. H., Krantz, D. S., Kop, W. J., Hedges, S. M., Klein, J., Gottdiener, J. S., & Rozanski, A. (1996). Triggers of myocardial ischemia during daily life in patients with coronary artery disease: Physical and mental activities, anger, and smoking. *Journal of the American College of Cardiology, 27,* 585–592.

18. Krantz, D. S., Hedges, S. M., Gabbay, F. H., Klein, J., Falconer, J. J., Merz, C. N., Gottdiener, J. S., Lutz, H., & Rozanski, A. (1994). Triggers of angina and ST-segment depression in ambulatory patients with coronary artery disease: Evidence for an uncoupling of angina and ischemia. *American Heart Journal, 128,* 703–712.

19. Krittayaphong, R., Light, K. C., Golden, R. N., Finkel, J. B., & Sheps, D. S. (1996). Relationship among depression scores, beta-endorphin, and angina pectoris during exercise in patients with coronary artery disease. *Clinical Journal of Pain, 12,* 126–133.

20. Mittleman, M. A., Maclure, M., Sherwood, J. B., Mulry, R. P., Tofler, G. H., Jacobs, S. C., Friedman, R., Benson, H., & Muller, J. E. (1995). Triggering of acute myocardial infarction onset by episodes of anger. *Circulation, 92,* 1720–1725.

21. Mittleman, M. A., Maclure, M., Nachnani, M., Sherwood, J. B., & Muller, J. E. (1997). Educational attainment, anger, and the risk of triggering myocardial infarction onset. *Archives of Internal Medicine, 157,* 769–775.

22. Verrier, R. L., & Mittleman, M. A. (1996). Life-threatening cardiovascular consequences of anger in patients with coronary artery disease. *Cardiology Clinics, 14,* 289–307.

23. Smith, T. W., & Allred, K. D. (1989). Blood pressure reactivity during social interaction in high and low cynical hostile men. *Journal of Behavioral Medicine, 11,* 135–143.

24. Suarez, E. C., & Williams, R. B. (1989). Situational determinants of car-

diovascular and emotional reactivity in high and low hostile men. *Psychosomatic Medicine, 51,* 404–418.

25. Suarez, E. C., Kuhn, C. M., Schanberg, S. M., Williams, R. B., & Zimmermann, E. A. (1998). Neuroendocrine, cardiovascular, and emotional responses of hostile men: The role of interpersonal challenge. *Psychosomatic Medicine, 60,* 78–88.

26. Suarez, E. C., Williams, R. B., Peoples, M. C., Kuhn, C. M., & Schanberg, S. M. (1991). *Hostility-related differences in urinary excretion rates of catecholamines.* Paper presented at the Annual Meeting of the Society for Psychophysiological Research, Chicago, IL.

27. Shiller, A. M., Suarez, E. C., Kuhn, C. M., Schanberg, S. M., Williams, Jr., R. B., & Zimmermann, E. A. (1997). The relationship between hostility and beta-adrenergic receptor physiology in healthy young males. *Psychosomatic Medicine, 59,* 481–487.

28. Veith, R. C., Lewis, N., Linares, O. A., Barnes, R. F., Raskind, M. A., Villacres, E. C., Murburg, M. M., Ashleigh, E. A., Castillo, S., Peskind, E. R., Pascualy M., & Halter, J. B. (1994). Sympathetic nervous system activity in major depression: Basal and desipramine-induced alterations in plasma norepinephrine kinetics. *Archives of General Psychiatry, 51,* 411–422.

29. Fukudo, S., Lane, J. D., Anderson, N. B., Kuhn, C. M., Schanberg, S. M., McCown, N., Muranaka, M., Suzuki, J., & Williams, R. B. (1992). Accentuated vagal antagonism of beta adrenergic effects on ventricular repolarization: Differential responses between Type A and Type B men. *Circulation, 85,* 2045–2053.

30. Sloan, R. P., Shapiro, P. A., Bigger, Jr., J. T., Bagiella, E., Steinman, R. C., & Gorman, J. M. (1994). Cardiovascular autonomic control and hostility in healthy subject. *American Journal of Cardiology, 74,* 298–300.

31. Carney, R. M., Rich, M., teVelde, A., Saini, J., Clark, K., & Freedland, K. E. (1988). The relationship between heart rate, heart rate variability and depression in patients with coronary artery disease. *Journal of Psychosomatic Research, 32,* 159–164.

32. Holsboer, F., van Bardeleben, U., Gerken, A., Stallag, K., & Muller, O. A. (1984). Blunted corticotrophin and normal response to human corticotrophin-releasing factor in depression. *New England Journal of Medicine, 311,* 1127.

33. Pope, M. K., & Smith, T. W. (1991). Cortisol excretion in high and low cynically hostile men. *Psychosomatic Medicine, 53,* 386–392.

34. Fleming, R., Baum, A., Gisriel, M. M., & Gatchel, R. J. (1982). Mediating influences of social support on stress at Three Mile Island. *Journal of Human Stress, 8,* 14–22.

35. Schnall, P., Pieper, C., Schwartz, J. E., Karasek, R. A., Schlussel, Y., Devereux, R. B., Ganau, A., Alderman, M., Warren, K., & Pickering, T. G. (1990). The relationship between job strain, workplace diastolic blood pressure, and life ventricular mass. *Journal of the American Medical Association, 263,* 1971–1972.

36. Luecken, L. J., Suarez, E. C., Kuhn, C. M., Barefoot, J. C., Blumenthal, J. A., Siegler, I. C., & Williams, R. B. (1997). Stress and employed

women. I. Impact of marital status and children at home on neurohormone output and home strain. *Psychosomatic Medicine, 59,* 352–359.

37. Siegler, I. C., Peterson, B. L., Barefoot, J. C., & Williams, R. B. (1992). Hostility during late adolescence predicts coronary risk factors at midlife. *American Journal of Epidemiology, 136,* 146–154.

38. Scherwitz, K. W., Perkins, L. L., Chesney, M. A., Hughes, G. H., Sidney, S., & Manolio, T. A. (1992). Hostility and health behaviors in young adults: The CARDIA study. Coronary Artery Risk Development in Young Adults Study. *American Journal Epidemiology, 136,* 136–145.

39. Glassman, A. H., Helzer, J. E., Covey, L. S., Cottler, L. B., Stetner, F., Tipp, J. E., Johnson, J. (1990). Smoking, smoking cessation, and major depression. *Journal of the American Medical Association, 264,* 1546–1549.

40. Hartka, E., Johnstone, B., Leino, E. V., Motoyoshi, M., Temple, M. T., & Fillmore, K. M. (1991). A meta-analysis of depressive symptomatology and alcohol consumption over time. *British Journal of Addiction, 86,* 1283–1298.

41. Mermelstein, R., Cohen, S., Lichtenstein, E., Baer, J. S., & Kamarck, T. (1986). Social support and smoking cessation and maintenance. *Journal of Consulting and Clinical Psychology, 54,* 447–453.

42. Williams, C. A., Beresford, S. A., James, S. A., LaCroix, A. Z., Strogatz, D. S., Wagner, E. H., Kleinbaum, D. G., Cutchin, L. M., & Ibrahim, M. A. (1985). The Edgecombe County High Blood Pressure Control Program, III: Social support, social stressors, and treatment dropout. *American Journal of Public Health, 75,* 483–486.

43. Kaplan, J. R., Petterson, K., Manuck, S. B., & Olsson, G. (1991). Role of sympathoadrenal medullary activation in the initiation and progression of atherosclerosis. *Circulation, 94*(Suppl VI), VI-23–VI-32.

44. Adams, D. O. (1994). Molecular biology of macrophage activation: A pathway whereby psychosocial factors can potentially affect health. *Psychosomatic Medicine, 56,* 316–327.

45. Rozanski, A., Bairey, C. N., Krantz, D. S., Friedman, J., Resser, K. J., Morell, M., Hilton-Chalfen, S., Hestrin, L., Bietendorf, J., & Berman, D. S. (1988). Mental stress and the induction of silent myocardial ischemia in patients with coronary artery disease. *New England Journal of Medicine, 318,* 1005–1012.

46. Jiang, W., Babyak, M., Krantz, D. S., Waugh, R. A., Coleman, R. E., Hanson, M. M., Frid, D. J., McNulty, S., Morris, J. J., O'Conner, C. M., & Blumenthal, J. A. (1996). Mental stress-induced myocardial ischemia and cardiac events. *Journal of the American Medicine Association, 275,* 1651–1656.

47. Ironson, G., Taylor, C. B., Boltwood, M., Bartzokis, T., Denis, C., Cesney, M., Spitzer, S., Segall, C. M. (1992). Effects of anger on left ventricular ejection fraction in coronary artery disease. *American Journal of Cardiology, 70,* 281–285.

48. Williams, R. B. (1994). Neurobiology, cellular and molecular biology, and psychosomatic medicine. *Psychosomatic Medicine, 56,* 308–315.

49. Williams, R. B. (1998). Lower socioeconomic status and increased mortality. Early childhood roots and the potential for successful interventions. *Journal of the American Medical Association, 279,* 1745–1746.
50. Lesch, K. P., Bengel, D., Heils, A., Sabol, S. Z., Greenberg, B., Petri, S., Benjamin, J., Muller, C. R., Hamer, D. H., & Murphy, D. L. (1996). Association of anxiety-related traits with a polymorphism in the serotonin transporter gene regulatory region. *Science, 274,* 1527–1531.
51. Friedman, M., Thoresen, C. E., & Gill, J. J. (1986). Alteration of type A behavior and its effect on cardiac recurrences in post myocardial infarction patients: Summary results of the Recurrent Coronary Prevention Project. *American Heart Journal, 112,* 653–665.
52. Blumenthal, J. A., Jiang, W., Babyak, M., Krantz, D. S., Frid, D. J., Coleman, R. E., Waugh, R., Hanson, M., Appelbaum, M., O'Conner, C. M., & Morris, J. J. (1997). Stress management and exercise training in cardiac patients with myocardial ischemia. *Archives of Internal Medicine, 157,* 2213–2223.
53. Fawzy, F. I., Fawzy, N. W., Hyun, C. S., Elashoff R., Guthrie, D., Fahey, J. L., & Morton D. L. (1993). Malignant melanoma: Effects of an early structured psychiatric intervention, coping, and affective state on recurrence and survival 6 years later. *Archives of General Psychiatry, 50,* 681–689.
54. Spiegel, D., Bloom, J. R., Kraemer, H. C., & Gottheil, E. (1989). Effect of psychosocial treatment on survival of patients with metastatic breast cancer. *Lancet, 2,* 888–890.
55. Williams, R. B., & Chesney, M. A. (1993). Psychosocial factors and prognosis in established coronary artery disease. The need for research on interventions. *Journal of the American Medical Association, 270,* 1860–1861.
56. Blumenthal, J. A., O'Connor, C., Hinderliter, A., Fath, K., Hegde, S. B., Miller, G., Puma, J. Sessions, W., Sheps, D., Zakhary, B., & Williams, R. B. (1997). Psychosocial factors and coronary disease. A National Multicenter Clinical Trial (ENRICHD) with a North Carolina focus. *North Carolina Medical Journal, 58,* 802–808.
57. Cummings, N. A., Pallak, M. S., Dorken, H., & Henke, C. W. (1991). The impact of psychological intervention on health care costs and utilization: The Hawaii Medicaid Project. *HCFA Contract Report # 11-C-983344/9.*
58. Williams, R. B., & Williams, V. P. (1993). *Anger kills: Seventeen strategies for controlling the hostility that can harm your health.* New York: Times Books/Random House. (Paperback edition, New York: Harper Perennial, 1994; 1998).
59. Williams, V. P., & Williams, R. B. (1997). *LifeSkills: Eight simple ways to build stronger relationships, communicate more clearly and improve your health.* New York: Times Books/Random House.
60. Bandura, A., & Cervone, D. (1983). Self-evaluative and self-efficacy mechanisms governing the motivational effects of goal systems. *Journal of Personality and Social Psychology, 45,* 1017–1028.
61. Antonovsky, A. (1993). The structure and properties of the sense of coherence scale. *Social Science in Medicine, 36,* 725–733.
62. Scheier, M. F., Carver, C. S., & Bridges, M. W. (1994). Distinguishing

optimism from neuroticism (and trait anxiety, self-mastery, and self-esteem): A reevaluation of the Life Orientation Test. *Journal of Personality and Social Psychology, 67,* 1063–1078.

63. Beck, J. (1995). *Cognitive therapy: Basics and beyond.* New York: Guilford Press.

64. Gidron, Y., Davidson, K., & Bata I. (1999). The short-term effects of a hostility-reduction intervention in CHD patients. *Health Psychology, 18,* 416–420.

8

Comparing Favorably: A Cognitive Approach to Coping Through Comparison with Other Persons

Thomas Ashby Wills
James M. Sandy

I remember standing at the door of the unit, worried to death about what my baby would look like. When I walked over to the isolette, I just fell apart completely. But then I looked around and saw several babies who were smaller than mine. And there was one baby whose head was bigger than his body. In a way, that helped calm me down. (1)

I had just a comparatively small amount of surgery on the breast, and I was so miserable because it was so painful. How awful it must be for women who have had a mastectomy. . . . I just can't imagine it; it would seem to be so difficult. (2)

In this chapter, we consider how people may use social comparison to cope with psychological distress arising from sources such as negative life events, failure experiences, and threats to self-esteem. Comparison-oriented coping is a cognitive process of comparing one's attributes with those of another person, so as to improve subjective well-being. Through favorable comparisons, individuals may come to feel better about their situation, coping, or worth as a person; these enhancements of subjective well-being can help individuals to avoid destructive or self-defeating responses to a problem and to remain motivated to cope with the stressor.

In theory, people may engage in three different types of social comparison. They may compare their own situation or attributes with those of other persons who are better off than the self, a process that is termed *upward comparison*. They may compare with another person at the same level, a process termed *lateral comparison*, or they may compare with others who are worse off than the self, a process termed *downward comparison*. These types of comparison are posited to be used for different reasons and to have different effects (3, 4). We will focus on downward comparison as a coping mechanism because it frequently has been linked to efforts to restore or enhance subjective well-being. This does not mean that upward or lateral comparisons are irrelevant for coping; indeed, in select situations, persons may use upward comparisons to generate optimism about the possibility of recovery or self-improvement (5, 6). We will consider how a balancing of downward and upward comparisons, together with other types of coping mechanisms, may be involved in the process of coping with an ongoing problem.

Comparison-oriented coping is a theory-based area, and in beginning this chapter we outline the theories that have generated predictions about social comparison. Then we discuss several different types of downward comparison mechanisms and consider their potential costs and benefits for coping with various types of stressors. In the next section we discuss some current issues in research on social comparisons: whether favorable comparison is an "automatic" process and, if so, what implications this has for coping, whether comparison-oriented coping differs for strictly cognitive comparisons versus actual affiliation with other persons; how use of social comparison is linked to self-esteem; and the role of social comparisons in depression and its maintenance or alleviation. In a final section we discuss questions about the effectiveness of favorable comparison as a coping mechanism and consider implications for prevention and treatment.

The Theory of Social Comparison

Festinger's Theory of Social Comparison

In articulating the theory of social comparison, Leon Festinger's (1954) aim was to outline how people use social information to obtain accurate self-evaluations (7). Festinger's original insight was based on the recognition that there are important domains of life where objective standards are not available: If a person questions, for example, how physically attractive he or she is, or how good a coper, there are no truly objective standards available. In such situations, Festinger reasoned, people can self-evaluate through making comparisons with other persons and, from the information available, determine where they rank on the particular dimension. In this way, people can obtain evaluations of their own attributes which, in turn, may assist them in adaptation.

Festinger's perspective was that people were basically motivated by a need for achievement and self-improvement; hence, the theory predicted that people would predominantly compare with better-off others in order to help reach the others' level. The specific prediction was that people would prefer to compare with someone who was slightly better off than the self, because information about others at a very different level is not really informative (e.g., a beginning tennis player would not compare with John McEnroe, but instead would compare with someone who was slightly more experienced); this is known as the principle of slight upward comparison. Furthermore, persons engaging in upward comparison were postulated to become more confident about their abilities in the domains under consideration. Once an accurate self-evaluation had been obtained, the comparison process was seen as completed because persons would be satisfied with obtaining the self-evaluation and better prepared to face whatever tasks confronted them.

Support for the Theory   The typical paradigm offering support for Festinger's theory placed participants (primarily college students) in a task situation with other persons, gave them data about the ranking of the other persons on the task, and then allowed for the selection of detailed information about at least one other person (for a review, see reference number 8). Indeed, participants tended to select slightly upward comparisons (e.g., 9, 10). Additionally, upward comparison increased participants' certainty about their level on the attribute (11). With its clearly stated predictions initially confirmed, Festinger's theory had considerable impact on social psychology.

Unresolved Issues

The theory of upward comparison had notable strengths, but there were several issues that received less attention. One was the assumption that all persons were motivated for continual self-improvement. While this might be true for persons at the higher end of the continuum of achievement and social status, such as the college students who participated in the original studies, there was the question of whether persons with lesser abilities and resources would have the same motivation. Also, the supporting studies mostly involved situations where comparison had little cost for self-esteem, because the subjects believed that they could become like the better-off others. There was less evidence from the more typical coping situation, where people were under threat and questioning their abilities, so there were grounds for wondering whether persons in such situations really were interested in a totally accurate self-evaluation (12).

The Theory of Downward Comparison

Another "branch" of social comparison theory was developed to address situations where people are experiencing problems that are not easily solved through instrumental action. For this condition of self-esteem threat and potential lack of control, it was proposed that persons would compare *with others who are at a lower level than the self on the attribute in question* (13). In this scenario, the aim of the comparison is to restore subjective well-being via comparisons showing others as being in worse conditions than the self.

The basic prediction was that downward comparison would be most prevalent in situations where persons perceived that they were not doing well. In such situations, it was predicted that the use of downward comparison would increase subjective well-being. Downward comparison theory did not necessarily predict that people would become more confident about the accuracy of their self-evaluation, however, because the posited goal of the comparison was different—feeling better about the self rather than achieving veridical feedback. It also was suggested that people would be somewhat ambivalent about use of downward comparison because they believed that it was undesirable to derive self-aggrandizement from the misfortunes of others; yet, when things were not going well, this ambivalence about downward comparison could be overridden by its potential benefits for self-enhancement.

Support for the Theory   Support for the theory initially came from research on comparison selection, projection, aversive environmental events, humor, and gossip. For example, studies on affiliation showed that individuals who were fearful preferred to affiliate with persons who were even more fearful; studies of projection showed that threatened subjects who made derogatory ratings of a target person showed improvements in subjective well-being (13). Laboratory studies showed that persons experiencing self-esteem threat tended to select information about worse-off others (e.g., 14); also, mood improvement was observed after downward comparison, and occurred primarily among persons who initially had negative mood (e.g., 15–17). In contrast to the several paradigms showing downward comparisons related to more favorable self-conceptions, forced upward comparisons on dimensions such as adjustment or physical attractiveness appear to evoke negative affect (17–21).

As predicted by downward comparison theory, persons use different social comparison patterns for controllable and uncontrollable problems (22, 23); and threat or failure experiences alter peoples' use of social comparison information (e.g., 24–27). In addition, persons with chronic and uncontrollable physical illness are found to use downward comparisons (e.g., 2, 28, 29). Overall, therefore, there is considerable support for the role of downward comparison as a coping mechanism (1, 30).

Unresolved Issues   While evidence suggests that downward comparisons may improve subjective well-being, several unresolved issues remain. For example, comparison with others was not always directly observed but was sometimes inferred from subjects' responses (e.g., in field research), so it was not always clear whether downward comparisons were with real persons or possibly with mentally constructed images of others (cf. 2). As there was little research on target preferences, the possibility remained that downward comparisons could turn threatening if the target was too similar to the subject, and, we do not know much about what kinds of targets people might prefer for favorable comparisons (32). Another general issue is that enhancement of subjective well-being in the absence of other efforts to resolve problems might not result in the most effective coping, and this issue is not directly addressed in much of the literature (cf. 33, 34).

Mechanisms of Downward Comparison

The original concept has been elaborated to include various ways in which downward comparisons occur (31, 33, 35, 36). In this section, we discuss several conceptually distinct ways in which downward comparison may occur, along with possible benefits and costs.

Active Selection of a Target

This approach to making a downward comparison theoretically requires three steps: (1) identifying a particular target who is worse off than the self on the attribute in question; (2) gathering information relevant to the target's standing on the attribute; and (3) mentally focusing on that part of the information which indicates the target is worse off than the self. The predicted result is improvement in subjective well-being. This type of comparison process is modeled in laboratory studies in which individuals experiencing a particular problem, such as adjusting to college, are given information about a person who also is experiencing difficulty in adjusting to college. Relevant results show improvement on self-ratings of mood, self-esteem, and perceived competence when persons are exposed to this type of information (e.g., 15, 37).

Costs and Benefits   The benefits are improved mood and perceived self-competence. The costs are that this approach is somewhat effortful, requiring active selection and processing of information. Also, information requirements are restrictive because a specific target must be identified who is potentially worse off on the specific attribute in question, and this prediction must be verified in order to produce a downward comparison. A search failure at any of these points would terminate the coping process, and a poor target choice might produce an unfavorable comparison. It is possible that persons become so skilled at comparisons that these issues are irrelevant, but this is a largely unexplored issue (17, 38).

Implications   While effortfulness per se may not be a limiting factor, the information requirements for this process are sufficiently demanding that there are grounds for questioning how common this approach is in everyday life. A possible way to circumvent information restriction issues would be to select a reasonably promising target and then compare on any dimension that happened to produce a downward comparison. This type of process has been suggested in some field studies (2).

Utilizing a Target of Opportunity

Another type of comparison may occur through exposure to a description of another person who is worse off than the self. Such "passive comparisons" may occur through observation in daily life or through examples presented in newspapers, magazines, or television. Accordingly, an individual could attend to information about worse-off others without necessarily having actively sought out such information. The mass media frequently present information about worse-off others; in fact, the development of downward comparison theory began with a colloquium on *why* there is so much bad news in newspapers (39). The prevalence of such information could vary across media sources; for example, it would be unusual to find many downward comparisons in magazines such as *Field and Stream* or *Scientific American*; but the reader can surely think of tabloid magazines or newspapers whose content is heavily loaded with gore, mayhem, and misfortunes to others, or television soap operas whose plots consist of recurring dilemmas, disappointments, and betrayals for the characters.[1] Persons who habitually followed the latter type of media presentations would find many opportunities to engage in downward comparison if they were so inclined. There is interesting evidence of such a process in media studies; Heath (40) showed that persons who read newspapers reporting high rates of crime in other cities felt better about their own city. In theory, it is likely that a proportion of individuals would not pay much attention to downward comparison information that they happened to encounter, but some individuals who were currently anxious or distressed about a problem would be primed to attend to information about worse-off others.

Costs and Benefits   From the standpoint of benefits, the opportunity for passive downward comparisons could be quite frequent in everyday life if a prediagnosed person read or viewed media presentations that were weighted in this direction. Also, such comparisons do not require much effort, which is a benefit from the cognitive processing standpoint, because the comparer needs only to maintain a minimal level of attention to the ongoing flow of information and focus on that information that meets downward comparison needs. A potential cost is that the comparison examples are unsystematic and unselected, so a specific comparison dimension of interest to an individual might be infrequently represented in media presentations. In practice, this might not be a major cost because the large volume of information available would, in the long run, provide sufficient examples of a particular comparison dimension that the information would be useful.

Implications   Theory points out that the presentation of comparison information in mass media may facilitate coping by providing some individuals with opportunities for favorable comparisons. Research on downward comparison through mass media raises a question about how precise the matching has to be between an individual's current problem and the information available through newspapers or television. If impactful favorable comparisons depend on a precise matching, then this mechanism might not be very important in daily life. However, it is possible that matching of dimensions is not crucial, and a downward comparison might be obtained on dimensions quite remote from an individual's current problem; for example, individuals concerned about their health might conceivably focus on information about individuals having problems with their jobs. There has been little reported research on this issue.

Constructed Comparisons

Although the theory of social comparison assumed that individuals make comparisons with specific persons, perhaps the target of comparison is mentally constructed in some sense. For example, Wood et al. (2) noted that patients frequently made reference to husbands who left their wives after an illness was diagnosed, but statistical data suggested that this was actually a rare occurrence. This raises the question of whether persons may construct mental images of worse-off others, and then make a favorable comparison with the constructed image (cf. 41). Another mechanism is that individuals may exaggerate the perceived attributes of other persons in a direction that is favorable to the self (42–44). In this vein, Beauregard and Dunning (24) noted that "people might be more creative than previously assumed in their ability to find esteem-enhancing comparisons. When people have no choice about whom they are able to compare themselves with, they are quite good at taking a person and construing his/her standing as worse off" (p. 619).

Costs and Benefits   Constructed comparisons have the potential benefit of producing a favorable comparison without requiring much cognitive effort, and descriptive reports suggest that persons can easily imagine prototypical worse-off others for several different comparison dimensions (41). Thus, in terms of cognitive load, this mechanism might appear to have some benefits for coping. A potential cost is that an individual taking this approach may be encouraged to play fast and loose with social perception. Whereas upward comparisons in theory are based on a need for accurate evaluation, constructed downward comparisons leave open the possibility of a departure from reality that could have negative implications for adjustment (e.g., failing to accurately perceive a real health risk). Several investigators have noted that subjects' perceptions are constrained in departing too far from known reality (44); but the tendency to be concerned with relative standing rather than absolute standing could be counterproductive in health contexts, where the absolute level of behavior (e.g., cigarette smoking, risky sexual behavior) may be the only important consideration (44–46).

Implications If comparisons are based to some extent on constructed images, this would suggest a different perspective on coping than a theory presuming that self-enhancing comparisons are tied (though perhaps not tightly) to comparisons with actual persons. It seems important to ask when comparisons are based on real people and when they aren't and to try to identify the consequences for people of using these different types of comparisons. Because constructed comparisons are not overt and visible, it may be necessary to use indirect methods designed to demonstrate their existence, as done by Perloff and Fetzer (41).

Derogation of an Outgroup

A different mechanism has been suggested in which people create a favorable comparison for themselves through exaggerating negative aspects of another group, thus increasing the social distance between the self and the outgroup. At the individual level, this mechanism has been demonstrated in laboratory studies showing that subjects presented with esteem threats make more negative ratings of another participant (e.g., 47). This mechanism has been extended to the group level with the proposition that derogation of social outgroups also may derive from a self-enhancing comparison process that is operative under threat conditions (48).[2] Laboratory studies have indicated that experimental subjects show enhancement on self-esteem measures following comparison with or derogation of an outgroup (51–53). Field research has also linked ethnic prejudice to status concerns. Ethnic prejudice is most prevalent among individuals with low social status, particularly those whose status is declining (54, 55), and prejudiced and authoritarian attitudes in the U.S. population have varied historically with national levels of threat as indexed from census data (56). Thus, there is evidence that people may sometimes deal with threat or status issues through derogation of socially defined outgroups.

Costs and Benefits Although this mechanism may yield some temporary esteem enhancement for an individual, the social costs of this mechanism are more prominent. If persons learn to habitually cope with problems through derogating others, this could lead to more negative perceptions of other persons and hence could affect interpersonal relations through encouraging distrust of and/or hostile behavior toward others. At the group level, comparative perceptions with outgroups might have some benefit for enhancing collective self-esteem (57), but seem likely to increase intergroup tensions over the long term. Although mild self-enhancement in social perceptions is a fairly common process that does not have obvious costs (48), more extreme forms of outgroup derogation seem likely to have harmful effects at the intergroup level.

Implications   Perhaps the frequency and extremity of this coping approach have implications for adjustment. Though a mild self-enhancing tendency in perceiving others may help maintain self-esteem, frequent derogation of target persons could lead to group tensions and the undermining of supportive relationships (cf. 58). We note that there are some empirical paradoxes in this area, because studies of college students sometimes show derogation (indexed through increase in the self-other differential in personality ratings) to be more prevalent among persons labeled as high self-esteem (59). This issue will be discussed in more detail in the section on social comparison and self-esteem.

Construction of Worse Alternatives (Counterfactual Thinking)

Another coping approach, following a negative outcome, is to imagine a comparable situation with an even worse outcome; this provides a downward comparison that is within-individual rather than interpersonal. This process, termed counterfactual thinking, has received considerable attention in the fields of cognitive and social psychology (e.g., 60–62). Analogous to the mood-enhancement effect resulting from downward social comparisons, subjects instructed to engage in downward counterfactual thinking (i.e., imagining a worse outcome) have improved in mood as compared with those instructed to engage in upward counterfactuals (e.g., 62, 62).

Costs and Benefits   This mechanism seemingly would have considerable benefits for coping because it is not cognitively effortful (simply taking an existing situation and imagining a worse variant), does not invoke a search for a specific target and does not involve considering negative information about others. There is some doubt, however, about how often this approach actually is used as a comparison-oriented coping mechanism. For one thing, recent thought-listing studies suggest that upward counterfactuals are much more prevalent than downward counterfactuals (61); these findings fit a self-improvement interpretation in that people may imagine more favorable outcomes so as to be mentally rehearsed for coping better the next time the situation occurs (cf. 4). In addition, several studies have shown a paradoxical process, in which persons with objectively better performance feel dissatisfied because of upward counterfactual thinking. For example, studies of Olympic Games winners found that silver medalists (second place) were less happy than bronze medalists (third place); this occurred because silver medalists engaged in upward counterfactual thinking about what they could have done to become first-place gold medalists whereas people in third place were happy that they got a medal (64, 65).

Implications   While counterfactual thinking seems credible as a coping mechanism, little research has been conducted on its use in naturalistic situations. It has been reported that downward counterfactuals improve mood after experiencing an initial failure situation but may result in worse performance when the situation is encountered a second time (61); therefore, interesting questions are raised about the balance between self-enhancement and self-improvement. Moreover, laboratory studies show that downward counterfactual thinking is used more often in high perceived-control situations (66), which is the opposite of findings from studies where type social comparison information selected is the dependent variable; accordingly, questions remain about the status of counterfactual thinking as a comparison-oriented coping mechanism. Also, a study conducted with naturalistic situations of a serious nature (automobile accidents) found that persons who were more distressed after the incident tended subsequently to engage in more counterfactual thinking about what they could have done to prevent it (67); this is consistent with the idea that self-blame may be more prevalent in situations with serious consequences (cf. 68, 69).

Summary

Downward social comparison appears to be a flexible process. Several mechanisms of downward comparison are theoretically possible, and many targets are potentially available. Five different mechanisms of downward comparison have been discussed: active selection of a target; using a target of opportunity; constructed comparisons; derogation of a target; and imagining worse outcomes. These mechanisms have somewhat different cost and benefit profiles, either to the individual or to society as a whole, so it is not possible to say that one mechanism is more or less adaptive. There is a substantial body of evidence, demonstrating the operation of each mechanism, and the findings are largely consistent with the predictions generated by downward comparison theory.

Current Issues in Social Comparison Research

In this section we consider three of the major current research issues: the level of consciousness at which comparison occurs, the relation between comparison preferences and actual affiliations, and the role of social comparison in self-esteem and depression.

Is Downward Comparison an Automatized Process?

The original conceptions of both upward comparison and downward comparison assumed that comparison was an effortful, conscious process in which people gathered social information, considered the available information, and selected others for comparison. However, based on cognitive research in recent years, there has been increasing emphasis on "automatized" processes—those *not* requiring a high level of attention or cognitive effort (e.g., 70, 71). From this latter perspective, the focus is on how persons routinely respond to a background of social comparison information that is always present.

Research by Gilbert, Giesler, and Morris (38) explored this question using information processing paradigms. Through conditions in which subjects' attention was occupied or not occupied, they showed that an unfavorable comparison with a confederate who performed better made subjects feel worse about their own competence; however, this effect was reversed when subjects had sufficient mental capacity to reverse the upward comparison effect through finding reasons to discount the confederate's performance. Although subjects asserted that they had been unaffected by the comparison, the data showed they had actually undergone changes in mood states, which faded by the end of the experiment, indicating that in some way the unwanted comparison had been "undone" so as to leave no net change in mood. The authors concluded, "Social comparisons can sometimes be so natural and easy that people may make them even when they don't really want to, and when that happens, they may have little choice but to mentally undo the [upward] comparisons they have made" (p. 232).

The concept that comparisons may have an immediate affective impact is complemented by findings from studies by Tesser, Millar, and Moore (72), who used unobtrusive observational measures of comparison and affect and noted that downward comparisons had a short-term impact for increasing positive affect. This is conceptually consistent with survey studies indicating that school students in settings where others' abilities are relatively low tend to have higher self-esteem than those in settings where the majority of others have relatively high ability (e.g., 73, 74). Automaticity research suggests that the general positivity bias in self-ratings may be produced in everyday life through an unobtrusive impact of downward comparisons and an undoing of upward comparisons (see 74, 75).

Is There a Divergence Between Evaluation and Affiliation Processes?   Another recent development concerns the prediction of affiliation preferences among persons with serious illness. Clinical observations have indicated that cancer patients express discomfort about being around other patients (e.g., in a clinical waiting room) who had severe and advanced disease (76, 77). This presented a challenge to a naive formulation of downward comparison theory, which some investigators read as predicting that comparison with any worse-off other would necessarily lead to increases in subjective well-being. The coping formulation, though, delineates the fact that the primary need of persons with serious illness is for information indicating that they are going to get better or at least not get worse (cf. 78, 79). When information is provided indicating that a similar person with the same disease is deteriorating, or has had a similar operation but is not recovering, threat rather than comfort is likely to be aroused (31).

A theoretical formulation by S. Taylor and Lobel (6) aimed to reconcile the clinical, "waiting room" observations with evidence that cancer patients often make self-evaluation statements that reflect downward comparisons. They suggested a divergence in affiliation and evaluation processes among threatened persons, such that actual affiliation choices would be guided by improvement motives, and threatened persons would prefer affiliation with patients who were doing relatively well (to provide optimism and hope for improvement); in contrast, comparative evaluations would be based on worse-off targets so as to provide a relatively favorable image of one's personality and adjustment. This formulation has now been supported in studies with cardiac patients (29) and cancer patients (80). A support group intervention study with cancer patients also found that affiliation was a significant issue for recruitment because some patients were reluctant to be in a group which they thought would include others with severe disease. Thus, there is evidence for the proposition that threatened persons may not necessarily benefit from being in forced close contact with similar others who are worse off.

The work on affiliation has interesting linkages to other areas. With respect to the studies by Gilbert et al. on unfavorable comparison (38), it is likely that being in direct contact with a similar but worse-off other is difficult to cognitively undo, because the social information is concrete and vivid. With respect to coping models, the concept that comparison may contribute to optimism is relevant (82). While upward comparison has been construed as generating optimism, several studies have suggested that downward comparisons can increase optimism if the other is perceived as similar and worse off, but likely to improve (30, 31). Thus, when persons are engaged in effortful coping, comparison information may be scanned to derive implications for the future.

Self-Esteem and Downward Comparison

The original postulate that downward comparison would be used primarily by persons with low self-esteem (13) has been modified somewhat by recent research, which has shown some interesting complexities about how high- and low-esteem individuals deal with threatening situations. One theme in this research concerns the question of whether persons with low esteem respond differently from persons with high esteem when exposed to downward comparison information. Findings from experimental studies show that mood improvement after exposure to downward comparison information is consistently observed among *low* self-esteem subjects who are *currently* experiencing threat or distress. For example, Gibbons and Boney-McCoy (47) did a study in which college students, previously selected to be low versus high on self-esteem, were either threatened or not threatened by false personality feedback; all subjects were then exposed to downward comparison information through hearing a tape about a student who was described as having difficulty adjusting to college. Improvement in mood was observed only among low self-esteem subjects who had been threatened; high self-esteem subjects showed no mood change in response to the downward comparison information (see also 15, 17, 82, 83). Parallel results were obtained by Lyubomirsky and Ross (17) in a study where subjects were selected for being generally happy or generally unhappy; here, comparison information was obtained through observing a peer who performed better or worse on a task. Differential increase in positive mood was found for unhappy subjects who had done poorly and observed a peer who performed even worse. Thus, in all these studies mood improvement was observed only among low-esteem (or dysphoric) subjects, particularly threatened ones, who were exposed to downward comparison information.

One complexity of this research is the different patterns of responding on measures reflecting derogation of a target. For example, Gibbons and Boney-McCoy (47) also had subjects make ratings of the personality characteristics of the comparison student presented in the tape. They found that ratings of the target were particularly negative among high-esteem subjects who were threatened; a gender difference also was noted in this effect, with males tending to derogate the target on achievement-related dimensions, whereas females tended to derogate the target on socially related dimensions. Parallel results were found by Beauregard and Dunning (24) for ratings of a target person's intelligence. These results are conceptually similar to findings from various studies on outgrouping (59) and health behavior (84).

Do these apparently contradictory observations mean that high self-esteem persons are the only ones who use favorable comparison to enhance subjective well-being, and low self-esteem persons don't engage in self-enhancement? A resolution has been proposed by several investigators (85, 86), who have suggested that high and low self-esteem persons engage in differing kinds of self-enhancement processes. The lows use more indirect forms of self-enhancement, whereas the highs use more active self-aggrandizement, exaggerating their own abilities and efforts and derogating those of others. The proposed reason for the difference is that there is some reality basis for self-esteem. Though there is considerable variance in self-perceptions, on average, persons with low esteem tend to score lower on various competencies. Thus, the self-enhancement approach among lows is to some extent bounded by reality constraints. Lows would like to get positive information about the self but cannot go too far in interpreting social information without stretching their own credibility (or that of their social audience), whereas highs—being pretty sure of their competencies—have more latitude regarding their self-aggrandizement in processing information about others. These dual processes have been supported in several kinds of research (86–88).

Depression and Social Comparison

"Depression" refers to a constellation of symptoms, including dysphoric mood, decreased interest and motivation, feelings of hopelessness and low self-worth, and vegetative symptoms such as sleep and appetite disturbance. The primary questions at issue here concern whether onset of depression is attributable to a particular use of social comparison, and whether favorable comparison may be used to help recover from an episode of depression.[3] We note that in studies of social comparison and depression, the subjects typically are college students with elevated scores on self-report scales of dysphoric mood, rather than subjects diagnosed with clinical depression; so there is some concern about whether this research is indexing unique predictors of depression, versus its component of low self-esteem. Nonetheless a number of studies have been conducted in this area (see 89, 90) and their findings are of interest for a coping formulation.

One hypothesis is that depressives may be more sensitive to social comparison information, so that (a) they seek it out more frequently and /or (b) are more influenced by comparisons that do occur. Accordingly, depressives would become exposed to more upward comparisons and would react more strongly (and unfavorably) to these, with resultant negative mood and lowered self-evaluations. Studies of depressed (or dysphoric) individuals do suggest that they tend to select more comparison information, particularly after failure and when the social information is complex (91–94).

Another hypothesis is that depressed persons may fail to use self-enhancing comparisons, and this could help maintain depression over time. Here the evidence is more mixed. Gibbons (95) found that depressive subjects differentially chose downward targets and improved in mood as a result so they are not lacking in ability for self-enhancing comparison. Elsewhere, distressed subjects exposed to downward comparison information also show mood improvement (e.g., 15, 47). Also, depressed individuals may preferentially focus on a dimension where they are particularly competent, in order to maintain a balanced sense of esteem (96), though they are unlikely to obtain self-enhancement through exaggerated perceptions of their own abilities.

From this discussion, we could propose that depressed persons sometimes become depressed in part through overreliance on social comparison information in combination with a tendency to react unfavorably to upward comparisons, which serves to exacerbate their already low self-worth. Whether depressives use downward comparison to help alleviate negative moods and to enhance self-image depends in part, we think, on what type of comparison mechanism is employed. There is considerable evidence that depressive-type individuals show mood improvement when passively exposed to information about a worse-off other. However, such persons show no tendency to derogate others in order to produce mood improvement. We think the desire for self-enhancement is usually present among depressed persons, but that only under certain conditions will such individuals tend to use social comparison information in attempts to self-enhance.

Summary

In this chapter we have outlined the postulates of the theory of social comparison, considered mechanisms through which people may cope through downward comparisons, and discussed some of the ongoing issues in this active research area. Our presentation has emphasized the flexible nature of downward comparison processes, showing that there are several ways in which people in adverse circumstances can arrive at relatively favorable perceptions of themselves. The cumulative weight of the research suggests that downward comparison is a fairly common coping mechanism, and that self-enhancement processes may be adaptive for contributing to better adjustment if more positive views of the self motivate people to remain engaged in efforts to actively cope with problems (31, 36, 97, 98).[4]

A primary question about any coping mechanism is whether it is effective. This question does not always have as clear an answer as one would like, because much of the research on coping is cross-sectional and hence does not provide clear inferences about whether coping precedes changes in adjustment. However, there is enough prospective evidence in the broader literature on coping to conclude that active types of coping are related to improved adjustment, whereas avoidant and angry types of coping are related to worse adjustment (98, 102). In the literature on downward comparison there are relatively few prospective studies (though see references 20, 103, 104, 105, for exceptions), so conclusions must be more qualified.

It should be clear from the preceding sections, however, that blanket assertions about whether a coping mechanism is effective or ineffective may serve to obscure real complexities in the process that relates coping to adjustment.[5] We have discussed, for example, how persons with high versus low self-esteem may use very different types of comparison-oriented coping strategies; so any statements about the effectiveness of downward comparison must state exactly what type of comparison mechanism is employed. We have noted that downward comparison in some conditions not only improves mood but also helps generate optimism and positive expectations about future success, intermediates that are important prerequisites for sustained, effective coping efforts. There is some suggestion in the literature that an excessive focus on self-enhancement, without investing effort in coping with problems, could interfere with subsequent performance (104, 105). These findings are troubling, yet the results are from a specific context, academic comparison level, and there is little good evidence so that conclusions about either benefits or possible harmful effects must be tentative. What is needed is the accumulation of a body of evidence from well-designed studies that use the complementary advantages of laboratory experimentation and longititudinal field research. We have tried to suggest some potential costs and benefits for each type of downward comparison mechanism, and further research may help to clarify these types of questions.

We think the research discussed in this chapter supports several suggestions that could be tested in clinical research and practice. For example, consistent with cognitive-behavioral therapy of depression (108), one approach is to train clients to identify irrational upward comparisons when they make them, and to generate alternative, more adaptive cognitions that could include rational downward comparisons about their present situation. Also, judicious use of rational downward comparisons may be useful for helping persons cope with blows to self-esteem. Our analysis suggests that social comparisons, perhaps with available or constructed targets, would be preferable to encouraging devaluation of others' attributes, which in any event does not seem to be pursued by low-esteem persons. Another therapeutic approach to comparison might involve emphasizing its potential for generating optimism about recovery through observing, empathizing, and learning from the experiences of other persons. The therapist should be alert to the possibility of overreliance on self-enhancing comparisons, and could encourage clients to balance appropriate use of downward comparison with an eventual focus on more difficult upward comparisons, in order to identify goals and provide realistic models of positive adjustment (cf. 109). Here, the therapist can give attention to addressing irrational beliefs that the others' status is unreachable and building the belief that the client can become like the upward comparison targets. A different approach would be to help some clients reduce their oversensitivity to any type of social comparison information, so that their self-concepts ultimately would be tied more to the match between their own aspirations and abilities rather than comparisons with others (17).

We believe the work presented in this chapter provides a demonstration of the richness of social comparison theory, which has generated a variety of questions about how comparison may be used for self-evaluation and self-enhancement. Many questions still remain to be answered, and some are only beginning to be addressed. For example, it is plausible that use of comparative approaches to coping is grounded in relatively stable personality characteristics (see 21, 110). Another intriguing question is whether a focus on defensive self-aggrandizement is more characteristic of Western cultures, whereas a focus on self-acceptance and internal harmony is more characteristic of Eastern cultures; recent studies provide some evidence to suggest that this focus may be true (111). Implications about the role of social comparison for group therapy and support processes also are being examined (81, 112). Such questions will, we think, continue to shed light on the roles of social comparison processes in coping with problems and adjusting to one's life circumstances.

Acknowledgments
Preparation of this chapter was facilitated by a Research Scientist Development Award #K02 DA00252 from the National Institute on Drug Abuse and by grant #R21 CA81646 from the National Cancer Institute. Thanks are extended to Frederick X. Gibbons for useful comments on an early draft.

Notes

1. Of course, there are other reasons for having negative information in the media; persons may need information about conflicts or events that could have instrumental implications for them. It remains that the proportion of bad news in newspapers, for example, varies widely, and there are grounds for believing that coping functions are part of the explanation.

2. It is also the case that persons show a marked tendency to perceive the world in terms of distinctions between ingroups and outgroups. Ingroup-outgroup perceptions can be established with minimal manipulations and are accompanied by preferential behavior toward ingroup members. Whether this basic process of social perception is grounded in a self-enhancement mechanism remains controversial (48). Some evidence has indicated that ingroup-outgroup distinctions are responsive to esteem-relevant manipulations (49), but it has been noted that identification with a group can serve many functions, including access to wealth and power (50).

3. Here we are making an implicit assumption that depression is not identical to low self-esteem. This same question has been raised about self-esteem and general happiness or optimism (17). Differences in comparison between dysphoric and nondysphoric subjects might be due to differences in self-esteem, but this question has not been clearly tested in the research we discuss, and remains to be clarified in further studies.

4. Note that there are other cognitive models of self-enhancement: self-affirmation (99), self-consistency (100), and Tesser's model of comparison/reflection (101). Extended discussion is beyond the scope of this chapter, but this does not reflect disinterest in these important models.

5. It should be noted that the concept that positive mood is equivalent to adjustment is not universally accepted, and this issue is still a source of some controversy (see 106, 107)

References

1. Affleck, G., & Tennen, H. (1991). Social comparison and coping with major medical problems. In J. Suls & T. A. Wills (Eds.), *Social comparison: Contemporary theory and research* (pp. 369–393). Hillsdale, NJ: Erlbaum.
2. Wood, J. V., Taylor, S. E., & Lichtman, R. R. (1985). Social comparison in adjustment to breast cancer. *Journal of Personality and Social Psychology, 49*, 1169–1183.
3. Helgeson, V. S., & Mickelson, K. D. (1995). Motives for social comparison. *Personality and Social Psychology Bulletin, 21*, 1200–1209.
4. Wood, J. V., & Taylor, K. (1991). Serving self-relevant goals through social comparison. In J. Suls & T. A. Wills (Eds.), *Social compari-

son: *Contemporary theory and research* (pp. 23–49). Hillsdale, NJ: Erlbaum.

5. Collins, R. L. (1996). The impact of upward social comparison on self-evaluations. *Psychological Bulletin, 119,* 51–69.

6. Taylor, S., & Lobel, M. (1989). Social comparison activity under threat: Downward evaluation and upward contacts. *Psychological Review, 96,* 569–575.

7. Festinger, L. (1954). A theory of social comparison processes. *Human Relations, 7,* 117–140.99.

8. Goethals, G. R., Arrowood, A. J., Wills, T. A., Suls, J., & Wheeler, L. (1986). Social comparison theory: Lost and found. *Personality and Social Psychology Bulletin, 12,* 261–299.

9. Miller, C. T. (1982). The role of performance-related similarity in social comparison of abilities: A test of the related-attributes hypothesis. *Journal of Experimental Social Psychology, 18,* 513–523.

10. Suls, J., Gastorf, J., & Lawhon, J. (1978). Social comparison choices for evaluating a sex-and age-related ability. *Personality and Social Psychology Bulletin, 4,* 102–105.

11. Radloff, R. (1966). Social comparison and ability evaluation. *Journal of Experimental Social Psychology, 2* (Supplement 1), 6–26.

12. Brickman, P., & Bulman, R. J. (1977). Pleasure and pain in social comparison. In J. M. Suls & R. M. Miller (Eds.), *Social comparison processes: Theoretical and empirical perspectives* (pp. 149–186). Washington, DC: Hemisphere.

13. Wills, T. A. (1981). Downward comparison principles in social psychology. *Psychological Bulletin, 90,* 245–271.

14. Smith, R. H., & Insko, C. A. (1987). Social comparison choice during ability evaluation: The effects of comparison publicity, performance feedback, and self-esteem. *Personality and Social Psychology Bulletin, 13,* 111–122.

15. Aspinwall, L. G., & Taylor, S. E. (1993). Effects of social comparison direction, threat, and self-esteem on affect, self-evaluation, and expected success. *Journal of Personality and Social Psychology, 64,* 708–722.

16. Gibbons, F. X., & Gerrard, M. (1989). Effects of upward and downward social comparison on mood states. *Journal of Social and Clinical Psychology, 8,* 14–31.

17. Lyubomirsky, S., & Ross, L. (1997). Hedonic consequences of social comparison: A contrast of happy and unhappy people. *Journal of Personality and Social Psychology, 73,* 1141–1157.

18. Brown, J., Novick, N., Kelley, A., & Richards, J. (1992). When Gulliver travels: Social context, psychological closeness, and self-appraisals. *Journal of Personality and Social Psychology, 62,* 717–727.

19. Kenrick, D. T., Montello, D. R., Gutierres, S. E., & Trost, M. R. (1993). Effects of physical attractiveness on affect and perceptual judgements: When social comparison overrides social reinforcement. *Personality and Social Psychology Bulletin, 19,* 195–199.

20. Gibbons, F. X., Benbow, C. P., & Gerrard, M. (1994). From top dog to bottom half: Social comparison strategies in response to poor performance. *Journal of Personality and Social Psychology, 67,* 638–652.

21. Smith, R. H., Parrott, W. G., Diener, E. E., Hoyle, R. H., & Kim, S. H. (1999). Dispositional envy. *Personality and Social Psychology Bulletin, 25,* 1007–1020.
22. Major, B., Testa, M., & Bylsma, W. H. (1991). Responses to upward and downward comparisons: The impact of esteem-relevance and perceived control. In J. Suls & T. A. Wills (Eds.), *Social comparison: Contemporary theory and research* (pp. 237–260). Hillsdale, NJ: Erlbaum.
23. Michinov, N., & Monteil, J-M. (1997). Upward or downward comparison after failure: The role of diagnostic information. *Social Behavior and Personality, 25,* 389–398.
24. Beauregard, K. S., & Dunning, D. (1998). Turning up the contrast: Self-enhancement motives prompt egocentric contrast effects in social judgments. *Journal of Personality and Social Psychology, 74,* 606–621.
25. Brown, J., & Gallagher, F. (1992). Coming to terms with failure: Private self-enhancement, public self-effacement. *Journal of Experimental Social Psychology, 28,* 3–22.
26. Pyszczynski, T., Greenberg, J., & LaPrelle, J. (1985). Social comparison after success and failure: Biased search for information consistent with a self-serving conclusion. *Journal of Experimental Social Psychology, 21,* 195–211.
27. Suls, J., & Wan, C. K. (1987). In search of the false-uniqueness phenomenon: Fear and estimates of social consensus. *Journal of Personality and Social Psychology, 52,* 211–217.
28. Blalock, S., DeVellis, B., & DeVellis, R. (1989). Social comparison among individuals with rheumatoid arthritis. *Journal of Applied Social Psychology, 19,* 665–680.
29. Helgeson, V. S., & Taylor, S. (1992). Social comparisons and adjustment among cardiac patients. *Journal of Applied Social Psychology, 23,* 1171–1195.
30. Gibbons, F. X., & Gerrard, M. (1991). Downward comparison and coping with threat. In J. Suls & T. A. Wills (Eds.), *Social comparison: Contemporary theory and research* (pp. 317–345). Hillsdale, NJ: Erlbaum.
31. Wills, T. A. (1991). Similarity and self-esteem in downward comparison. In J. Suls & T. A. Wills (Eds.), *Social comparison: Contemporary theory and research* (pp. 51–78). Hillsdale, NJ: Erlbaum.
32. Bunk, B. P., & Ybema, J. F. (1997). Social comparison and occupational stress: The identification-contrast model. In B. P. Buunk & F. X. Gibbons (Eds.), *Health, coping, and well-being: Perspectives from social comparison theory* (pp. 359–388). Mahwah, NJ: Erlbaum.
33. Wills, T. A. (1992). Social comparison and self-change. In J. D. Fisher, J. Chinsky, Y. Klar, & A. Nadler (Eds.), *Self-change: Social-psychological and clinical perspectives* (pp. 231–252). New York: Springer-Verlag.
34. Wills, T. A. (1997). Modes and families of coping: An analysis of downward comparison in the structure of other cognitive and behavioral mechanisms. In B. Buunk & F. X. Gibbons (Eds.), *Health, coping, and social comparison* (pp. 167–193). Mahwah, NJ: Erlbaum.
35. Wills, T. A. (1987). Downward comparison as a coping mechanism. In C. R. Snyder & C. E. Ford (Eds.), *Coping with negative life events: Clin-*

ical and social-psychological perspectives (pp. 243–268). New York: Plenum Press.

36. Wills, T. A. (1991). Social comparison processes in coping and health. In C. R. Snyder & D. R. Forsyth (Eds.), *Handbook of social and clinical psychology* (pp. 376–394). Elmsford, NY: Pergamon.

37. DeVellis, R. F., Blalock, S. J., Holt, K., Renner, B. R., Blanchard, L. W., & Klotz, M. L. (1991). Arthritis patients' reactions to unavoidable social comparisons. *Personality and Social Psychology Bulletin, 17,* 376–384.

38. Gilbert, D. T., Giesler, R. B., & Morris, K. A. (1995). When comparisons arise. *Journal of Personality and Social Psychology, 69,* 227–236.

39. Wills, T. A. (1974, April). Why is there so much bad news in newspapers? Social comparison theory, the gambler's fallacy, and death on the highway. Colloquium presented at Department of Psychology, University of Oregon.

40. Heath, L. (1984). Impact of newspapers crime reports on fear of crime: Multimethodological investigation. *Journal of Personality and Social Psychology, 47,* 263–276.

41. Perloff, L. S., & Fetzer, B. K. (1986). Self-other judgments and perceived vulnerability to victimization. *Journal of Personality and Social Psychology, 50,* 502–510.

42. Dunning, D., & Cohen, G. L. (1992). Egocentric definitions of traits and abilities in social judgment. *Journal of Personality and Social Psychology, 63,* 341–355.

43. Dunning, D., Perie, M., & Story, A. L. (1991). Self-serving prototypes of social categories. *Journal of Personality and Social Psychology, 61,* 957–968.

44. Klein, W. M., & Kunda, Z. (1993). Maintaining self-serving social comparisons: Biased reconstruction of one's past behaviors. *Personality and Social Bulletin, 19,* 732–739.

45. Tigges, B. B., Wills, T. A., & Link, B. G. (1998). Social comparison, the threat of AIDS, and adolescent condom use. *Journal of Applied Social Psychology, 28,* 861–887.

46. Klein, W. M., & Weinstein, N. D. (1997). Social comparison and unrealistic optimism: About personal risk. In B. P. Buunk & F. X. Gibbons (Eds.), *Health, coping, and well-being: Perspectives from social comparison theory* (pp. 26–62). Mahwah, NJ: Erlbaum.

47. Gibbons, F. X., & Boney-McCoy, S. (1991). Self-esteem, similarity, and reactions to active versus passive downward comparison. *Journal of Personality and Social Psychology, 60,* 414–424.

48. Banaji, M. R., & Prentice, D. A. (1994). The self in social contexts. *Annual Review of Psychology, 45,* 297–332.

49. Brewer, M. B. (1979). Ingroup bias in the minimal intergroup situation: A cognitive-motivational analysis. *Psychological Bulletin, 86,* 307–324.

50. Abrams, D. (1994). Social self-regulation. *Personality and Social Psychology Bulletin 20,* 473–483.

51. Brewer, M. B., & Weber, J. G. (1994). Self-evaluation effects of interpersonal versus intergroup social comparison. *Journal of Personality and Social Psychology, 66,* 268–275.

52. Brown, J., Collins, R., & Schmitt, G. (1988). Self-esteem and direct versus indirect forms of self-enhancement. *Journal of Personality and Social Psychology, 55,* 445–453.
53. Major, B., Sciacchitano, A. M., & Crocker, J. (1993). In-group versus outgroup comparisons and self-esteem. *Personality and Social Psychology Bulletin, 19,* 711–721.
54. Brewer, M. B., & Campbell, D. T. (1976). *Ethnocentrism and intergroup attitudes: East African evidence.* New York: Halstead Press.
55. Smedley, J. W., & Bayton, J. A. (1978). Evaluative race-class stereotypes by race and class of subjects. *Journal of Personality and Social Psychology, 36,* 530–535.
56. Doty, R. M., Peterson, B. E., & Winter, D. G. (1991). Threat and authoritarianism in the United States, 1978–1987. *Journal of Personality and Social Psychology, 61,* 629–640.
57. Crocker, J., & Luhtanen, R. (1990). Collective self-esteem and ingroup bias. *Journal of Personality and Social Psychology, 58,* 60–67.
58. Lane, C., & Hobfoll, S. (1992). Loss creates anger that alienates potential supporters. *Journal of Consulting and Clinical Psychology, 60,* 935–942.
59. Crocker, J., Thompson, L. L., McGraw, K. M., & Ingerman, C. (1987). Downward comparison and evaluations of others: Effects of self-esteem and threat. *Journal of Personality and Social Psychology, 52,* 907–916.
60. Miller, D. T., Turnbull, W., & McFarland, C. (1990). Counterfactual thinking and social perception. In L. Berkowitz (Ed.), *Advances in experimental social psychology* (Vol. 23, pp. 305–331). San Diego, CA: Academic Press.
61. Roese, N. J. (1997). Counterfactual thinking. *Psychological Bulletin, 121,* 133–148.
62. Roese, N. J. (1994). The functional basis of counterfactual thinking. *Journal of Personality and Social Psychology, 66,* 805–818.
63. Markman, K. D., Gavanski, I., Sherman, S. J., & McMullen, M. N. (1993). The mental simulation of better and worse possible worlds. *Journal of Experimental Social Psychology, 29,* 87–109.
64. Medvec, V. H., Madey, S. F., & Gilovich, T. (1995). Counterfactual thinking and satisfaction among Olympic medalists. *Journal of Personality and Social Psychology, 69,* 603–610.
65. Medvec, V. H., Savitsky, A. (1997). When doing better means feeling worse: Effects of categorical cutoff points on counterfactual thinking and satisfaction. *Journal of Personality and Social Psychology, 72,* 1284–1296.
66. Markman, K. D., Gavanski, I., Sherman, S. J., & McMullen, M. N. (1995). The impact of perceived control on the imagination of better and worse possible worlds. *Personality and Social Psychology Bulletin, 21,* 588–595.
67. Davis, C. G., Lehman, D. R., Wortman, C. D., Silver, R., & Thompson, S. (1995). The undoing of traumatic events. *Personality and Social Psychology Bulletin, 21,* 109–124.
68. Schulz, R., & Decker, S. (1985). Long-term adjustment to physical disability. *Journal of Personality and Social Psychology, 48,* 1162–1172.

69. Tennen, H., Affleck, G., & Gershman, K. (1986). Self-blame among parents of infants with perinatal complications: The role of self-protective motives. *Journal of Personality and Social Psychology, 50,* 690–696.

70. Gilbert, D. T. (1991). How mental systems believe. *American Psychologist, 46,* 107–119.

71. Schwartz, N., & Bless, H. (1992). Constructing reality and its alternatives: An inclusion-exclusion model of assimilation and contrast effects in social judgment. In L. L. Martin & A. Tesser (Eds.), *The construction of social judgments* (pp. 217–245). Hillsdale, NJ: Erlbaum.

72. Tesser, A., Millar, M., & Moore, J. (1988). Some affective consequences of social comparison: The pain and pleasure of being close. *Journal of Personality and Social Psychology, 54,* 49–61.

73. Marsh, H. W., & Parker, J. W. (1984). Determinants of student self-concept: Is it better to be a relatively large fish in a small pond even if you don't learn to swim as well. *Journal of Personality and Social Psychology, 47,* 213–231.

74. Marsh, H. W., Kong, C-K., & Hau, K-T. (2000). Longitudinal multilevel models of the Big-Fish-Little-Pond effect on academic self-concept: Counterbalancing contrast and reflected-glory effects in Hong Kong schools. *Journal of Personality and Social Psychology, 78,* 337–349.

75. Hagerty, M. R. (2000). Social comparisons of income in one's community: Evidence from national studies of income and happiness. *Journal of Personality and Social Psychology, 78,* 764–771.

76. Molleman, E., Pruyn, J., & van Knippenberg, A. (1986). Social comparison process among cancer patients. *British Journal of Social Psychology, 25,* 1–13.

77. Rofe, Y., Lewin, I., & Hoffman, M. (1987). Affiliation patterns among cancer patients. *Psychological Medicine, 17,* 419–424.

78. Kulik, J. A., & Mahler, H. I. M. (1987). Effects of preoperative roommate assignment on preoperative anxiety and postoperative recovery from coronary-bypass surgery. *Health Psychology, 6,* 525–543.

79. Kulik, J. A., Mahler, H. I. M., & Moore, P. J. (1996). Social comparison and affiliation under threat: Effects on recovery from major surgery. *Journal of Personality and Social Psychology, 71,* 967–979.

80. Stanton, A. L., Danoff-Burg, S., Cameron, C. L., Snider, R., & Kirk, S. B. (1999). Social comparison and adjustment to breast cancer: An experimental examination of upward affiliation and downward evaluation. *Health Psychology, 18,* 152–158.

81. Helgeson, V. S., Cohen, S., & Schulz, R. (in press). Group support interventions for people with cancer: Benefits and hazards. In A. Baum & B. Andersen (Eds.), *Psychosocial interventions and cancer.* Washington, DC: American Psychological Association.

82. Aspinwall, L. G. (1997). Future-oriented aspects of social comparisons: A framework for studying health-related comparison activity. In B. Buunk & F. X. Gibbons (Eds.), *Health, coping, and social comparison* (pp. 125–165). Mahwah, NJ: Erlbaum.

83. Reis, T. J., Gerrard, M., & Gibbons, F. X. (1993). Social comparison and the pill: Reactions to upward and downward comparison of contraceptive behavior. *Personality and Social Psychology Bulletin, 19,* 13–20.

84. Boney-McCoy, S., Gibbons, F. X., & Gerrard, M. (1999). Self-esteem, compensatory self-enhancement, and the consideration of health risk. *Personality and Social Psychology Bulletin, 25,* 954–965.
85. Baumgardner, A. H., Kaufman, C. M., & Levy, P. E. (1989). Regulating affect interpersonally: When low esteem leads to greater enhancement. *Journal of Personality and Social Psychology, 56,* 907–921.
86. Wood, J. V., Giordano-Beech, M., & Ducharme, M. J. (1999). Compensating for failure through social comparison. *Personality and Social Psychology Bulletin, 25,* 1370–1386.
87. Brown, J., & Dutton, K. (1995). Self-esteem and people's emotional reactions to success and failure. *Journal of Personality and Social Psychology, 68,* 712–722.
88. Olson, B. D., & Evans, D. L. (1999). The role of the Big Five personality factors in the direction and affective consequences of everyday social comparisons. *Personality and Social Psychology Bulletin, 25,* 1498–1508.
89. Ahrens, A. H., & Alloy, L. B. (1997). Social comparison processes in depression. In B. Buunk & F. X. Gibbons (Eds.), *Health, coping, and social comparison* (pp. 389–410). Mahwah, NJ: Erlbaum.
90. Wood, J. V., & Lockwood, P. (1997). Social comparisons in dysphoric and low self-esteem people. In R. M. Kowalski & M. R. Leary (Eds.), *The social psychology of emotional and behavioral problems: Interfaces of social and clinical psychology* (pp. 97–135). Washington, DC: American Psychological Association.
91. Ahrens, A. H. (1991). Dysphoria and social comparison: Combining information regarding others' performances. *Journal of Social and Clinical Psychology, 10,* 190–205.
92. Swallow, S. R., & Kuiper, N. A. (1990). Mild depression, dysfunctional cognitions, and interest in social comparison information. *Journal of Social and Clinical Psychology, 9,* 289–302.
93. Swallow, S. R., & Kuiper, N. A. (1992). Mild depression and frequency of social comparison behavior. *Journal of Social and Clinical Psychology, 11,* 167–180.
94. Swallow, S. R., & Kuiper, N. A. (1993). Social comparison in dysphoria and nondysphoria: Differences in target similarity and specificity. *Cognitive Therapy and Research, 17,* 103–122.
95. Gibbons, F. X. (1986). Social comparison and depression: Company's effect on misery. *Journal of Personality and Social Psychology, 51,* 140–148.
96. Pelham, B. W. (1991). On the benefits of misery: Self-serving biases in the depressive self-concept. *Journal of Personality and Social Psychology, 61,* 670–681.
97. Carver, C. S., Scheier, M. F., & Weintraub, J. K. (1989). Assessing coping strategies: A theoretically-based approach. *Journal of Personality and Social Psychology, 56,* 267–283.
98. Wills, T. A., & Hirky, A. E. (1996). Coping and substance abuse. In M. Zeidner & N. S. Endler (Eds.), *Handbook of coping: Theory, research, and applications* (pp. 279–302). New York: Wiley.
99. Steele, C. M. (1988). The psychology of self-affirmation. In L. Berkowitz

(Ed.), *Advances in experimental social psychology* (Vol. 21, pp. 261–302). New York: Academic Press.

100. Swann, W. B. Jr., Griffin, J. J., Jr., Predmore, S. C., & Gaines, B. (1987). The cognitive-affective crossfire: When self-consistency confronts self-enhancement. *Journal of Personality and Social Psychology, 52,* 881–889.

101. Tesser, A. (1991). Emotion in social comparison and reflection processes. In J. Suls & T. A. Wills (Eds.), *Social comparison: Contemporary theory and research* (pp. 115–145). Hillsdale, NJ: Erlbaum.

102. Zeidner, M., & Saklofske, D. (1996). Adaptive and maladaptive coping. In M. Zeidner & N. S. Endler (Eds.), *Handbook of coping: Theory, research, and applications* (pp. 505–531). New York: Wiley.

103. Affleck, G., Tennen, H., Pfeiffer, C., & Fifield, J. (1988). Social comparisons in rheumatoid arthritis: Accuracy and adaptational significance. *Journal of Social and Clinical Psychology, 6,* 219–234.

104. Blanton, H., Buunk, B. B., Gibbons, F. X., & Kuyper, H. (1999). When better-than-others compare upward: Choice of comparison and comparative evaluation as predictors of academic performance. *Journal of Personality and Social Psychology, 76,* 420–430.

105. Gibbons, F. X., Blanton, H., Gerrard, M., Buunk, B. P., & Eggleston, T. (2000). Does social comparison make a difference: Optimism as a moderator of the relation between comparison level and academic performance. *Personality and Social Psychology Bulletin, 26,* 637–648.

106. Colvin, C. R., & Block, J. (1994). Do positive illusions foster mental health? An examination of the Taylor and Brown formulation. *Psychological Bulletin, 116,* 3–20.

107. Taylor, S., & Brown, J. D. (1994). Positive illusions and well-being revisited. *Psychological Bulletin, 116,* 21–27.

108. Beck, A. T., & Young, J. E. (1985). Depression. In D. Barlow (Ed.), *Clinical handbook of psychological disorders* (pp. 206–244). New York: Guilford Press.

109. Ruble, D. N., & Frey, K. S. (1991). Changing patterns of comparative behavior as skills are acquired: A functional model of self-evaluation. In J. Suls & T. A. Wills (Eds.), *Social comparison: Contemporary theory and research* (pp. 79–113). Hillsdale, NJ: Erlbaum.

110. Gibbons, F. X., & Buunk, B. P. (1999). Individual differences in social comparison: Development of a scale of social comparison orientation. *Journal of Personality and Social Psychology, 76,* 129–142.

111. Heine, S. J., & Lehman, D. R. (1999). Culture, self-discrepancies, and self-satisfaction. *Personality and Social Psychology Bulletin, 25,* 915–925.

112. Gerrard, M., Gibbons, F. X., & Sharp, J. (1985, August). *Social comparison in a self-help group for bulimics.* Paper presented at the meeting of the American Psychological Association, Los Angeles.

9

Self-Focused Attention and Coping: Attending to the Right Things

Nancy A. Hamilton
Rick E. Ingram

Few concepts in psychology are more fundamental than attention and coping. For example, from the earliest experimental psychology approaches to cognition to the most recent cognitive sciences concepts, researchers have consistently emphasized the central role that attention plays in virtually all human (as well as nonhuman) endeavors. Likewise, from the more clinical side of the equation, scholars view coping as central to virtually all theoretical, empirical, and applied features of the mental health professions. Although there have been some attempts in the past (1) to more formally unite cognitive and applied concepts such as attention and coping, these paradigms and their corresponding theories and data have typically developed in isolation from one another, a situation that parallels a large dissociation between cognitive science and clinical psychology in general (2, 3).

Despite this relative isolation, we believe that theory and research on attention and coping have much to offer each other. Elsewhere, we have discussed what clinical efforts such as coping can offer to cognitive science (4). Here, we focus on how theory and research on attention can inform our understanding of effective coping. Although we do not claim that examination of attentional factors will lead to answers for all coping questions, we do believe that the theories and data on attentional focus may help to improve coping efforts for clients in psychological treatment. In addition, to the extent that information on coping can be widely promulgated, we believe that an emphasis on attentional processing may help improve the coping efforts of individuals in the larger population.

Attention: Definitions and Chapter Overview

The concept of attention can encompass numerous attributes. Although several of these attributes may be appropriate to our exploration of coping, we believe that *self-focused attention* is especially useful in explicating coping variables. We begin with a definition of self-focused attention, which Carver (5), a pioneer of theory and research in this area, defined in this way:

> When attention is self-directed, it sometimes takes the form of focus on internal perceptual events, that is, information from those sensory receptors that react to changes in bodily activity. Self-focus may also take the form of an enhanced awareness of one's present or past physical behavior, that is, a heightened cognizance of what one is doing or what one is like. Alternatively, self-attention can be an awareness of the more or less permanently encoded bits of information that comprises, for example, one's attitudes. It can even be an enhanced awareness of temporarily encoded bits of information that have been gleaned from previous focus on the environment; subjectively, this would be experienced as a recollection or impression of that past event. (p. 1255)

As can be seen from Carver's definition, self-focused attention is typically thought to reflect a focus on internal information (e.g., thoughts, beliefs, expectancies, etc.) rather than a focus on other information derived through sensory receptors ("external information"). We do not imply here that self-focus excludes external information, for indeed, external information is critical to functioning and has significant effects on self-focus; rather, because our capacity for attention is limited, individuals tend to be self-focused in that their attention is primarily captured by internal factors. In this chapter, we propose that some types of self-focusing play important roles in the emotional distress to which coping must be directed, and hence, that alterations in the self-focus process may have important implications for effective coping.

To provide a context for our exploration of attention and coping, we discuss clinical theories in which attentional factors are prominently featured. We note in this regard that disturbances in attentional functioning appear to be ubiquitous among numerous forms of psychopathology (1). Nowhere, however, are the ideas of attentional functioning so well developed as in depression theories and, to a lesser degree, in theories of anxiety states. For the most part then, the theories we examine focus on depression. Although our decision to focus on depression may seem too specific for a chapter on coping, depression theorists are inclined to describe factors that characterize generalized psychological or emotional distress; that is, although many of the variables that these theories emphasize are intended to explain depression, they also are just as likely to explain generalized distress as well (6). These theories have broad applicability across numerous human facets of human functioning that involve distress, and arguably are thus related to coping.

Following our discussion of theoretical factors, we next turn to a burgeoning literature on attentional variables in treatment. Again, the focus in much of this treatment is on depression, but the targeted factors have wide applicability across the treatment of numerous forms of emotional distress. Finally, we conclude the chapter by bringing together diverse literatures and perspectives on attention and coping—our goal being to contribute to a better understanding of coping and copers.

Theories Incorporating Attentional Variables: Theoretical Perspectives on Self-Focus and Distress

Many theories of depression focus on cognitive functioning. In our estimation, the theories that have the most applicability for elucidating attentional factors are those proposed by Beck (7, 8), Teasdale (9, 10), Ingram (6, 11), Nolen-Hoeksema (12, 13), and Pyszczynski and Greenberg (14, 15). Additionally, while not proposed as a theory per se, Kendall (16, 17) also has offered important theoretical ideas on the specificity of attentional functioning in different affective states. We examine these theoretical ideas in general and concentrate in particular on what they have to say about attention-related variables.

Schemas and Automatic Thinking

Beck (7, 8) was among the first to propose a psychological theory of depression, and he almost certainly was the first to propose a theory of depression with an emphasis on cognitive factors (18). The central element of Beck's and indeed of many cognitive theories (6) is the *schema*. There are numerous definitions of schemas, but for our proposes, schemas are conceptualized as cognitive structures that guide the processing of information. More specifically, schemas structurally constitute the cognitive residual of our past interactions in the form of stored experiences that establish a "relatively cohesive and persistent body of knowledge capable of guiding subsequent perception and appraisal" (19, p. 147). Although it is important to note that the idea of an organizational information processing structure such as a schema was not originally developed by Beck, it was Beck's work that propelled the idea of schemas into much of clinical psychology and thus into a psychological domain concerned with coping (see 20).

In addition to guiding our perceptual activity, schemas also underlie a number of other cognitive functions. For example, theories propose, and research shows, that negatively oriented self-schemas become activated in emotional distress (21) and that they lead to a perceptual negative cognitive triad. In such a triad, individuals tend to see themselves, others, and their world in a negative fashion. Part of these negative appraisals stem from attentional variables; as schemas evidence an increasingly negative organization, attention correspondingly is devoted to negative situations and appraisals. Based on various clinical conceptualizations of schemas, it also appears that these structures perpetuate themselves in that the information that is processed becomes increasingly organized within these negative structures, which in turn provides access to similarly toned negative information.

Automatic Thinking: Interpretation   Although there are numerous cognitive functions ascribed to schemas in contemporary accounts of emotional distress, for our purposes, schema-linked cognition has one extremely important function: automatic thinking. Automatic thinking, in turn, has two important attentional attributes: it filters the interpretation of events, which we will briefly describe here, and it has a ruminative nature, upon which we more exclusively focus in this chapter.

Sometimes referred to as cognitive self-statements (22), *automatic thinking* refers to ongoing internal dialogues that occur at the periphery of awareness for individuals. Such peripheral awareness, however, does not mean that these thoughts cannot reach awareness; in fact, they can and do come into awareness. More important, however, automatic thoughts underlie our reactions to stressful events—they guide how we interpret the things that happen to us. As a result, the interpretation of events through automatic thinking can have an enormous effect on both human emotions and behaviors. In the face of stressful events, for example, individuals who are vulnerable to exacerbated emotional distress engage in a dialogue that is negative, maladaptive, and, quite possibly, unrealistic and distorted (6). In such a case, the thoughts that automatically accompany stressful events are negative and self-defeating, and effective coping is consequently impaired by such thoughts.

To illustrate, consider a common experience among virtually all professionals that requires coping—a presentation at a conference or meeting. In the case of ineffective coping, emotional dysregulation at the prospect of this presentation is fueled by a self-focus on the *potential* negatives of the experience (e.g., "What if this doesn't go well?"; "What if people think I'm stupid?"; or "What if I don't have much to say?"). Maladaptive self-statements also can darken our appraisals of the *actual* event (e.g., "The yawning in the back of the room means I'm boring"; "The person whispering to the other is making disparaging remarks about me"). These negative self-statements, in turn, lead to emotional distress, that may have little correspondence to actual performance. Our point is that it is not the actual events *but the interpretation of the event that determines the emotional reaction*. This point virtually all cognitive theorists emphasize; in the parlance of Beck's theory, it is the automatic thinking that leads to stress, not the event per se.

Let us offer one more definition of the power of automatic thinking to determine our emotional reactions to events. One of the most convincing definitions and illustrations of this process is found in Freud's distinction between mourning (normal mood reactions) and melancholia (dysfunctional mood reactions). In mourning, the person's predominant thought is "this is bad" while in melancholia, the predominant thought is "I am bad." It is easy to see how these different automatic thoughts lead to fundamentally different emotional and behavioral paths.

Automatic Thinking: Rumination   Although Beck alluded to the importance of ruminative processes, he originally focused more exclusively on the content of thoughts, and how that content influenced the interpretation of events. Although the interpretation of events is important in determining stressful reactions, we believe that the real power of cognitive variables such as automatic thinking in creating stress lies in the rumination that occurs *after* the stressful event has occurred; automatic thinking does not only refer to the content of thoughts, but also to their recurrence, repetition, and persistence. Thus, while emotional reactions to difficult life events are certainly linked to the thoughts that greet their occurrence, the continual rumination that follows these events amplifies and extends the negative emotional reactions to such events. Indeed, it may be that there is more stress linked to the rumination than to the interpretational aspects of automatic thinking. Thus, in our example of the stress associated with a conference presentation, it is less maladaptive to interpret the situation as suggesting incompetence and to then "cognitively move on," but quite another to continue these dysfunctional automatic thoughts long after the talk is over.

In our previous discussion we do not mean to downplay the importance of initial appraisal processes in interpreting stressful events, nor to suggest that coping does not need to accompany these actual events in order to function effectively and avoid acute emotional distress. Rather, *we believe that the long-term emotional effects of these events are the most psychologically problematic aspects of stress.* This distinction has yet to receive widespread attention in the coping literature. Moreover, such chronic negative effects may initiate a new set of persistent dysfunctional thoughts; "It went badly, and I am therefore incompetent or stupid" (see our earlier example of Freud's conception of melancholia). No doubt, this ruminative process influences the short-term processes for future stressful events which, in turn, may amplify and extend long-term negative consequences. Ruminative processes thus give rise to a vicious cognitive-emotional cycle that can prove difficult, but not impossible, to escape.

Differential Activation Processes

Beck's theoretical ideas have spawned a host of related theories of depression and emotional distress. Although the proponents of these theories adopt the major elements of Beck's theory, many have clarified, amplified, augmented, or extended Beck's propositions. Of interest in the current context, the ideas proposed by Teasdale have contributed substantially to the theoretical understanding of cognition and emotional distress, and by extension, coping with emotional distress.

In particular, Teasdale (9) and Teasdale and Barnard (10) have proposed the "Interacting Cognitive Subsystems" (ICS) model to examine the cognitive and emotional features of emotional distress and their interaction. Although Teasdale and Barnards' models describes a number of quite complex cognitive relationships and functions, for our purposes it is important to note that they suggest that rumination is linked to the maintenance of dysfunctional emotional states. For example, Teasdale and Barnard argue that "The ICS analysis suggests that (extended emotional distress) . . . depends, to a considerable extent, on the establishment of self-perpetuating processing configurations that continue to regenerate depressogenic schematic models" (3, p. 33), or within the rubric of automatic thinking, emotional distress "seems to be maintained, not so much by negative environmental events, as by persistent streams of negative ruminative thoughts" (3, p. 33). Thus, negative automatic thinking is again proposed to play a powerful role in coping (or the lack thereof) with stressful events, long after the actual event has passed.

Teasdale has also suggested that *differential activation* is an important aspect of this process that leads to severely dysfunctional emotional states (such as depression). All individuals experience negative mood states. Such mood states may be quite uncomfortable, but they are typically resolved in a relatively short period of time, perhaps through effective coping. For some individuals, however, these states lead to dysfunctional cognitive processes. Thus, by suggesting differential activation Teasdale argues that negative mood states in certain individuals initiate negative cognitive processes that lead to a downward spiral into clinically severe emotional distress. Although this downward spiral is quite similar to that proposed by Beck, Teadale's differential activation hypothesis provides a more detailed description of the underlying mechanisms that are responsible for this spiral and for whom it will affect.

Associative Network Models

Teasdale's original cognitive model (9) appeared in 1983 and was based heavily on both Beck's work and that of cognitive psychologist Bower (23). Independent of Teasdale, in 1984 Ingram (11) proposed a cognitive model of depression that also was based on Bower's proposals, as well as on models developed by other cognitive psychologists (e.g., 24, 25, 26). In brief, Ingram (6, 11) suggested that emotionally and distressing events activate various affective and cognitive structures that, in turn, produce spreading activation throughout the cognitive system. This spread of activation is proposed to have a number of effects on exacerbating or maintaining emotional distress.

One key aspect of spreading activation is the creation of a "cognitive loop" in which thoughts and memories associated with the person's predominant mood state become continually accessible. Such "cognitive recycling" also occupies the individual's limited cognitive capacity, leaving fewer possibilities for attending to external events (e.g., attending to the information necessary to successfully perform tasks). Ingram (11) suggested that individuals phenomenologically experience this cognitive looping process as the occurrence of memories and thoughts that are negative, continual, intrusive, and difficult to inhibit—a process that serves to maintain the person's negative emotional state. Such a process is conceptually identical to several aspects of self-focused attention (1) in that ". . . individuals . . . have a high degree of attention focused upon themselves and their cognitions as available capacity becomes increasingly occupied by spreading activation" (11, p. 455). Thus, this model clearly implicates automatic thinking, and self-focused attention, in dysfunctional emotional responsivity to events. By extension, it is easy to see how such heightened self-focused attention impedes effective coping.

Ruminative Response Styles

Nolen-Hoeksema (12, 27), in an approach she has termed the *response styles theory*, has proposed that individuals who are vulnerable to the maintenance of negative affective states differ in their responses to aversive situations from people who cope effectively with these situations. In particular, she suggests that people who tend to ruminate are more likely to maintain negative affect than are those who are able to cognitively individuals distract themselves. Those who focus their attention externally are thus more able to engage in adaptive activities and to cope effectively. Again, we see in Nolen-Hoeksema's theory that rumination response styles is posited to cause and intensified dysfunctional emotional responses. The response styles theory is, we suggest, highly similar to self-focused attention models of affective distress.

Self-Regulatory Perseveration

In their *self-regulatory perseveration* model, Pyszczynski and Greenberg (14, 15) also accord a central role to self-focused attention in the onset and maintenance of emotional distress. Although they proposed a number of variables that are linked to the exacerbation and maintenance of emotional states such as depression, for our purposes, the important point is the emphasis on self-focused attention. Specifically, Pyszczynski and Greenberg suggested that when experiencing a stressful event in a life domain that is central to self-worth, the person begins a self-focusing processing that is linked to self-evaluation. It is posited that emotionally distressed individuals perseverate in this self-focusing process; in turn, individuals with this attentional style have limited cognitive access to positive information and unfettered access to negative information. As such, self-focused people have both impaired coping and perpetuated emotional distress.

Self-Statement Specificity in Emotional Distress

A final set of theoretical ideas that we briefly examine concerns the specificity of automatic thinking in emotional states. Although the previous theories that we have reviewed were developed specifically to account for depression, their applicability is not necessarily limited to depression. Moreover, most theorists and researchers acknowledge the tremendous overlap in varying forms of emotional disorders. For example, anxiety commonly cooccurs with depression, as do other dysfunctional psychological states (20, 29). In several respects, such comorbidity (where emotional states frequently occur in conjunction with one another [30]) provides greater generality across psychological conditions.

Despite the frequent comorbidity of many emotional states such as depression and anxiety, in some situations these states occur relatively independently of each other (31, 32, 33, 34). Correspondingly, at least some theoretical explanation is necessary for such specificity (1). On this point Kendall (16, 17) differentiates between the statements seen primarily in anxiety versus those seen primarily in depression. In particular, Kendall suggests that the *form* of these self-statements differ, with depressive self-statements having a declarative nature ("I am incompetent") and anxiety self-statements taking the form of questions ("Am I incompetent?"). This distinction prompted Kendall to label this latter process *automatic questioning*. It is important to note, however, that these questions should be differentiated from the healthy and adaptive ones when attempting to effectively handle various stressors. Kendall argues that automatic questioning occurs with such rapidity that it prevents the requisite thoughtful reflection necessary to answer such questions and to then formulate a plan of action based on a lucid understanding of the situation. As such, persons experiencing automatic questioning retain a sense of uncertainty in situations that continues to arouse anxiety and inhibit effective coping strategies. Although different in form, both automatic thoughts and automatic questioning precipitate heightened self-focus and a consequent inability to cope effectively.

Converging Theories and Ideas: Self-Focus and Coping with Distress

We believe that two important points emerge from our review of cognitive theories of emotional distress. First, although differing in some theoretical details, the proponents of these theories argue that cognitions play a central role in precipitating and maintaining emotional distress. Moreover, the defining features of these problematic cognitions are not only that they are negative and self-defeating, but also that they are persistent.

A second point is that these negative and persistent cognitions can be understood within the framework of self-focused attention. It is important to note at this juncture, however, that not all self-focused attention is dysfunctional. Indeed, self-focusing can be a healthy cognitive process that is part of adapting successfully to changing circumstances. What the authors of each of these theories either implicitly or explicitly suggest, however, is that self-focused attention that is heightened, tends to be negative, is less flexible, and because it is sustained over a relatively lengthy period of time, is not adaptive (1).

As such, self-focused attention can be seen as a *mediator of the coping process*. That is, to the extent that self-focusing is not too lengthy, elevated, or overly negative, it should enhance problem solving and coping efforts. Conversely, when self-focused attention is extremely heightened, persistent, negative, and intransigent, it becomes a cognitive impediment to effective coping; moreover, in the wake of stressful events, this type of self-focused attention sustains emotional distress and interferes with cognitions and behaviors that are necessary for adaptation. We thus propose that self-focused attention at least partially regulates the effectiveness of coping.

Our discussion of the mediational role of self-focused attention in relation to coping is a significant departure from the norms in much of the current coping theory and research. Coping research tends to be event based; that is, researchers frequent emphasis on coping is in the context of relatively discrete stressful events. But as we have concluded from the literature on emotional dysfunction, what is so problematic about the emotional distress that sometimes leads to psychological disorders, is not the distress per se, *but the fact that it lasts for an extended period of time.* For example, depression can result from a significant loss in an individual's life. What is problematic about this depression, however, is not that it occurs, but that it can and often does last for many months (and sometimes years) after the loss. As another example, Post-Traumatic Stress Disorder (PTSD), based on a single traumatic event, can remain for years. In this case, coping with the trigger event is less important than the coping that needs to take place to help alleviate the PTSD. Thus, we strongly believe that long-term effects or "emotional half-life" of aversive events need to be addressed in the coping literature. We have proposed one mechanism—self-focused attention—that we can use to better our understanding of how distress is experienced, as well as how it influences coping, sometimes well after the stressful event has occurred.

Steps Toward Effective Coping:
Self-Focused Attention, Distraction, and
Mindfulness

Now that we have examined some of the ways in which self-focusing processes are linked to the distress that surrounds the occurrence and afterlife
of stressful events, what can we suggest for understanding and improving
effective coping? We think that several provocative and potentially exciting
answers to these questions can be derived from a recently burgeoning theoretical and research literature.

De-Self-Focusing: Distraction and Coping

The natural answer to a problem of too much self-focused attention is less
self-focused attention. Such de-self-focusing can be found under the rubric
of *distraction*. As we shall see, however, distraction is not merely a matter
of consciously diverting attention elsewhere, but rather as a strategy for
effective coping to occur, the person must figure out how best to accomplish
this diversionary task. We will focus on distraction as it affects the psychological states that are caused by stress, which as we have seen, means emotional distress.

We start by asking two simple questions: "What is distraction?" and "Is
distraction effective for mood management or for coping with stress?" The
answer to the first question is fairly simple and straightforward. Distraction,
as a method for managing noxious internal states such as a negative mood,
rests on the assumption that attentional capacity is finite (35). Because we
can only attend to a limited amount of information, attention focused outwardly toward others, or on more positive elements of ourselves, reduces
the amount of attention that we can devote to a negative mood state.

The answer to the second question is a bit more complex. Researchers
examining distraction probably would concur with the conclusion that
some forms of distraction are effective some of the time. The effectiveness
of distraction as a mood management strategy seems to vary depending on
the nature of the distractor, the strength of the stressor, and the intensity of
the emotional response. In the following sections we will review research
on these variables. Specifically, we will examine how researchers have
characterized effective distractors as positive events and cognitions (13),
internal sensations, (36, 37), and cognitively demanding tasks (38).

Positive Events and Cognitions   Pleasurable distractions may be particularly
effective in regulating affect in the face of uncontrollable stressors. Nolen-
Hoeksema (13) defines such distraction as enjoyable activities and cognitions that focus attention away from the current mood and self-focus. To
illustrate, in an interesting study of distraction to a severe stressor, Nolen-
Hoeksema studied San Francisco residents' responses to the Loma Prieta
earthquake and discovered that pleasurable distractions were associated

with less psychological distress for up to 10 days following the quake (27). Distraction was not related to adjustment seven weeks after the earthquake, but this finding must be viewed with caution because only 25% of the original sample could be located and assessed again. Based on Nolen-Hoeksema's data, however, some immediate relief seems to be related to decreasing self-focusing; more specifically, pleasurable distraction can be used to effectively cope with stress.

Goal Directed Self-Regulation of Mood   Based on data indicating that reducing self-focus through distraction may be an effective coping method, we might reasonably conclude that distraction may be the mood change strategy of choice when people cope with a negative event. When the need for coping arises, therefore, does it make sense to simply decide not to think about the negative effects of stressful events? Probably not; effective distraction entails more than simply deciding not to think about negative things. Analogous to the notion that nature abhors a vacuum, one cannot simply instruct oneself to "not be in a bad mood" or "not think about a distressing event." Instead, one must think of a specific distractor or try to invoke a different mood (via distracting thoughts).

Some may see distraction as an attempt to "will" one's self into a different mood or to suppress distressing thoughts. Research has indicated, however, that these attempts may not only be ineffective, but they may also have unintentional or *ironic* effects (36, 37, 39). For example, Wegner (39) has shown that attempting to suppress the thoughts that are associated with a given mood may in fact lead, ironically, to an increase rather than a reduction in these thoughts. To illustrate, in a well-known set of experiments, Wegner asked research participants specifically *not* to think about a white bear. Demonstrating the ironic effect of attempted suppression, Wegner's participants overwhelmingly reported *thinking about* a white bear. Thus, distraction via suppression seems to be a particularly poor coping method.

It also is important to note that not all distractors are created equal. Although suppression is not a good coping strategy, other types of distractions, such as focusing on cognitively demanding external tasks, may be more effective coping strategies. For example, Erber (40, 41) suggested that certain types of non-self-focused distractions "absorb" mood. Erber argued that moods are maintained via working memory. When working memory becomes occupied by a demanding external task, negative mood-related cognitions cannot be processed efficiently. Mood is thus attenuated or "absorbed" by the externally focused cognitive task. Erber emphasized, however, that not all tasks (or distractors) absorb mood. Simple distractors (e.g., watching a movie) require little in terms of cognitive processing and leave plenty of working memory free to process mood-related information. In contrast, demanding distractors may promote effective coping with negative affect because they occupy a significant amount of working memory. For example, exercise, a demanding task by most accounts, has been found to help manage moods (42).

Turning Self-Focus into an Adaptive State: Mindfulness Meditation   As an alternative to traditional distraction in which attention is focused on external stimuli, Cioffi (35) advocates somatic awareness. Somatic awareness is the active ingredient in a coping paradigm known as *mindfulness meditation* (43, 44). Although perhaps counterintuitive from the perspective of research on the dysfunctional effects of self-focused attention, proponents of this strategy characterize sensory awareness as a form of distraction (35). Mindfulness meditation involves focusing attention on the here and now, to the exclusion of all metacognition or thoughts about one's cognitions. From a clinical coping perspective, mindfulness meditation has demonstrated measurable success as a method for treating chronic pain (43, 44). Additionally, in conjunction with phototherapy and photochemotherapy, mindfulness meditation has been used as a treatment for psoriasis (45).

As described by Kabat-Zinn (43), mindfulness meditation involves focusing attention on thoughts, affect, and bodily sensations *without* evaluation or infusion with meaning. The goal is to become a detached observer of one's own conscious experience. Clinical training in mindfulness meditation involves two steps. Students first learn to focus on breathing. As thoughts or moods come into consciousness, they are acknowledged and attention is returned to breathing. The second step involves expanding attention to include awareness of thoughts, affect, physical sensations, and external events as they occur in time. If a practitioner becomes aware of evaluative or meaning-oriented thoughts, these thoughts are acknowledged and attention is returned to breathing. After such attention is "stabilized," attention is again allowed to expand to other sensations, moods, cognition, and external events. Kabat-Zinn refers to the state of nonevaluative self-observance as "bare attention." By giving only bare attention to internal and external events, practitioners report being able to separate physical sensations from affect and cognition.

We have referred to mindfulness meditation as a type of distraction (35). Traditional forms of distraction involve directing attention away from somatic and affective states and toward another external event. The goal of mindfulness meditation is to call attention toward somatic and affective states and, by doing so, to reduce the processing space for other types of evaluative processing such as self-focused rumination and catastrophizing. Thus, the practice of mindfulness meditation is a form of distraction in the sense that intensive attention to the here and now prevents (distracts) one from rumination, or from the self-focused thoughts that tend to worsen the mood-producing results of stressful events.

In addition to diverting attention from maladaptive self-focused thoughts, another way to understand mindfulness is to contrast it with a state of "mindlessness" (43). Kabat-Zinn argues that mindlessness is a state in which attention is diffusely focused on here-and-now events, evaluations of the event, memories of similar events, and expectations for the future (i.e., self-focused attention). In a mindless state, here-and-now events are not fully experienced and are likely to be biased by affective states, memory, and speculation. In contrast, the goal of mindfulness meditation is to keep attention strictly in the moment and, by so doing, distracting oneself from the dysfunctional processes that exacerbate emotional responses to stress. Recall, for instance, that we noted that one of the cognitive functions of the schemas associated with depression is to produce the cognitive triad in which people see themselves, others, and their world, in a negative manner. By staying in the here and now, mindfulness promotes a type of attention that helps to diffuse this dysfunctional triad.

Mindfulness meditation has several advantages over other forms of distraction. First, mindfulness meditation emphasizes acceptance of moods, cognitions, and somatic states and eschews goal (or future) oriented cognition. Because the emphasis is on acceptance, mindfulness meditation should not trigger the negative effects seen in efforts to suppress thinking or to will oneself into a positive mood (39). Second, mindfulness meditation is a general strategy and can be used in any context and as a method for coping with a range of life-stressors from pain management to job-stress (43). Third, the practice of mindfulness meditation actually should enhance the performance of other activities. Traditional distraction involves turning attention away from distressing situations. Although active distractions such as taking a walk in the park or cognitive distractions such as daydreaming may have long-term benefits, these strategies are more costly in the short term, temporarily halting or inhibiting progress on other activities. Fourth, Kabat-Zinn (43) theorized that the practice of mindfulness meditation is likely to prevent "thoughtless coping." As a result of the here and now focus of mindfulness meditation, what we ordinarily think of as coping responses are temporarily *inhibited*. Taking time to meditate before responding to an event may prevent the use of habitual and dispositional coping strategies that are inconsistent with a flexible response to stress (46). Thus, mindfulness meditation may, in some cases, be superior to other forms of distraction.

Some Clinical Coping Applications of Mindfulness Meditation   Clinically oriented researchers recently have developed a model that integrates mindfulness meditation training with an information processing model of mood and mood-change (47). Recall our discussion of the ICS model proposed by Teasdale and Barnard (3, 10). In this model it is suggested that mood is the outcome of implicit meanings attached to visual, acoustic, and somatic stimuli (what we see, hear, and feel). In addition, within the ICS model for those vulnerable to negative affect states such as depression, negative events trigger the "depressive interlock" of two interrelated feedback loops involving negative implicit meanings, negative mood states, low somatic arousal, and negative automatic thoughts. Or, in other words, depressive interlock occurs when individuals experience "persistent streams of negative ruminative thoughts."

In accordance with these ideas, three methods for changing mood are specified in the ICS model. First, distraction can prevent depressive interlock by redirecting cognitive resources (e.g., working memory) away from stressful situations and toward positive or neutral stimuli. Second, cognitive restructuring can be used so that people can reconceptualize stressful circumstances into less psychologically threatening situations, and also can reconceptualize the potentially long-term effects of stressful events into more realistic and manageable situations. Third, somatic and behavioral responses to depressogenic stimuli can be modified directly.

Applying the ICS model to mindfulness meditation, Teasdale has suggested that mindfulness meditation would be likely to have immediate effects as a distractor and would serve as a method for altering somatic and behavioral responses and delayed effects on cognitive schemas (47). Specifically, bare attention to sensations, perceptions, and affective responses as they occur in real time requires all available processing space, effectively "jamming" the feedback loops that maintain emotional distress. In addition, the practice of mindfulness meditation is relaxing, a state that is inconsistent with emotional upset and with dysfunctional self-focused attention. Finally, learning to observe rather than evaluate stimuli may fundamentally change implicit belief systems about what is meaningful and important. In all, mindfulness meditation may be a method to take the "dysfunctional" out of dysfunctional self focused attention.

Summary and Conclusions

In this chapter we have summarized the theory and research showing the negative implications of self-focused attention. We have reviewed several theories that, although differing in their terminology (automatic thoughts, self-statements, rumination, depressive interlock, etc.), all converge on the idea that self-focused attention can produce maladaptive negative affect in the face of stressful events. Perhaps more important, we have examined the fact that self-focused attention can serve to maintain negative affect over an extended period of time. We then argued that attempts to reduce this state have significant implications for ideas on how we cope, and we also suggested that a focus on self-focus, and the long-term consequences of stressful events, takes us into a fundamentally different arena than is typically addressed by coping researchers. That is, coping researchers typically emphasize coping around some discrete stressful event(s). To the contrary, however, we believe that coping with the extended effects of these events is where the real coping action needs to be.

We also suggested some ways to conceptualize coping from these longer term perspectives and argued that one (but certainly not the only) way to effectively cope was to reduce the chronic, heightened self-focusing that comes with the type of emotional distress that is produced by stress. Although many researchers in this area have focused on individuals who are vulnerable to severe emotional reactions from stress, we believe that these processes are also applicable for the coping efforts of all people as they attempt to negotiate life's vicissitudes. Based on theory and research in the realm of self-focused attention, we suggest that one way to quiet the emotional distress that is maintained via self-focus is to reduce the self-focus through external distraction. Although we do not believe that this method alone is a sufficient answer for individuals who are severely distressed, we believe that it is one of the many cognitive, emotional, and behavioral methods that can contribute to recovery from such states. Likewise, although there are numerous coping methods that may help people who are within the "normal" range of distress from negative life events, we believe that distractions can significantly help reduce negative mood states, and thus promote positive and adaptive living that was typical before stressful events took their psychological toll.

We briefly explored how various forms of distraction are not equally effective and discussed how some are downright ineffective. For example, suppressing, or just not thinking about negative things, may be a "common-sense" coping strategy, but based on theory and research we conclude that such efforts may in fact increase negative affect. Finally, we discussed a coping paradigm that is beginning to receive a great deal of interest in the clinical literature—mindfulness meditation.

Mindfulness meditation may seem counterintuitive to our discussion of self-focused attention because it increases self-focus. Indeed, this is the case, but it is designed to increase self-focus in a way that reduces the maladaptive aspects of this process. Although early in this chapter we noted that while self-focus contributes to many kinds of psychopathology, we also emphasized that self-focus *can* be adaptive. Mindfulness meditation offers, we believe, one method to help transform such a condition into a state that is not only more adaptive, but also perhaps necessary when difficult situations are encountered. Certainly under the right circumstances, self-focus is probably necessary for the self-reflection and problem solving that must contribute to the resolution of the many problems in our lives. And, in fact, researchers have found great promise in mindfulness meditation for helping to alleviate clinically significant emotional mood states. Moreover, mindfulness meditation is currently being explored by investigators as a means to not only treat these states, but also to help prevent their relapse and recurrence. In mindfulness meditation, then, we may find one way to help us attend to the right things in life.

References

1. Ingram, R. E. (1990). Self-focused attention in clinical disorders: Review and a conceptual model. *Psychological Bulletin, 107*, 156–176.
2. Ingram, R. E. (Ed.). (1986). *Information processing approaches to clinical psychology*. Orlando: Academic Press.
3. Teasdale, J. D. (1998). Clinically relevant theory: Integrating clinical insight with cognitive science. In P. M. Salkovskis (Ed.), *Frontiers of cognitive therapy* (pp. 26–47). New York: Guilford Press.

4. Ingram, R. E., & Kendall, P. C. (1986). Cognitive clinical psychology: Implications of an information processing perspective. In R. E. Ingram (Ed.), *Information processing approaches to clinical psychology* (pp. 3–21). Orlando: Academic Press.

5. Carver, C. S. (1979). A cybernetic model of self-attention processes. *Journal of Personality and Social Psychology, 37*, 1251–1281.

6. Ingram, R. E., Miranda, J., & Segal, Z. V. (1998). *Cognitive vulnerability to depression.* New York: Guilford Press.

7. Beck, A. T. (1967). *Depression: Causes and treatments.* Philadelphia: University of Pennsylvania Press.

8. Beck, A. T. (1987). Cognitive model of depression. *Journal of Cognitive Psychotherapy, 1*, 2–27.

9. Teasdale, J. D. (1983). Negative thinking in depression: Cause, effect, or reciprocal relationship. *Advances in Behaviour Research and Therapy, 5*, 3–25.

10. Teasdale, J. D., & Barnard, P. J. (1993). *Affect, cognition, and change: Re-modelling depressive thought.* Hillsdale, NJ: Erlbaum.

11. Ingram, R. E. (1984). Toward an information processing analysis of depression. *Cognitive Therapy and Research, 8*, 441–477.

12. Nolen-Hoeksema, S. (1987). Sex differences in unipolar depression: Evidence and theory. *Psychological Bulletin, 101*, 259–282.

13. Nolen-Hoeksema, S. (1991). Responses to depression and their effects on the duration of depressive episodes. *Journal of Abnormal Psychology, 100*, 569–582.

14. Pyszczynski, T., & Greenberg, J. (1987). Self-regulatory perseveration and the depressive self-focusing style: A self-awareness theory of reactive depression. *Psychological Bulletin, 102*, 1–17.

15. Pyszczynski, T., & Greenberg J. (1992). *Hanging on and letting go: Understanding the onset, progression and remission of depression.* New York: Springer-Verlag.

16. Kendall, P. C. (1985). Toward a cognitive-behavioral model of child psychopathology and a critique of related interventions. *Journal of Abnormal Child Psychology, 13*, 337–353.

17. Kendall, P. C., & Ingram, R. E. (1989). Cognitive-behavioral perspectives: Theory and research on negative affective states. In P. C. Kendall & D. Watson, (Eds.), *Anxiety and depression: Distinctive and overlapping features* (pp. 27–53). San Diego: Academic Press.

18. Haaga, D. A. F., Dyck, M. J., & Ernst, D. (1991). Empirical status of cognitive theory of depression. *Psychological Bulletin, 110*, 215–234.

19. Segal, Z. V. (1988). Appraisal of the self-schema construct in cognitive models of depression. *Psychological Bulletin, 103*, 147–162.

20. Salkovskis, P. M. (1998). Cognitive therapy and Aaron Beck. In P. M. Salkovskis (Ed.), *Frontiers of cognitive therapy* (pp. 531–539). New York: Guilford Press.

21. Segal, Z. V., & Ingram, R. E. (1994). Mood priming and construct activation in tests of cognitive vulnerability to unipolar depression. *Clinical Psychology Review, 14*, 663–695.

22. Hollon, S. D., & Kendall, P. C. (1980). Cognitive self-statements in depression. Development of an automatic thoughts questionnaire. *Cognitive Therapy and Research, 4*, 363–375.

23. Bower, G. H. (1981). Mood and memory. *American Psychologist, 36,* 131–148.
24. Collins, A. M., & Loftus, E. F. (1975). A spreading-activation theory of semantic processing. *Psychological Review, 82,* 387–408.
25. Norman, D. A. (1986). Toward a theory of memory and attention. *Psychological Review, 75,* 522–536.
26. Shiffrin, R. M., & Schneider, W. (1977). Controlled and automatic human processing: Perceptual learning, automatic attending and a general theory. *Psychological Review, 84,* 127–190.
27. Nolen-Hoeksema, S., & Morrow, J. (1991). A prospective study of depression and posttraumatic stress symptoms after a natural disaster, the 1989 Loma Prieta earthquake. *Journal of Personality and Social Psychology, 61,* 115–121.
28. Ingram, R. E., & Hamilton, N. A. (1999). Evaluating precision in the social psychological assessment of depression: Methodological considerations, issues, and recommendations. *Journal of Social and Clinical Psychology, 18,* 160–180.
29. Smith, T. W., & Rhodewalt, F. T. (1991). Methodological challenges at the social/clinical interface. In C. R. Snyder & D. R. Forsyth (Eds.), *Handbook of social and clinical psychology: The health perspective* (pp. 737–752). New York: Pergamon Press.
30. Klein, D., & Riso, L. P. (1993). Psychiatric disorders: Problems of boundaries and comorbidity. In C. G. Costello (Ed.), *Basic issues in psychopathology* (pp. 19–66). New York: Guilford Press.
31. Clark, D. A. (1986). Cognitive-affective interaction: A test of the "specificity" and "generality" hypotheses. *Cognitive Therapy and Research, 10,* 607–623.
32. Clark, D. A., Beck, A. T., & Brown, G. (1989). Cognitive mediation in general psychiatric outpatients: A test of the content-specificity hypothesis. *Journal of Personality and Social Psychology, 56,* 958–964.
33. Ingram, R. E., Kendall, P. C., Smith, T. W., Donnell, C., & Ronan, K. (1987). Cognitive specificity in emotional distress. *Journal of Personality and Social Psychology, 53,* 736–740.
34. Ingram, R. E., & Malcarne, V. L. (1995). Cognition in depression and anxiety: Same, different, or a little of both? In K. D. Craig & K. S. Dobson (Eds.), *Anxiety and depression in adults and children* (pp. 37–56). Newbury Park: Sage Publications.
35. Cioffi, D. (1991). Beyond attentional strategies: A cognitive-perceptual model of somatic interpretation. *Psychological Bulletin, 109,* 25–39.
36. Wegner, D. M., Erber, R., & Zanakos, S. (1993). Ironic processes in the mental control of mood and mood-related thought. *Journal of Personality and Social Psychology, 65,* 1093–1104.
37. Wenzlaff, R. M., Wegner, D. M., & Klein, S. B. (1991). The role of thought suppression in the bonding of thought and mood. *Journal of Personality and Social Psychology, 60,* 500–508.
38. Erber, R. (1996). The self-regulation of moods. In L. L. Martin & T. Abraham (Eds.), *Striving and feeling: Interactions among goals, affect, and self-regulation* (pp. 251–275). Hillsdale, NJ: Erlbaum.
39. Wegner, D. M. (1994). Ironic processes of mental control. *Psychological Review, 101,* 36–52.

40. Erber, R. (1996). The self-regulation of moods. In L. L. Martin & T. Abraham (Eds.), *Striving and feeling: Interactions among goals, affect, and self-regulation* (pp. 251–275). Hillsdale, NJ: Erlbaum.

41. Erber, R., & Tesser, A. (1992). Task effort and the regulation of mood: The absorption hypothesis. *Journal of Experimental Social Psychology, 30,* 319–337.

42. Prochaska, J. O. (2000). Change at differing stages. In C. R. Snyder & R. E. Ingram (Eds.), *Handbook of psychological change: Psychotherapy processes and practices for the 21st century* (pp. 109–128). New York: Wiley.

43. Kabat-Zinn, J. (1982). An outpatient program in behavioral medicine for chronic pain patients based on the practice of mindfulness meditation. *General Hospital Psychiatry, 4,* 31–47.

44. Kabat-Zinn, J., Lipworth, L., & Burney, R. G. (1985). The clinical use of mindfulness meditation for the self-regulation of chronic pain. *Journal of Behavioral Medicine, 8,* 163–190.

45. Kabat-Zinn, J., Wheeler, E., Light, T., Skillings, A., Scharf, M. J., Cropley, T. G., Hosmer, D., & Bernhard, J. D. (1998). Influence of a mindfulness meditation-based stress reduction intervention on rates of skin clearing in patients with moderate to severe psoriasis undergoing phototherapy (UVB) and photochemotherapy (PUVA). *Psychosomatic Medicine, 60,* 625–636.

46. Suls, J., David, J. H., & Harvey, J. H. (1996). Personality and coping. *Journal of Personality, 64,* 711–736.

47. Teasdale, J. D., Segal, Z., & Williams, M. G. (1994). How does cognitive therapy prevent depressive relapse and why should attentional control (mindfulness) training help? *Behavior Research Therapy, 31,* 25–37.

10

Dealing with Secrets

Anita E. Kelly
Jennifer E. Carter

Most people know how much of a burden it can be to keep secrets from others, especially those whom they respect. They know the torture of hiding feelings of discontentment from their boyfriends or girlfriends, poor grades from their parents, infidelities from their spouses, and indiscretions from their employers. They want others to know them but do not want to be reminded of the things that make them feel bad or ashamed. What can be done to alleviate this anguish? What are the factors that should enter into making a wise decision to reveal a secret? These are two of the central questions to be addressed in this chapter on dealing with troubling, personal secrets (i.e., ones that directly involve the secret keeper).

We begin by defining secrecy and looking at the negative views of secrecy among psychotherapists dating back to Freud. Then, we describe the evidence to support the notion that secrecy might make people sick. We also explore how revealing secrets in an anonymous setting can lead to health benefits and explain why these health benefits may occur. Most important, we describe those instances when the revealing of secrets to various confidants can backfire and specify a model for when people might benefit from revealing their personal secrets.

Nature of Secrecy

Keeping secrets involves deliberately hiding information from other people (1), and it often has the negative connotation of being a form of deception (e.g., 2). Secrets always have a social context and are only meaningful in relation to the people from whom they are kept. Secret relationships can involve only one person's knowledge of the relationship, such as in the case when someone has a secret crush on a colleague or classmate (3). But even in such cases, the very existence of the secret depends on the secret keeper's awareness of another person.

In understanding the nature of secrecy, it is important not only to keep in mind that secrets always have a social context, but also to distinguish secrecy from privacy. Whereas privacy connotes the expectation of being free from unsanctioned intrusion, secrecy does not. Secrecy involves active attempts to prevent such intrusion or leaks, and the secret keeper exerts this energy, in part, because he or she perceives that other people may have some claim to the hidden information. For example, the sexual practices between a wife and husband are considered to be private in American society because people agree that theses practices are not for public display. However, a parent's hidden sexual molestation of his child would be considered secret because society has a right or obligation to intervene in such cases. Also, the hiddon rituals that are required in order to join a particular organization may be considered secret rather than private, because members of the organization understand that the broader society does not necessarily expect such rituals to be confidential.

The distinction between secrecy and privacy is not a small one, and it helps to explain why the recent Clinton-Lewinsky affair was so controversial. President Clinton may have lied under oath about his having had sexual relations with Monica Lewinsky to protect what he perceived as his privacy. In contrast, the Independent Counsel, Ken Starr, may have seen Clinton's perjurious actions as a means of protecting a secret to which the public was entitled access, because the facts surrounding the affair may have had some bearing on the Paula Jones's sexual harassment case. That many Americans viewed the Lewinsky affair as a matter of privacy may account partly for why Clinton's job-approval ratings remained so high even throughout his impeachment trial.

What may start out as a healthy form of privacy potentially can lead to secrecy in the context of a particular relationship. This shift is especially likely in relationships in which the partners have different expectations concerning how much personal information they should tell each other. For example, in a budding romantic relationship, a young man might expect full disclosure about such things as how many previous sexual partners his new girlfriend has had. He might feel deceived if she omits such disclosures. In contrast, the girlfriend may consider such information either irrelevant or private and thus may refuse to disclose the information. Even if she initially considered it to be her right to keep such information private, the fact that she is aware that he expects revelation might cause her to exert energy in hiding that information from him. This expenditure of energy occurs because in deciding that this information should be kept a secret, she must constantly monitor information that is consistent with the state of mind that she wishes to maintain, as well as monitor the information that she wishes to hide from others (3). It is not easy for people to engage in these dual processes: "The secret must be remembered, or it might be told. And the secret cannot be thought about, or it might be leaked" (3, p. 288). Hence, what was once merely private information can become secret information (that requires energy to keep) in the context of that relationship.

What kinds of secrets do people tend to keep? The most embarrassing, disturbing, or traumatic personal experiences often are concealed. Most secrets are likely to involve negative or stigmatizing information that pertains to the secret keepers themselves. Examples of secrets include those about a person's being gay or lesbian, having been raped, cheating on his or her income taxes, and being a drug user. Secrecy also has been called *self-concealment* (e.g., 4) and *active inhibition of disclosure* (e.g., 5).

Psychoanalytic Views of the Detriments of Secrecy

Psychoanalysts long have viewed secrecy as problematic. The revelation of secrets through hypnosis was the basis of the cathartic method that was developed by Breuer in the late 1800s and later expanded by Freud (6). Breuer and Freud (7) observed that patients' revealing their secrets allowed them to relive their repressed or buried traumatic experiences. This reliving in the safety of the psychoanalytic sessions, or abreaction, was typically followed by a reduction in the patients' symptoms.

Based on these and other case observations, Freud (8) developed his *fundamental rule of psychoanalysis*, which required patients to reveal as much about themselves as possible, no matter how silly, inappropriate, or anxiety-provoking those secrets seemed to them (see 9). Likewise, Jung (10) encouraged patients to face those things that they typically kept hidden from themselves. He made patients' revelations of these secrets the focus of his psychoanalytic sessions. Cathartic treatment required a thorough confession, including a retelling of the facts and a release of suppressed affect (10). Jung stated that "every personal secret has the effect of sin or guilt. If we are conscious of what we conceal, harm is less than if we do not know what we are repressing" (p. 34).

Even though they educated their patients about the importance of revealing their secrets in treatment, Freud and Jung observed that their patients resisted complete openness (11). Freud concluded that neurotics are instinctively, biologically motivated to strive for competing ends. On the one hand, neurotics wish to be cured through revealing themselves completely. On the other hand, they want to avoid being cured through keeping their unconscious impulses and images buried in the deeper regions of their minds (8). This phenomenon has been described as a tension between the urge to retain such material and the urge to expel it (9). The patients fear penetration, and yet they long for extraction of their secrets (12). When patients refuse to explore their secrets in psychoanalysis, they are perceived to be defensive and resistant (12, 13).

Psychoanalysis as a form of treatment thus developed as a means of overcoming patients' resistance to revelation of buried material (14). Although analysts do not rush or outwardly force patients to reveal their deepest secrets (12), they believe that by examining the manner in which patients disclose a secret, they can gain great insight into their psychological development and conflicts (15).

Psychoanalysts try to remove obstacles to confession by hypothesizing what the patient's secret might be, observing resistance in the patient, and then making a conjecture about the hidden content to the patient (14). The analyst's comments and actions are intended to create an encouraging environment that decreases the patient's discomfort or shame (16). The primary psychoanalytic techniques of dream analysis and free association (i.e., in which the analyst presents a series of words, and the patient blurts out words that immediately come to mind) are utilized to extract hidden, unconscious material (17). For example, Jung relied heavily on dream analysis to draw out the patient's inner psyche when the patient had trouble accessing his or her inner, personal world (11). Freud compared the psychoanalyst's intense efforts to elicit private information to criminal investigation procedures in which the investigator obtains a confession (18). Psychoanalysis relies on the search for unspeakable, sealed-off trauma; "behind an emotion expressed, behind a symptom manifested, there lurks a contrary, repressed emotion" (19, p. 18).

From the psychoanalytic perspective, if patients are not willing or able to share their secrets, the energy they spend keeping secrets repressed might become represented in compulsive behavior or other symptoms (8, 19, 20, 21, 22, 23). For instance, a patient's denial or repression of a trauma supposedly may contribute to the development of psychological disorders such as multiple personality disorder, bipolar disorder, anorexia, and melancholia (19). Presumably, only through the confession of secrets can the treatment of these disorders succeed and the symptoms be reduced (19). Such confession is considered particularly beneficial when the patient has been unaware of his or her secrets (21).

There are many case studies (i.e., examinations of one or a few individuals in depth) that have supported the claim that the confession of secrets is crucial in psychoanalysis. In one well-known case, for example, Freud employed a strategy of identifying and reconstructing the traumatic childhood experience of a woman named Dora (24). Freud believed that the source of Dora's illness was her childhood masturbation. He drew out her confession that she had masturbated, and her migraine headaches and depression diminished. Another case involved a 41-year-old man who suffered from alcoholism and drug abuse. Essential components of his analysis included the emergence of his previously withheld sexual history and his confession of gay sexual feelings for the analyst (25). The patient reached his treatment goals after seven years of analysis. His addictive behaviors were gone, and he was leading a contented life with his wife and children. In yet another case, the patient "Mrs. C." revealed her guilt and fear about her own sexual power in her therapy sessions. Afterward, she demonstrated greater cooperative and assertive behavior (26).

Why Revealing Is Critical for Therapeutic Progress

There are several, interrelated reasons that psychoanalysts have offered for why revealing secrets is essential for therapeutic progress. First, patients seem to have an intense yearning to reenact a past traumatic event to resolve unfinished business (27). Traumatized patients "fear the return of the trauma, yet they tend to retraumatize themselves though repeated actions symbolizing aspects of the trauma" (28, p. 452). Confession allows an emotional reliving of the original trauma and thus provides partial gratification of the patient's impulses and drives (22). In particular, confession allows the overcoming of anxiety or guilt, and presumably gratifies one's masochistic need for punishment (22, 29).

Second, revealing the secret is believed to allow a discharge of pent-up emotions such as shame, guilt, and anger that previously blocked creative growth (9). Hymer (30) theorized that revealing private information is worth any risk of doing so: "The initial embarrassment of confessing is frequently outweighed by the relief that comes with the verbalization of the darker, secretive aspects of the self" (p. 131).

Third, the disclosure of secrets may help a patient develop his or her identity (30). The revealing of a secret makes it less foreign to one's sense of self and allows integration of the positive and negative aspects of oneself (30). In one case study (31), a psychiatric inpatient kept secret the fact that he had killed one of his parents. The patient later reported feeling isolated from the other patients on his ward as a result of hiding this information from them. Schwartz (31) recommended that patients reveal their secrets to other patients at a stage in their treatment when they feel ready to do so. This revealing allows them to rid themselves of an uncomfortable moral burden of deceptiveness and to experience a more integrated sense of self.

Underlying all of these explanations is the notion that revealing secrets to a noncondemning analyst instead of to rejecting parents is a corrective emotional experience (1). In contrast to past experiences, presumably the analyst will not reveal the secret, will not take sides, and will not use the information against the patient (unless the analyst is legally required to reveal the secret, such as in cases when patients threaten to harm other people). Through confessing the buried impulses and the mechanisms driving toward repression of these impulses, a better adjustment to reality may replace the process of repression. Confession offers a more realistic meaning for the repressed wishes and the possibility for greater self-understanding (22).

Summary

Psychoanalysis developed as a means of helping patients reveal themselves to the analyst and confess their secrets. A number of case studies from the psychoanalytic literature have pointed to the notion that keeping secrets in treatment prevents patients from benefiting from the treatment. These cases have shown that recovery typically follows an important confession or re-telling of previously suppressed or repressed material.

However, the findings from these case studies, as with all case reports, must be interpreted with caution. Such studies are particularly vulnerable to the biases of the investigators. Psychoanalysts are likely to have expected to find that secrecy in sessions is problematic. For example, they may not have documented the times when revealing a secret backfired, because that result so contradicted their expectations. Furthermore, the psychoanalytic researchers could not have documented the times when secret keeping was associated with healthy outcomes, because they would not have known when secrets had been kept from them.

Family Therapists' Views of the Detriments of Secrecy

Although psychoanalysts were the first modern-day psychotherapists to emphasize the importance of unearthing secrets in therapy, family thera-pists perhaps have had the most to say about the dysfunctional nature of secrecy. A common view among family therapists is that the strain of keep-ing a secret is typically the source of clients' problems. Symptoms are con-sidered to be mere by-products of the secret keeping (e.g., 32), such as in cases where a child exhibits symptoms as a diversion from the family's denied or secret problems (33). It is thought that parents bring a child into therapy because it is easier to blame the child than to look at their own problems (34). Case reports indeed have linked secret keeping to psychotic symptoms in children (32).

Some therapists have construed the central function of therapy as help-ing the family with their secrets, while also helping them find a way to stay together (35). Secrets are thought to shackle family members to one another by making them feel a guilty sense of obligation to one another (35). It has been suggested that when one family member wants to separate from the secretive family, these families often are driven into therapy (36).

Consistent with these negative views of secrecy, research on secrets within the family has shown that there is a negative relationship between family satisfaction and family members' reports of the number of secrets that the family keeps in relation to other families (37). However, Vangelisti (37) also found that the actual estimated number of secrets that family mem-bers reported was not correlated with their family satisfaction. It is possible that dissatisfied family members may be inclined to believe that their fam-ilies are unusually secretive, even if the families actually are not secretive (37).

The types of secrets that family members keep from one another include those about incest (38), extramarital affairs (39), the sexual orientation of one or more family members (40), and death (41). In the following sections we describe the theories and research advocating the revelation of these various types of secrets in couples' and family therapy. We have organized the section in this manner because the rationales for the sharing of family secrets vary somewhat as a function of the types of secrets that the family is keeping.

Incest

In cases where father-daughter incest has occurred, secrecy is thought to isolate the family from the outside world, thereby contributing to the father's abusive dominance in the family (42). The incest is maintained by secrecy (43), and repression or denial are typical responses to the incest experience (44, 45). The child feels isolated and different from other children her age (46). A critical part of therapy is to diminish the daughter's sense of isolation by encouraging her to break the silence surrounding the incest trauma (42, 47). The daughter understands that revealing her secret could destroy her family and could result in her removal from it (38). As such, there is tremendous pressure on her to maintain the secrecy (38).

Incest victims have reported that they fear abandonment (48), not being believed (49), punishment (50), and being blamed for complying with the incestuous activity (51, 52, 53, 54). Despite these fears, Swanson and Biaggio (38) argue that the victim must reveal the secret during therapy sessions. The victim also must ultimately discuss the incest with someone other than the therapist so as to dispel her feelings of isolation (see 50, 54, 55).

Some family therapists have proposed that even though the initial relief of revealing family secrets in therapy may be followed by feelings of guilt and exacerbation of symptoms, the revealer ultimately will experience symptom reduction. Three documented cases involving family sexual secrets showed this pattern (32). In each case, an adolescent was hiding information about the inappropriate sexual conduct of one or more family members and was encouraged to reveal this secret in therapy. After complying, the adolescents experienced some immediate reduction in their presenting psychotic symptoms of paranoia, acting out, and severe depression. However, these symptoms became worse during the days immediately following the disclosure. After more time had passed, their symptoms abated once again. The authors suggested that this pattern was due to the patients' initial feelings of disloyalty to the family for having revealed their secrets. Then, the patients regained a sense of equilibrium after coming to terms with this disloyalty, even though their families dissolved.

Extramarital Affairs

A number of marriage and family therapists have indicated that it is essential for a marital partner who has had an affair to confess to the other spouse (e.g., 39, 56, 57). Presumably, it is not the extramarital sex that causes problems, but rather the secrecy surrounding the sex (57). Keeping such a secret requires omitting truths or telling lies, and this deception may undermine a person's sense of self-worth (39). The guilt and shame of the secret affair may become unbearable for the person who is having the affair (39).

Moreover, the "other woman" (or the "other man") also may suffer from secrecy surrounding the affair (58). Interviews with 65 women who were involved with married men showed that the relationships typically were perpetuated by mutual efforts to keep them hidden. This secrecy created intense feelings of togetherness for the secretive partners. However, the secrecy seemed to reduce the woman's power within the relationship and protect the interests of the married man (58).

Some marital therapists have asserted that secret extramarital affairs should be revealed, even if they were brief and happened a long time ago, because "hiding it means holding back a piece of oneself" (56, p. 138). Brown (56) indicated that when clients bring up the affairs to the therapist, it is evident to the therapist that the affairs still are having an impact. The reason that therapists are encouraged to work toward getting clients to reveal the affairs to them (56) is that, lacking this information, the therapists obviously cannot readily assess the effects of the previous affairs on the present marital relationship. The therapists presumably need to be aware of the affairs to try to understand their impact (59).

One case example involved a couple who had the vague goal of improving their marriage. In an individual therapy session with the husband, the therapist learned indirectly about the affair (56). Just before the next session, the wife canceled their treatment. The therapist interpreted this abrupt termination to mean that the wife and husband were both trying to avoid facing the affair, and that they could have benefited from an open discussion of the infidelity (56).

Sexual Orientation

The literature on revealing one's gay or lesbian identity to others suggests that having an open identity across all spheres of life is associated with improved self-esteem (e.g., 60, 61, 62). Coming out to important others, parents in particular, is considered to be central to lesbian women's self-acceptance (63). Revealing her lesbian identity allows the daughter to avoid the isolation from her parents that her secrecy can create (64). Before the disclosure to parents, "what closeness exists is considered pseudocloseness, because a relevant piece of information is missing" (40, p. 49).

Many gay men and lesbians who have come out to their parents, however, have reported parental disapproval of their sexual orientation (65, 66, 67). For example, a survey of twenty lesbians in committed relationships who had come out to their parents showed that 70% of the women reported parental disapproval (40). At the same time, respondents in that study also reported feeling relieved that they did not have to hide an important aspect of their lives. Thus, Murphy concluded that the negative effects of coming out were outweighed by the positive aspects of having parents know about the nature of the couple's relationship.

Murphy (40) recommended that, in therapy with lesbian couples, the therapist should help the clients engage in "identity management," or help them balance the effects of secrecy against the consequences of coming out. In particular, Murphy recommended that therapists should help the couple prepare for the effects of coming out to parents. Another recommendation was that the therapist should help the couple grieve over the loss of "heterosexual privilege" in the family of origin.

Death and Loss

After conducting two family therapy case studies of families whose secret was that a family member had died or was about to die, Evans (68) concluded that the dysfunctional secret contributed to the development of symptoms in one child in each family. The secret surrounding death seemed to intensify feelings of alienation among the members of each family. The treatments specifically aimed at bringing the secret out in the open and resolving it seemed to lead to substantial improvements in the clients' functioning.

It has been proposed that families in crisis, such as in the case of an impending death, necessarily have secret or denied emotions that members often project onto one scapegoated (i.e., unduly blamed) family member (41). It is believed that such secrets need to be addressed head-on in therapy (41). A case of several families treated in multifamily group therapy offers an illustration of this phenomenon (41). For one family in the group, the suicidal ideation of John, the son, was viewed by therapists as part of the effort to keep the secret of his father's terminal illness from the father. "It became apparent that the strain of hiding his serious illness from Mr. Henry had produced frantic behavior in the family, leading to reinforced scapegoating of John" (p. 43). With the therapist's encouragement, the family told the father of his illness. Although John's self-esteem improved after the disclosure, the family abruptly terminated treatment in a move led by the parents. The authors indicated that if they had stayed in treatment, they might have ultimately developed healthier and more open patterns of interaction.

Another example of the emphasis on resolving secrets is offered by a case study in which an asthmatic 10-year-old son engaged in play therapy. He revealed his secret wish that his divorced father would come back to the family or would at least befriend his mother (33). Shortly after such discussions, the boy's symptoms lessened. His 12-year-old brother, however, subsequently developed some acting-out behaviors at home and at school. Despite these mixed findings, Eaker concluded that, although families may resist revealing their secrets, they often are helped by such open discussions (33). Play therapy is seen as a "cushion" that can allow the family to tolerate the anxiety associated with the revealing, because many families drop out after secrets emerge in standard family therapy (see 69).

Research on families with a member who has AIDS suggests that the families expend a great deal of energy keeping the secret because of the social stigma associated with the disease (e.g., 70, 71, 72). Two case studies of families dealing with HIV-infected members showed that, regardless of how the disease was contracted (i.e., because of hemophilia or promiscuous sexuality), both families expended a great deal of energy hiding the disease from others (72). Moreover, extensive interviews of eleven significant others of persons who died of AIDS showed that all eleven reported that there was some attempt to keep the AIDS a secret from others. Forty four percent of the families of the AIDS victims reported that it was stressful for them to maintain the secrecy (71). It seemed that the burden of the secret, over time, left these significant others feeling isolated from their own support networks (71). Thus, it is believed that the first major recurring theme to which a therapist should attend is the secrecy of the illness (70). The therapist should discuss who could be told about the illness to address feelings of loneliness and isolation (70).

Greif and Porembski (71) provided a more cautious perspective on revealing the secret of AIDS by indicating that, despite these negative effects of secret keeping, secrecy may be the best way for the person with the disease to deal with his or her immediate crisis. Contending with the disease itself is so stressful that the patient may not have the resources to cope with the added strain of managing other people's reactions to the disease.

Summary

As with the psychoanalytic literature, there is a preponderance of theoretical work that suggests the revealing of secrets is a critical part of family therapy. Yet the evidence supporting this claim has been composed almost entirely of case reports which offer limited generalizability. In the next section, we review the empirical evidence of the link between secrecy and health problems.

Research Supporting the Link Between Secrecy and Health Problems

It is clear from recent health-psychology research that people who tend to keep secrets have more physical and mental complaints, on average, than people who do not. For example, researchers found that human services workers' tendencies to keep personal secrets from others were related to greater anxiety, depression, and bodily symptoms, such as back pain and headaches (73). Moreover, these relationships between self-concealment and symptoms remained even after removing the shared variance related to the participants' traumatic experiences and distress, disclosure of the trauma, social support, social network, and self-disclosure (73). Greater self-concealment also was correlated with more depression (74), anxiety, shyness, and low self-esteem among samples of undergraduates (75), and with an array of physical and psychological symptoms among a sample of therapy outpatients (76). Likewise, in a study of survivors of childhood traumas, those who did, as compared to those who did not, discuss the traumas with others tended to develop more problems such as hypertension, cancer, and influenza (77).

Based on recent research, it appears that gay men who conceal their sexual orientation from others are at a greater risk for cancers and infectious diseases than those men who do not conceal their orientation. Specifically, one study involved 80 gay men who were HIV-seropositive, but otherwise healthy, at the beginning of the study (78). These men were assessed at six-month intervals for the nine years for signs of HIV progression. The measures included how long it took for the men to develop a critically low ED T lymphocyte level, to receive an AIDS diagnosis, and to die from AIDS. The findings were that the men who concealed their homosexual identity experienced a more rapid progression of these negative outcomes than did the men who were more "out of the closet." In describing these results, the researchers posited that it is stressful to inhibit the expression of one's sexual identity, and that such stress can lead to negative health effects. The researchers were able to rule out competing explanations for these remarkable findings by statistically controlling for various demographic characteristics, health practices, sexual behaviors, antiretroviral therapy, depression levels, anxiety levels, and degree of social support.

In another study, the investigators examined the incidence of cancer and infectious diseases among 222 HIV-seronegative gay men (79). They found that those who concealed their homosexual identities, relative to those who did not, experienced a significantly higher incidence of cancer and several infectious diseases (i.e., pneumonia, bronchitis, sinusitis, and tuberculosis) over a five-year follow-up period. After ruling out counterexplanations related to differences in age, ethnicity, socioeconomic status, health-relevant behavioral patterns (e.g., drug use, exercise), anxiety, depression, or reporting biases (e.g., negative affectivity, social desirability), the researchers speculated that inhibiting the expression of something as important as one's sexual orientation is stressful and can take a toll on one's health.

Just as people who are high in self-concealment appear to have more problems, researchers also have shown that talking or writing about private traumatic experiences is associated with health benefits. For example, spouses of suicide and accidental-death victims were surveyed, and those who reported that they had talked about the loss of their spouses with family and friends suffered fewer health problems the year after the loss than did those participants who did not speak with others (80). (This difference held up even when taking into account the number of friends these individuals had before and after the loss of the spouse.) In another study, patients with advanced breast cancer, who were randomly assigned to a group that was designed to encourage them to talk about their emotions, survived twice as long as patients who were assigned to a routine oncological care group (81).

In a laboratory experiment with undergraduates, writing anonymously about the facts and emotions surrounding a personal traumatic event, as compared with writing about either the emotions or the facts alone, led to fewer health-center visits during the six months after the writing experience (82). Similarly favorable results were obtained in an experiment in which undergraduates wrote about personal traumatic events or superficial topics for four days (83). The trauma-writing group had significantly higher proliferative responses of lymphocytes (white blood cells) to stimulation of a mitogen (substance foreign to the body) by the end of the writing intervention than did the students who wrote about superficial topics. In another experiment, medical students were randomly assigned to write about either private traumatic events or control topics for four consecutive days and then were vaccinated against hepatitis B (84). The group that wrote about traumatic events had significantly higher antibody levels against hepatitis B at the four- and six-month follow-up periods than did the control group. From these findings, one may infer that the emotional expression of traumatic experiences can lead to improved immune functioning.

In sum, people who tend to be high rather than low in self-concealment also tend to be more sick. Furthermore, revealing private negative experiences in anonymous, confidential settings leads to health benefits. It is important to note, however, that despite the documented association between secrecy and problems, *to date there is no direct (i.e., experimental) evidence that keeping secrets causes these problems.* There is only direct evidence that through keeping a secret, a person misses out on the potential health benefits of revealing.

Why Revealing Is Helpful

Recent explanations offered by leading health-psychology researchers for the health benefits of revealing secrets resonate with some aspects of the psychoanalytic and family-therapy explanations described earlier. In particular, Pennebaker (85) has proposed that revealers gain new insights into their traumatic experiences and no longer have to expend cognitive and emotional resources actively hiding them. Polivy (86) also has suggested that by attaining catharsis (i.e., expressing pent-up emotions behaviorally), one's level of emotional arousal surrounding a troubling event may be lessened. Polivy has been careful to note, however, that the question of whether catharsis actually purges emotions is visited by both confirming and disconfirming results (86).

Because of the competing explanations for why revealing secrets leads to health benefits, members of our research team conducted a pair of studies in which we compared the effects of gaining new insights with the effects of gaining catharsis (87). In our first study, we examined undergraduates' reports of what they had gained from revealing their most private secrets to their confidants in the past. We found that gaining new perspectives on their secrets was positively related to the participants' feeling better about the secrets now, whereas experiencing catharsis actually was associated negatively with recovery from the secrets. In addition, participants' ratings of the expertness of their confidants (i.e., their preparedness and their abilities to help) were associated with the participants' gaining insights into their secrets (87, Study 1).

In the second study, we directly compared the effects of gaining catharsis with the effects of gaining new insights into one's troubling secrets (87, Study 2). Undergraduates ($N = 85$) were randomly assigned to write about their: (a) secrets while trying to gain new insights; (b) secrets while trying to gain catharsis; or (c) previous day. The new-insights group felt significantly better about their secrets than did the other groups, thereby supporting that idea that the key to recovery from troubling secrets comes via gaining new insights. Based on additional analyses conducted on the content of the writing, it appeared that participants' coming to terms with their secrets mediated the relation between their gaining new insights and feeling better about them. In other words, it was only through coming to terms with their secrets that participants seemed to benefit from gaining new insights into them. These findings are consistent with the results from a series of writing-about-trauma studies in which participants' increased use of words associated with insightful and causal thinking was linked with improved physical health (88, Study 1).

The reason why gaining new insights is likely to be curative is that people may be able to put closure on their secrets and avoid what has been termed the *Zeigarnik effect* (89, see also 87.) This effect refers to the fact that people think more about and remember better their uncompleted as compared to completed tasks. One might infer from our findings (87, Study 2) that revealing secrets with the explicit intention of gaining new perspectives may help people feel a sense of completion or resolution about the secrets, so that they can put the secrets behind them.

Self-Presentation and the Role of the Confidant

Almost all of the experiments (i.e., studies that involve random assignment of participants to treatment and control groups) conducted to date have involved anonymous, confidential revealing. As such, researchers have not paid enough attention to the role of the confidant in influencing the outcomes of revealing secrets. Given that secrecy always has a social context, it is crucial to study the role of the confidant in assessing the outcomes of revealing secrets. Indeed, the health benefits observed in those experiments may not generalize to circumstances in which people reveal unfavorable or stigmatizing information about themselves to important audiences (e.g., their coworkers or friends) in their everyday interactions. In these interpersonal circumstances, the revealers may perceive that that they are being rejected by and alienated from the listeners.

Revealing one's gay or lesbian identity, for example, might backfire because one's confidants may not be emotionally prepared to deal with such information. For instance, in a well-publicized incident involving the videotaping of an episode of the Jenny Jones show, called "Secret Crushes on People of the Same Sex," a gay man proclaimed his attraction to a male neighbor (who appeared on the show hoping to learn of a woman's attraction to him). Shortly thereafter, the emotionally unstable neighbor murdered the gay man. Even though this example obviously is an extreme one, we suggest that it is premature to conclude that for most gay men and lesbians, the reported relief from revealing is necessarily worth the costs of being rejected by some friends, colleagues, and family members. In this latter regard, consider the results from a nine-year longitudinal study of initially healthy HIV-positive gay men. For those men who were sensitive to social rejection, those who concealed their sexual orientation from others experienced a *slower* progression of HIV-related symptoms than did those who revealed it to others (90). These findings run counter to the earlier pattern discovered by these same researchers, in which gay men who concealed their sexual orientation were at a greater risk for cancer and infectious diseases.

Turning to a Psychotherapist for Help

Perhaps turning to a psychotherapist for help is a way around the risks associated with revealing one's secrets to others. Therapy sessions are confidential, similar to the laboratory experiments in which the health benefits of revealing secrets were demonstrated. Also, therapists are experienced at giving people new insights into their personal problems.

However, we suggest that because the therapists' opinions of the clients are so important to the clients, the clients may be reluctant to make such revelations in psychotherapy. Even though clients openly admit to their feelings of depression and low self-esteem at intake, they nevertheless try to look like good people to their counselors (91). Even long-term therapy clients appear to keep secrets from their therapists (92). For example, Hill et al. (92) asked individual therapy clients, averaging 86 sessions, to indicate whether they were keeping any secrets from their therapists. Forty-six percent reported keeping secrets from their therapists. The clients' most frequently listed reason for their secrecy was shame or embarrassment at sharing them. The themes to their secrets concerned sex, failure, and mental-health issues (92), which are similar to the themes of the secrets described by encounter-group and group-therapy members in previous research (93, 94). Also noteworthy is the fact that clients' length of time in therapy was not related to the number of secrets kept (92). Because so many of the clients reported keeping secrets from their therapists, Hill et al. (92)

recommended that therapists try to help clients feel more comfortable and less embarrassed about revealing secrets. It should be noted, however, that secret keeping was not significantly related to the clients' satisfaction with therapy, and symptom reduction was not assessed in that study.

Not only are some clients reluctant to reveal their secrets, but also revealing secrets in therapy might backfire. Kelly conducted a study which tested the relation between secret keeping in therapy and symptom reduction with a sample of 42 clients who had received an average of 11 therapy sessions (76). Over 40% of the clients reported keeping relevant secrets (i.e., ones that they perceived to be related to their presenting problems) in therapy. Among their most frequently listed reasons were: fear of expressing feelings, shame or embarrassment, or concern that the therapist would see how little progress they had made (76). After adjusting for clients' social desirability scores (i.e., a measure of their trying to look good on the surveys) and self-concealment scores, Kelly found that keeping relevant secrets in therapy was associated with a *reduction* in symptoms since the intake, as reported by the clients. (She adjusted for self-concealment scores, are which quantify the tendency to keep negative or distressing personal information to oneself [4], to see if keeping particular secrets from the therapists was associated with a reduction in symptoms above and beyond the effects of the clients' general tendencies to keep secrets.) The results support the idea that clients who conceal some unfavorable aspects of themselves from their therapists may benefit more from therapy than those who do not (76). Perhaps hiding the most unfavorable aspects of themselves from their therapists helps clients feel better because the clients can create desirable images of themselves before this important audience (76).

Self-Presentation Research

The essence of the problem with revealing personal, undesirable information to anyone is that the revealers may come to see themselves in undesirable ways if others—even their therapists—know their stigmatizing secrets. A number of experiments from the self-presentation literature have demonstrated that describing oneself as having undesirable qualities, such as being depressed or introverted, to various audiences leads to shifts in one's self-beliefs and behaviors in the negative direction of the self-presentations (e.g., 95, 96, 97, 98). So, the question remains: If even revealing secrets in therapy has the potential of causing people to see themselves more negatively, when should people reveal their secrets?

When to Reveal Secrets

In this section, we explain how making the decision to reveal one's personal secrets to others involves a trade-off between: (a) feeling better by revealing the secrets and gaining new insights into them; and (b) avoiding looking bad before important audiences (such as one's boss or therapist) by not revealing (99). *The key to making a wise decision to reveal one's personal secrets is finding an appropriate confidant* (99, 100). An appropriate confidant is one who is discreet, is perceived by the secret keeper to be nonjudgmental, and is able to offer new insights into the secrets (99, 100). We also suggest that people should reveal their secrets to others only if keeping the secrets is troubling or is actually causing the internal stress and negative effects described by various researchers (e.g., 2, 5, 73, 101, 102). See Figure 10.1 for a depiction of this model developed by Kelly and McKillop (100). We elaborate on each of these parts of the model in the following paragraphs.

Troubling Secrets

One problem with these recommendations is that the secret keeper cannot always tell if a secret is troubling. The secret keeper may have to infer that the secret is troubling if she is spending a considerable amount of time mulling over the secret and is upset by such thoughts, or if she is experiencing the kinds of symptoms (e.g., depression, ulcers, and headaches) that have been found to be associated with secret keeping (e.g., 73). In those instances, the secret keeper should talk about the secrets with an appro-

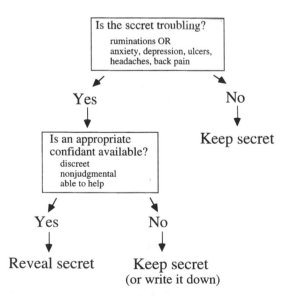

Figure 10.1. Decision-making for revealing secrets. Copyright © 1996 by the American Psychological Association. Reprinted with permission.

priate confidant who is likely to react positively to such revelations. On the one hand, if the secret is indeed causing the troubling symptoms and the secret keeper reveals to an appropriate confidant, then the secret keeper should benefit from revealing. On the other hand, if the secret is not causing the symptoms, the secret keeper is still unlikely to be harmed by revealing to an appropriate confidant.

Features of Helpful Confidants

What makes an appropriate confidant or one to whom secret keepers would benefit from revealing? As mentioned earlier, we suggest that if a troubled secret keeper has a confidant who is (a) discreet and can be trusted not to reveal a secret; (b) perceived by the secret keeper to be nonjudgmental; and (c) able to offer new insights into the secret, then the secret keeper should reveal the secret to that person.

Discreet   Assuring people of the confidentiality of their disclosures generally leads to greater revealing of private information (103, 104). Trusting the confidant not to reveal the secret to others may be the most important factor in determining whether someone should reveal to that person. When one can be assured that only the confidant will know a secret, then that person can assess how the confidant is reacting and can make a decision about whether to continue the relationship with the confidant.

Unfortunately, a problem associated with the revealing of one's secrets is that confidants often cannot be trusted to keep the secrets or to protect the revealer's identity. In a survey of college students, when someone had disclosed an emotional event to them, they in turn revealed the emotional disclosure to others in 66% to 78% of the cases—despite the fact that the participants were intimates of the original revealers in 85% of the cases (105). Furthermore, when the original disclosure was of a high as compared to low or moderate emotional intensity, participants reported that they had shared it with others even more frequently and had told more people (i.e., more than two other people). In another study, in 78% of the cases in which the original event was disclosed to others, the name of the original revealer was explicitly mentioned. Taking what is obviously a most conservative position on this issue, Christophe and Rime recommended that if people do not want others to learn about their emotional experiences, then they should avoid sharing the experiences with others altogether (105). It is important to note, though, that these researchers did not specifically ask the confidant-participants if they had been sworn to secrecy. Also, the participants were of college age, and it is possible that more mature participants would have been more discreet.

In situations in which confidentiality is not guaranteed, the former secret keeper loses a sense of control and may be victimized by others who are privy to the secrets (106). The person may begin to construct a negative identity for himself or herself by imagining—or actually hearing—the judgments others will make upon learning about the secret (see 107). Given these negative possibilities, we recommend that a secret keeper avoid revealing secrets to any confidants who cannot or will not refrain from passing the secrets on to others.

Nonjudgmental   The idea that it is important for a confidant to be nonjudgmental is supported by Carl Rogers's (108, 109) theoretical work on the benefits of having an accepting therapist or close friend with whom one can sort out personal problems. Rogers (108, 109) proposed that the primary role of the therapist is to provide clients with a safe environment (i.e., one free from conditions of worth or judgments from the therapist), so clients can learn to trust their inner experiencing.

Supporting the notion that establishing trust and offering warmth are important curative factors are the findings from a review of what psychotherapy researchers across 50 publications believed to be the effective elements of therapy. The review showed the most frequently proposed factor (56% of all authors) was the development of a therapeutic relationship or working alliance between the therapist and client (110). These authors' beliefs are backed by the findings from psychotherapy studies which have shown that establishing a positive alliance is associated with therapy success (see 111). Similarly, in their review of the effects of a variety of therapist variables on counseling outcome—most of which showed no consistent relations to outcomes—Beutler, Machado, and Neufeldt (112) concluded that "a warm and supportive therapeutic relationship facilitates therapeutic success" (p. 259). Moreover, in his study of brief counseling, Elliott (113) found that clients rated their therapists' encouraging a new perspective on the clients' problems as being particularly helpful, along with the therapists' offering understanding, assurance, personal contact, etc. Elliott (113) concluded that what the clients deemed to be helpful went beyond the therapists' accurate following of client material to include the clients' experiencing the therapist as being "on the client's side" (p. 319). The principal findings from all these studies on what is helpful in counseling are consistent with the idea that being nonjudgmental is an important element of being a good confidant.

The reason why having a nonjudgmental confidant is so helpful is that such a confidant provides all the benefits associated with the unburdening of secrets described above (i.e., new insights about the secret and the corresponding health benefits), but none of the ramifications associated with receiving negative feedback (e.g., being rejected by and becoming isolated from others). In revealing to nonjudgmental others, the secret keeper can feel accepted and comforted by the fact that he or she is no longer carrying the secret burden alone (94). For instance, imagine that a former police officer tells his girlfriend that he shot and killed a woman on a routine traffic stop because he mistook her cellular phone for a gun. If his girlfriend conveys that she accepts him despite his actions, then he can feel relieved from his guilt. He can continue to construct a positive self-image by seeing himself through her eyes, rather than through the critical eyes of imagined others.

Able to Offer New Insights   A key factor in making a wise decision to reveal to a confidant seems to be whether that confidant is able to offer new perspectives on a problematic secret. As described earlier, research supports the notion that it is not so much catharsis as it is gaining new insights that helps people feel better about their secrets (87). In addition, in research that has examined all types of brief therapy interventions, interpretations made by the therapist have been found to be associated with client improvement (see 114). Apparently, this improvement occurs because the interpretations provide clients with new perspectives on their problems. Therefore, we suggest that if the secret keeper has a confidant who is particularly insightful and is able to provide new perspectives on the secret, then the person should reveal to that confidant.

Making a Wise Decision to Reveal

It is not easy to choose an appropriate confidant because secret keepers can never know how their confidants will react until after their secrets have been revealed. Research has shown that people often test their potential confidants by floating "trial balloons" before making serious and potentially damaging disclosures (115). They jokingly or hypothetically introduce the secret topics and gauge the confidants' reactions (116). For example, a husband who is considering revealing his hidden sexual infidelities to his wife might ask her if she would leave him if he were to have an affair. If she says yes, then he might decide that it is not worth telling her about the secret. Another way in which secret keepers are likely to test their confidants is to reveal less important secrets and see if the confidant is discreet, nonjudgmental, and insightful with those secrets. If the confidant passes such "tests," then the secret keeper should reveal to that person, while still remaining aware that there is some risk or uncertainty in sharing with another.

Conclusions

Consistent with psychoanalytic and family-therapy perspectives on the importance of addressing personal secrets, there is some exciting experimental evidence that revealing one's personal secrets leads to health benefits. It seems that gaining new insights into one's secrets is especially helpful and may be causing the health benefits. However, these findings must be viewed with caution because the benefits of such anonymous revealing may not generalize to everyday interactions with one's confidants. Researchers have not paid sufficient attention to the role of the confidant.

We have argued, as did Kelly and McKillop (100), that if a troubled secret keeper has a discreet, nonjudgmental, and insightful confidant, then the secret keeper should reveal secrets to that person. The rationale for taking such a risk is that even if the secrets are not actually causing the symptoms that have been found to be associated with secrecy, the secret keeper is unlikely to be harmed as a result of having revealed to an appropriate confidant.

A limitation to this recommendation for when to reveal secrets is raised by the findings from the recent (76) study on relevant secret keeping in outpatient therapy. It was found that even with trained therapists who apparently fit all of the positive qualities of confidants described above, clients who were keeping a relevant secret experienced greater symptom reduction than those who were not keeping one. The seeming contradiction between this finding and our recommendations can be resolved by the fact that we have stressed that the revealer's *perception* of the confidant as nonjudgmental is critical in his or her decision to reveal a personal secret (see 99). It is likely that at times clients may imagine, or accurately perceive, that their therapists are judgmental (see 117). This perception may occur particularly when the clients have committed unusually bad acts. In such instances, the clients' decision to avoid revealing some of their secrets to their therapists may not be problematic. It is possible that they may instead benefit from writing about the secrets in an effort to gain new insights into them.

Acknowledgments
We thank Mercedes R. Kelly for her helpful editorial comments.

References

1. Margolis, G. J. (1974). The psychology of keeping secrets. *International Review of Psycho-Analysis, 1*, 291–296.
2. Lane, J. D., & Wegner, D. M. (1995). The cognitive consequences of secrecy. *Journal of Personality and Social Psychology, 69*, 237–253.
3. Wegner, D. M., Lane, J. D., & Dimitri, S. (1994). The allure of secret relationships. *Journal of Personality and Social Psychology, 66*, 287–300.
4. Larson, D. G., & Chastain, R. L. (1990). Self-concealment: Conceptualization, measurement, and health implications. *Journal of Social and Clinical Psychology, 9*, 439–455.
5. Pennebaker, J. W. (1989). Confession, inhibition, and disease. *Advances in Experimental Social Psychology, 22*, 211–244.
6. Fancher, R. E. (1973). *Psychoanalytic psychology: The development of Freud's thought.* New York: W. W. Norton & Co.
7. Breuer, J., & Freud, S. (1975). *Studies in hysteria.* New York: Basic Books. (Original work published 1893–1895.)
8. Freud, S. (1958). *On the beginning of treatment: Further recommen-*

dations on the techniques of psychoanalysis. London: Hogarth Press. (Original work published 1913).

9. Hoyt, M. F. (1978). Secrets in psychotherapy: Theoretical and practical considerations. *International Review of Psycho-Analysis, 5,* 231–241.

10. Jung, C. G. (1933). *Modern man in search of a soul.* New York: Harvest Books.

11. Kaufman, Y. (1989). Analytical psychotherapy. In R. J. Corsini and D. Wedding (Eds.), *Current psychotherapies* (pp. 119–154). Itasca, IL: F. E. Peacock.

12. Rosenfeld, D. (1980). The handling of resistances in adult patients. *International Journal of Psychoanalysis, 61,* 71–83.

13. Minoff, L. A. (1992). A case of rape: Real and imagined. *Psychoanalytic Review, 79,* 537–553.

14. Bernfeld, S. (1941). The facts of observation in psychoanalysis. *The Journal of Psychology, 12,* 289–305.

15. Schoicket, S. (1980). Secrets. *American Journal of Psychoanalysis, 40,* 179–182.

16. Weiss, J. (1995). Bernfeld's "The facts of observation in psychoanalysis: A response from psychoanalytic research." *Psychoanalytic Quarterly, 64,* 699–716.

17. Handelman, S. (1981). Interpretation as devotion: Freud's relation to Rabbinic hermeneutics. *The Psychoanalytic Review, 68,* 201–218.

18. Welsh, A. (1994). *Freud's wishful dream book* (pp. 29–50). Princeton, NJ: Princeton University Press.

19. Abraham, N., Torok, M., & Rand, N. (1994). *The shell and the kernel: Renewals of psychoanalysis, Vol. 1.* Chicago, IL: University of Chicago Press.

20. Hesselman, S. (1983). Elective mutism in children 1877–1981: A literary review. *Acta Paedopsychiatrica, 49,* 297–310.

21. Margolis, G. J. (1966). Secrecy and identity. *International Journal of Psycho-Analysis, 47,* 517–522.

22. Reik, T. (1945). *The compulsion to confess: On the psychoanalysis of crime and punishment.* New York: Grove Press.

23. Wergeland, H. (1980). Elective mutism. *Annual Progress in Child Psychiatry & Child Development, 65,* 373–385.

24. Mahony, P. J. (1996). *Freud's Dora: A psychoanalytic, historical, and textual study.* New Haven, CT: Yale University Press.

25. Wallerstein, R. S. (1986). *Forty-two lives in treatment: A study of psychoanalysis and psychotherapy* (pp. 265–277). New York: Guilford Press.

26. Gassner, S., Sampson, H., Brumer, S., & Weiss, J. (1986). The emergence of warded-off contents. In J. Weiss, H. Sampson, & the Mount Zion Psychotherapy Research Group (Eds.), *The psychoanalytic process: Theory, clinical observation, and empirical research* (pp. 171–186). New York: Guilford Press.

27. Dushman, R. D., & Bressler, M. J. (1991). Psychodrama in an adolescent chemical dependency treatment program. *Individual Psychology, 47,* 515–520.

28. Bergmann, M. V. (1992). An infantile trauma, a trauma during analysis,

and their psychic connexion. *International Journal of Psycho-Analysis, 73*, 447–454.

29. Gillman, R. D. (1992). Rescue fantasies and the secret benefactor. *Psychoanalytic Study of the Child, 47*, 279–298.

30. Hymer, S. (1982). The therapeutic nature of confessions. *Journal of Contemporary Psychotherapy, 13*, 129–143.

31. Schwartz, R. S. (1984). Confidentiality and secret-keeping on an inpatient unit. *Psychiatry, 47*, 279–284.

32. Saffer, J. B., Sansone, P., & Gentry, J. (1979). The awesome burden upon the child who must keep a family secret. *Child Psychiatry and Human Development, 10*, 35–40.

33. Eaker, B. (1906). Unlocking the family secret in family play therapy. *Child and Adolescent Social Work, 3*, 235 253.

34. Pincus, L., & Dare, C. (1978). *Secrets in the family.* New York: Pantheon Books.

35. Avery, N. (1982). Family secrets. *Psychoanalytic Review, 69*, 471–486.

36. Gutheil, T., & Avery, N. (1977). Multiple overt incest as family defense against loss. *Family Process, 16*, 106–116.

37. Vangelisti, A. L. (1994). Family secrets: Forms, functions, and correlates. *Journal of Social and Personal Relationships, 11*, 113–135.

38. Swanson, L., & Biaggio, M. K. (1985). Therapeutic perspectives on father-daughter incest. *American Journal of Psychiatry, 142*, 667–674.

39. Shlien, J. (1984). Secrets and the psychology of secrecy. In R. Levant & J. Shlien (Eds.), *Client centered therapy and the person centered approach* (pp. 390–399). New York: Praeger.

40. Murphy, B. (1989). Lesbian couples and their parents: The effects of perceived parental attitudes on the couples. *Journal of Counseling & Development, 68*, 46–51.

41. Paul, N. L., & Bloom, J. D. (1970). Multiple-family therapy: Secrets and scapegoating in family crisis. *International Journal of Group Psychotherapy, 20(1)*, 37–47.

42. Hoorwitz, A. (1983). Guidelines for treating father-daughter incest. *Social Casework: The Journal of Contemporary Social Work, Nov.*, 515–524.

43. Hays, K. F. (1987). The conspiracy of silence revisited: Group therapy with adult survivors of incest. *Journal of Group Psychotherapy, Psychodrama, & Sociometry, 39*, 143–156.

44. Lindberg, F. H., & Distad, L. J. (1985) Survival responses to incest: Adolescents in crisis. *Child Abuse & Neglect, 9*, 521–526.

45. Russell, D. E. (1986). *The secret trauma: Incest in the lives of girls and women.* New York: Basic Books.

46. Lubell, D, & Soong, W. (1982). Group therapy with sexually abused adolescents. *Canadian Journal of Psychiatry, 27*, 311–315.

47. Black, C. (1981). Innocent bystanders at risk: The children of alcoholics. *Alcoholism*, 22–26.

48. Kaufman, I., Peck, A., & Tagiuri, C. (1954). The family constellation and overt incestuous relations between father-daughter. *American Journal of Orthopsychiatry, 24*, 266–279.

49. Butler, S. (1978). *Conspiracy of silence: The trauma of incest.* San Francisco: New Glide.
50. Herman, J. (1981). *Father-daughter incest.* Cambridge: Harvard University Press.
51. Geiser, R. (1979). *Hidden victims: The sexual abuse of children.* Boston: Beacon.
52. Goodwin, S. (1982). *Sexual abuse: Incest victims and their families.* Boston: John Wright.
53. Justice, B., & Justice, R. (1979). *The broken taboo: Sex in the family.* New York: Human Sciences Press.
54. Meiselman, K. C. (1978). *Incest.* San Francisco: Jossey-Bass.
55. Tsai, M., & Wagner, N. N. (1978). Therapy groups for women sexually molested as children. *Archives of Sexual Behavior, 7,* 417–427.
56. Brown, E. (1991). Dealing with secret affairs in psychotherapy. In E. Brown (Ed.), *From patterns of infidelity and their treatment* (pp. 53–73). New York: Brunner-Mazel.
57. Pittman, F. (1989). *Private lies.* New York: Norton.
58. Richardson, L. (1988). Secrecy and status: The social construction of forbidden relationships. *American Sociological Review, 53,* 209–219.
59. Westfall, A. (1989). Extramarital sex: The treatment of the couple. In G. R. Weeks (Ed.), *Treating couples* (pp. 163–190). New York: Brunner/Mazel.
60. Cass, V. (1979). Homosexual identity formation: A theoretical model. *Journal of Homosexuality, 4,* 219–235.
61. Hencken, J., & O'Dowd, W. T. (1977). Coming out as an aspect of identity formation. *Gay Academic Union Journal: Gai Saber, 1,* 18–22.
62. Ponse, B. (1978). *Identities in the lesbian world.* Westport, CT: Greenwood.
63. Sophie, J. (1988). Internalized homophobia and lesbian identity. In E. Coleman (Ed.), *Integrated identity for gay men and lesbians* (pp. 53–65). New York: Harrington Park.
64. Roth, S. (1985). Psychotherapy with lesbian couples: Individual issues, female socialization, and the social context. *Journal of Marital and Family Therapy, 11,* 273–286.
65. Chafetez, J., Sampson, P., Beck, P., & West, J. (1974). A study of homosexual women. *Social Work, 19,* 714–723.
66. Jay, K., & Young, A. (1979). *The gay report.* New York: Summit Books.
67. Mendola, M. (1980). *The Mendola Report: A new look at gay couples.* New York: Crown.
68. Evans, N. (1976). Mourning as a family secret. *Journal of the American Academy of Child Psychiatry, 15,* 502–509.
69. Winnicott, D. W. (1980). *Playing and reality.* New York: Penguin Books.
70. Bor, R., Miller, R., Scher, I., & Salt, H. (1991). The practice of counseling HIV/AIDS clients. *British Journal of Guidance and Counseling, 19,* 129–138.
71. Greif, G., & Porembski, E. (1988). Implications for therapy with significant others of persons with AIDS. *Journal of Gay & Lesbian Psychotherapy, 1,* 79–86.

72. Miller, R., Goldman, E., & Bor, R. (1994). Application of a family systems approach to working with people affected by HIV disease—two case studies. *Journal of Family Therapy, 16*, 295–312.

73. Larson, D. G., & Chastain, R. L. (1990). Self-concealment: Conceptualization, measurement, and health implications. *Journal of Social and Clinical Psychology, 9*, 439–455.

74. Kelly, A. E., & Achter, J. A. (1995). Self-concealment and attitudes toward counseling in university students. *Journal of Counseling Psychology, 42*, 40–46.

75. Ichiyama, M. A., Colbert, D., Laramore, H., Heim, M., Carone, K., & Schmidt, J. (1993). Self-concealment and correlates of adjustment in college students. *Journal of College Student Psychotherapy, 7*, 55–68.

76. Kelly, A. E. (1998). Clients' secret keeping in outpatient therapy. *Journal of Counseling Psychology, 45*, 50–57.

77. Pennebaker, J. W., & Susman, J. R. (1988). Disclosure of traumas and psychosomatic processes. *Social Science and Medicine, 26*, 327–332.

78. Cole, S. W., Kemeny, M. E., Taylor, S. E., Visscher, B. R., & Fahey, J. L. (1996). Accelerated course of human immunodeficiency virus infection in gay men who conceal their homosexual identity. *Psychosomatic Medicine, 58*, 219–231.

79. Cole, S. W., Kemeny, M. E., Taylor, S. E., & Visscher, B. R. (1996). Elevated physical health risk among gay men who conceal their homosexual identity. *Health Psychology, 15*, 243–251.

80. Pennebaker, J. W., & O'Heeron, R. C. (1984). Confiding in others and illness rate among spouses of suicide and accidental-death victims. *Journal of Abnormal Psychology, 93*, 473–476.

81. Spiegel, D., Bloom, J. H., Kraemer, H. C., & Gottheil, E. (1989). Effects of psychosocial treatment of patients with metastatic breast cancer. *Lancet, 2*, 888–891.

82. Pennebaker, J. W., & Beall, S. K. (1986). Confronting a traumatic event: Toward an understanding of inhibition and disease. *Journal of Abnormal Psychology, 95*, 274–281.

83. Pennebaker, J. W., Kiecolt-Glaser, J. K., & Glaser, R. (1988). Disclosure of traumas and immune function: Health implications for psychotherapy. *Journal of Consulting and Clinical Psychology, 56*, 239–245.

84. Petrie, K. J., Booth, R. J., Pennebaker, J. W., Davison, K. P., & Thomas, M. G. (1995). Disclosure of trauma and immune response to a hepatitis B vaccination program. *Journal of Consulting and Clinical Psychology, 63*, 787–792.

85. Pennebaker, J. W. (1997). *Opening up: The healing power of expressing emotions*. New York: Guilford Press.

86. Polivy, J. (1998). The effects of behavioral inhibition: Integrating internal cues, cognition, behavior, and affect. *Psychological Inquiry, 9*, 181–204.

87. Kelly, A. E., Klusas, J. A. von Weiss, R. T., & Kenny, C. (in press). What is it about revealing secrets that is beneficial? *Personality and Social Psychology Bulletin*.

88. Pennebaker, J. W., Maybe, T. J., & Francis, M. E. (1997). Linguistic predictors of adaptive bereavement. *Journal of Personality and Social Psychology, 72*, 863–871.

89. Zeigarnik, B. (1927). Uber das behalten von erledigten und unerledigten handlungen. *Psychologische Forschung, 9,* 1–85.
90. Cole, S. W., Kemeny, M. E., & Taylor, S. E. (1997). Social identity and physical health: Accelerated HIV progression in rejection-sensitive gay men. *Journal of Personality and Social Psychology, 72,* 320–335.
91. Kelly, A. E., Kahn, J. H., & Coulter, R. G., (1996). Client self-presentations at intake. *Journal of Counseling Psychology, 43,* 300–309.
92. Hill, C. E., Thompson, B. J., Cogar, M. C., & Denman, D. W. (1993). Beneath the surface of long-term therapy: Therapist and client report of their own and each other's covert processes. *Journal of Counseling Psychology, 40,* 278–287.
93. Norton, R., Feldman, C., & Tafoya, D. (1974). Risk parameters across types of secrets. *Journal of Counseling Psychology, 21,* 450–454.
94. Yalom, I. D. (1995). *The theory and practice of group psychotherapy (4th ed.).* New York: Basic Books.
95. Fazio, R. H., Effrein, E. A., & Falender, V. J. (1981). Self-perceptions following social interaction. *Journal of Personality and Social Psychology, 41,* 232–242.
96. Jones, E. E., Rhodewalt, F., Bugles, S., & Skelton, J. A. (1981). Effects of strategic self-presentation on subsequent self-esteem. *Journal of Personality and Social Psychology, 41,* 407–421.
97. Schlenker, B. R., Dlugolecki, D. W., & Doherty, K. (1994). The impact of self-presentations on self-appraisals and behavior: The power of public commitment. *Personality and Social Psychology Bulletin, 20,* 20–33.
98. Tice, D. M. (1992). Self-concept change and self-presentation: The looking glass self is also a magnifying glass. *Journal of Personality and Social Psychology, 63,* 435–451.
99. Kelly, A. E. (1999). Revealing personal secrets. *Current Directions in Psychological Science, 8,* 106–109.
100. Kelly, A. E., & McKillop, K. J. (1996). Consequences of revealing personal secrets. *Psychological Bulletin, 120,* 450–465.
101. Wegner, D. M. (1992). You can't always think what you want: Problems in the suppression of unwanted thoughts. In M. Zanna (Ed.), *Advances in experimental social psychology* (Vol. 25, pp. 193–225). San Diego, CA: Academic Press.
102. Wegner, D. M. (1994). Ironic processes of mental control. *Psychological Review, 101,* 34–52.
103. Kobocow, B., McGuire, J. M., & Blau, B. J. (1983). The influence of confidentiality conditions on self-disclosure of early adolescence. *Professional Psychology, 4,* 435–443.
104. Woods, K., & McNamara, J. R. (1980). Confidentiality: Its effect on interviewee behavior. *Professional Psychology, 11,* 714–721.
105. Christophe, V., & Rime, B. (1997). Exposure to the social sharing of emotion: Emotional impact, listener responses and secondary social sharing. *European Journal of Social Psychology, 27,* 37–54.
106. Henley, N. M. (1973). Power, sex, and nonverbal communication. *Berkeley Journal of Sociology, 18,* 1–26.
107. Schlenker, B. R. (1986). Self-identification: Toward an integration of

the private and public self. In R. Baumeister (Ed.), *Public self and private self* (pp. 21–62). New York: Springer-Verlag.

108. Rogers, C. R. (1951). *Client-centered therapy: Its current practice, implications, and theory.* Boston: Houghton Mifflin.

109. Rogers, C. R. (1957). The necessary and sufficient conditions of therapeutic personality change. *Journal of Consulting Psychology, 21,* 95–103.

110. Grencavage, L. M., & Norcross, J. C. (1990). Where are the commonalities among the therapeutic common factors? *Professional Psychology: Research and Practice, 21,* 372–378.

111. Horvath, A. O., & Luborsky, L. (1993). The role of the therapeutic alliance in psychotherapy. *Journal of Consulting and Clinical Psychology, 61,* 561–573.

112. Beutler, L. E., Machado, P. P. P., & Neufeldt, S. A. (1994). Therapist variables. In A. E. Bergin & S. L. Garfield (Eds), *Handbook of psychotherapy and behavior change* (4th ed., pp. 229–269). New York: John Wiley & Sons.

113. Elliott, R. (1985). Helpful and nonhelpful events in brief counseling interviews: An empirical taxonomy. *Journal of Counseling Psychology, 32,* 307–322.

114. Hill, C. E. (1992). Research on therapist techniques in brief individual therapy: Implications for practitioners. *The Counseling Psychologist, 20,* 689–711.

115. Miell, D. E., & Duck, S. W. (1986). Strategies in developing friendship. In V. J. Derlega & B. A. Winstead (Eds.), *Friendship and social interaction* (pp. 129–144). New York: Springer-Verlag.

116. Duck, S. W. (1988). *Relating to others.* Pacific Grove, CA: Brooks/Cole.

117. Regan, A. M., & Hill, C. E. (1992). Investigation of what clients and counselors do not say in brief therapy. *Journal of Counseling Psychology, 39,* 240–246.

11

A Look at the Coping Strategies and Styles of Asian Americans: Similar and Different?

Edward C. Chang

Where there is great doubt, there will be great awakening; small doubt, small awakening; no doubt, no awakening.

—Zen saying

Although we have learned a great deal about how individuals cope with stressful life situations, most of what we know is limited to individuals of European background. In fact, according to Graham (1), the authors publishing in some of America's leading and internationally respected psychology journals have continued over the past decade to focus on the behaviors of Caucasian Americans. Hence, despite the growth of minority populations and the increases in biracial and bicultural subpopulations in America today (2), there has been little apparent effort to study ethnically and racially diverse samples of people.

Given this limitation, I will focus on one minority group—Asian Americans—to see if and how their coping behaviors might differ from that of Caucasian Americans. Although the coping behaviors of other ethnic minorities also are worth examination, the coping behaviors of Asian Americans might be of particular interest because, unlike other ethnic minorities, they have been touted in American society as the "model minority" (3, 4). Yet, we know very little about this "model minority."

In this chapter, I will begin by noting some of the important issues and concerns in understanding Asian Americans. I then will examine the coping behaviors of Asian Americans based on my previous work related to their coping strategies and styles (5, 6). Finally, I will close by discussing the implications of these findings, as well as what we need to do subsequently in order to understand better the coping behaviors of Asian Americans.

Asian Americans: Not Just One

Just as it is incorrect to say that all Caucasian Americans look or act the same, it is important to realize that Asian Americans are a very diverse population. Although genetically influenced features such as the skin color of Asian Americans might indicate more racial similarity to each other than to other racial groups, they are not all the same. In fact, in regard to ethnic factors such as language and cultural practices, Asian Americans look and sound quite different from each other.

According to Uba (7), one can enumerate as many as 25 distinct Asian American ethnic groups living in the United States. Each of these ethnic groups differs across a number of important dimensions, including their history of living in the United States. For example, while Chinese and Japanese Americans typically have been members of American society for several decades (8), Korean and Vietnamese Americans have immigrated more recently (9).

Nonetheless, although sharing similar immigration histories, Chinese and Japanese Americans are not alike. As a tragic historical example, consider the treatments of Chinese and Japanese Americans in the United States during World War II. Unlike Chinese Americans, about 120,000 Japanese Americans, many of whom were U.S. citizens, were transported to internment camps. This prejudicial treatment experienced by many *Nisei* (second generation) Japanese Americans has profoundly influenced *Sansei* (third generation) Japanese Americans. According to Nagata (10), third generation Japanese Americans not only struggle with the same problems their parents did, but they also struggle to believe and trust in American society. For these reasons, some researchers have argued that the term Asian American itself is misleading and potentially harmful if important differences are not considered between and within the different ethnic groups (11, 12). In that regard, although I will talk about Asian Americans, I definitely am *not* implying that they are all the same.

In this chapter, I cannot explore the coping of each Asian American ethnic group because there is too little research on any specific Asian ethnic group. Hence, in keeping with this generalist framework, in the studies conducted over the past several years (some which I will present shortly), I typically have focused on studying Asian Americans in general (e.g., 13, 14, 15, 16). Moreover, while I believe that there are important differences that need to be illuminated within the Asian American population, there also are many important shared Asian American attributes that transcend those racial dissimilarities. A prime example that I will discuss subsequently in greater detail is the tendency of Asian American ethnic groups to value collectivism.

Cultural Roots of Individualism and Collectivism

In recent years, psychologists have joined anthropologists, sociologists, and even linguists in recognizing how cultural differences influence human behavior (17, 18). In particular, a growing number of psychologists have emphasized distinguishing between largely individualistic or collectivist cultures (19). Noteworthy, Western cultures have been described as individualistic, with individuals seeking independence from others by attending to self-based needs and desires (20). As an example, this Western individualism is reflected in doctrines such as the Declaration of Independence.

In contrast, the focus in Eastern cultures has been on the individual maintaining a fundamental relatedness with others (21). Hence, attending to others, harmonious interdependence, and fitting in not only are valued but also often are expected (4, 22). Within the Asian family, where order, hierarchy, and duty are expected and valued, there is the important notion of *filial piety*. Thus, Asian Americans are raised to have an almost unconditional respect for and duty to their parents, as well as to their other cherished elder figures. Similarly, the notion of *"loss of face"* often is a process experienced not just by the Asian individual but by an entire family. This collectivism also is consistent with the rich philosophical and religious traditions of Eastern cultures (23). For example, one of the Four Noble Truths in Buddhism is that all existence entails suffering. To reach a state of enlightenment, therefore, one need only to eliminate individual desires.

According to Markus and Kitayama (21), these Eastern and Western cultural differences not only promote two relatively distinct notions of the self, but they also differentiate the thoughts, feelings, and actions of individuals from such cultures. Indeed, given that much of the coping research has used Caucasian American research participants, one would expect different results with individuals from Eastern cultures (e.g., Asian Americans). An examination of how Asian Americans might differ in their coping behaviors from Caucasian Americans, however, also will depend on the specific coping model being considered. For example, in some models of coping, the emphases are on the importance of coping strategies that are based on responses to specific situations, whereas in other models, the foci are on general, dispositional-like tendencies related to coping behavior. Hence, I will look at the coping behaviors of Asian Americans across different coping models to obtain a more pluralistic view of their coping strategies and styles. I will begin with one of the most popular models of coping in the research literature.

Lazarus and Folkman's Stress and Coping Model

According to Lazarus and Folkman (24), *coping* refers to the behavioral and cognitive efforts that people use to manage the internal and external demands of a stressful situation. In their view, coping can be classified as either problem- or emotion-focused. *Problem-focused coping* involves activities focusing directly on changing elements of the stressful situation. For example, if I knew I had to prepare for a difficult exam, I would consider what I had to do to meet the challenge and take specific actions such as outlining my notes and memorizing key facts. *Emotion-focused coping* involves modifications made in one's internal reactions to the stressful situation. As in my example, rather than take any explicit action to prepare for the exam, I could decide to get my mind off of worrying by going out to have some fun with my friends.

Some psychologists, however, suggest that coping reflects approach versus avoidance behaviors. In this regard, Suls and Fletcher (25) define *approach* coping as the use of strategies that focus on both the source of stress and reactions to it, whereas *avoidant* coping is the use of strategies that place the focus away from both the source of stress and reactions to it. Approach and avoidance coping and problem-focused and emotion-focused coping, however, need not reflect mutually exclusive coping models. On this point, Tobin, Holroyd, Reynolds, and Wigal (20) conceptualized coping strategies so as to take into account all these elements. They accomplished this through the development of the Coping Strategies Inventory (CSI), a multidimensional coping measure of both engaged (approach) and disengaged (avoidance) problem-focused and emotion-focused coping strategies.

Asian American Coping Strategies

I now report on the data in which I compared the coping strategies of Asian and Caucasian Americans. In one study looking at cultural differences, coping, and adjustment, 45 self-identified Asian Americans and 49 self-identified Caucasian Americans completed several measures, including the CSI (26). All participants were college students from a large northeast public university.

Eight coping strategies are measured by the different CSI scales. Problem Solving is associated with efforts to engage in specific problem solving steps (e.g., "I made a plan of action and followed it"). Cognitive Restructuring involves efforts to think about the stressful situation in a more positive manner (e.g., "I looked at things in a different light and tried to make the best of what was available"). Express Emotions tap efforts to deal with stress by expressing one's emotions (e.g., "I let my emotions go"), similar to Freud's notion of catharsis. Social Support involves efforts to obtain emotional support from others (e.g., "I talked to someone about how I was feeling"). These four scales measure engaged and more adaptive coping efforts.

Problem Avoidance is associated with efforts to not deal with the problem situation at hand (e.g., "I wished that the situation would go away or somehow be over with"). Wishful Thinking involves efforts to think that a stressful situation simply will resolve itself (e.g., "I hoped a miracle would happen"). Self-Criticism gets at an excessive preoccupation with one's lack of ability to deal with the situation (e.g., "I criticized myself for what happened"). Social Withdrawal taps efforts to distance oneself from the problem and from others who might be able to help with the problem (e.g., "I avoided my family and friends"). These four scales represent disengaged and more maladaptive coping efforts.

In addition to responses on the CSI, participants also completed the Satisfaction With Life Scale or SWLS (27) to measure global life satisfaction, and the Beck Depression Inventory or BDI (28) to measure depressive symptoms. These two adjustment measures were used to examine the extent to which the relations between coping strategies and adjustment were similar or different for Asian and Caucasian Americans.

Based on the view that Asian and Caucasian Americans are guided by two differing notions of the self (viz., interdependent versus independent), each with different ways of thinking, feeling, and acting, it follows that these ethnic groups also may vary in their coping strategies. The results comparing the mean differences of the two ethnic groups on each of the CSI coping strategies are presented in Table 11.1.

As you can see, the two ethnic groups generally are similar on their reported use of specific coping strategies when dealing with a stressful situation, *with two exceptions*—Asian as compared to Caucasian Americans reported more Problem Avoidance and Social Withdrawal. Although one might interpret these findings as suggesting more maladaptive coping strategies for the Asian relative to the Caucasian Americans, remember that both samples were from a normal (i.e., nonclinical) college student population. Thus, what "works" for Asian relative to Caucasian Americans simply might be different, *not necessarily more ineffective*. Nonetheless, it also is important to realize that a simple examination of the mean differences reveals very little about how these coping strategies relate to other important variables. Therefore, I now present the relations between coping strategies and adjustment.

The correlations between the eight CSI scale scores and the scores on the SWLS and the BDI are presented in Table 11.2. As can be seen in this table, many similarities, as well as important ethnic differences, emerge in the relational patterns between coping strategies and outcomes. For both Asian and Caucasian Americans, greater Problem Solving efforts were associated significantly with greater life satisfaction, but not with significantly lower depressive symptoms. Conversely, greater Social Withdrawal for both ethnic groups was associated with greater depressive symptoms, but not with significantly lower life satisfaction.

On the other hand, despite the lack of a mean difference on Self-Criticism noted earlier, the use of this coping strategy was related significantly to lower life satisfaction and depressive symptoms for Caucasian Americans, but only to greater depressive symptoms for Asian Americans. Likewise, in comparison to Caucasian Americans, it is interesting to note that the Asian Americans' higher mean scores on Problem Avoidance were

Table 11.1 Mean Ethnic Differences Between Asian and Caucasian
Americans on the Coping Strategies Inventory (CSI)

	Ethnic Group		
CSI Scale	Asian	Caucasian	p
Problem Solving	27.07 (6.51)	26.16 (6.14)	ns
Cognitive Restructuring	27.04 (6.47)	27.47 (6.68)	ns
Express Emotions	23.87 (7.00)	25.18 (8.19)	ns
Social Support	27.24 (6.55)	29.04 (7.57)	ns
Problem Avoidance	21.91 (5.41)	18.02 (5.41)	<.01
Wishful Thinking	26.22 (6.92)	25.84 (8.78)	ns
Self-Criticism	22.80 (7.19)	20.00 (9.88)	ns
Social Withdrawal	22.82 (6.26)	18.16 (6.13)	<.001

Note. For Asian Americans, $n = 45$; for Caucasian Americans, $n = 49$.
Numbers in parentheses are standard deviations. ns = not significant.

Table 11.2 Relations Between Coping Strategies and Life Satisfaction and
Depressive Symptoms

CSI Scale	Life Satisfaction	Depressive Symptoms
Problem Solving	.36*	−.16
	(.36*)	(−.13)
Cognitive Restructuring	.41**	−.37**
	(.45***)	(−.23)
Express Emotions	.16	−.16
	(.07)	(.17)
Social Support	.19	−.29
	(.09)	(.05)
Problem Avoidance	.03	.05
	(−.12)	(.10)
Wishful Thinking	−.27	.24
	(−.28)	(.26)
Self-Criticism	−.25	.29*
	(−.46***)	(.43**)
Social Withdrawal	−.25	.30*
	(−.28)	(.29*)

Note. For Asian Americans, $n = 45$; for Caucasian Americans, $n = 49$.
Numbers in parentheses are for Caucasian Americans. CSI = Coping Strategies Inventory.
*$p < .05$; **$p < .01$; ***$p < .001$.

not related reliably to lower life satisfaction or greater depressive symptoms. Thus, the Asian Americans' heightened use of "disengaged" coping strategies was not associated with greater maladjustment.

Based on these CSI findings, taken together, one can discern differences in Asian and Caucasian Americans in their use of coping strategies, as well as the potential influences of these strategies on psychological adjustment.

Epstein's Constructive Thinking Model of Experiential Coping

In some ways similar to and yet distinct from Lazarus and Folkman's (24) coping model, Epstein (29, 30) has developed a model of coping that involves the way people generally respond to their external environments based on past experiences. In Epstein's (30) Cognitive-Experiential Self-Theory, or CEST, personality is composed of three relatively distinct conceptual systems: a rational; an experiential; and an associationist. The operations of the experiential system play a prominent role in facilitating effective coping with environmental stressors. Based on past experiences, one purported response to the environment is to maintain a balance of pleasure over pain. When people feel good, they continue the activities promoting such feelings. In contrast, when people feel bad, they discontinue any causative related activities. Accordingly, the experiential system is involved with the maintenance and promotion of positive well being. Moreover, the operations of this system are purported to be fast, influenced by experiences, and slow to change.

To measure attributes of this experiential system, Epstein and Meier (31) developed the Constructive Thinking Inventory (CTI). The CTI was developed to tap constructive and destructive thought patterns emerging from past experiences. Unlike the focus on particular coping strategies for specific stressful situations in the CSI, the CTI focuses on trait-like ways of thinking and coping. Based on recent studies conducted by Epstein and his associates (31, 32, 33), it appears that individuals who express greater constructive thinking (e.g., "I look at challenges not as something to fear, but as an opportunity to test myself and learn") are better able to cope with stressful situations than those who express greater destructive thinking (e.g., "I spend much more time mentally rehearsing my failures than remembering my successes"). Furthermore, if cultural differences influence how Asian and Caucasian Americans experience their worlds, then their experiential systems (as measured by the CTI) should be relatively distinct.

Constructive Thinking Styles of Asian Americans

In a study of cultural differences in constructive thinking and adjustment, 64 self-identified Asian Americans and 175 self-identified Caucasian Americans participated (all college students attending a large public university in the northeast; 6). Participants completed a version of the CTI tapping three constructive and four destructive thinking styles. Global Constructive Thinking involves elements from all of the other CTI scales, except Naive Optimism. In general, higher scores on the global scale reflect greater constructive thinking ability. Emotional Coping refers to the tendency not to take things personally, not to be sensitive to disapproval, and not to worry excessively about failure (e.g., "If I said something foolish when I spoke up in a group, I would chalk it up to experience and not worry about it"). Behavioral Coping is associated with the tendency to think in ways that promote effective action (e.g., "When I realize I have made a mistake, I usually take immediate action to correct it"). Both the Behavioral Coping and Emotional Coping scales are believed to tap distinct constructive dimensions of coping, similar to Lazarus and Folkman's (24) distinction between problem-focused and emotion-focused coping, respectively. Categorical Thinking involves the tendency to think in overly rigid and extreme ways (e.g., "There are two kinds of people in this world, winners and losers"). Superstitious Thinking refers to beliefs in personal superstitions (e.g., "I sometimes think that if I want something to happen too badly, it will keep it from happening"). Esoteric thinking is associated with beliefs related to matters such as astrology and ghosts (e.g., "I believe the moon or the stars can affect people's thinking"). Naive Optimism involves gross overgeneralizations following positive outcomes (e.g., "When something good happens to me, I feel that more good things are likely to follow"). These latter four scales reflect destructive dimensions of coping.

In the previously described study (5), in addition to obtaining responses on the CTI, participants also were asked to complete the SWLS and the BDI so as to examine whether the relations between constructive and destructive coping styles and adjustment were similar for Asian and Caucasian Americans. The results of comparing the means on the CTI scales for Asian Americans and Caucasian Americans are presented in Table 11.3. As can be observed in the table, the only similarity was on one scale—Behavioral Coping. Otherwise, Asian as compared to Caucasian Americans expressed lower scores on Emotional Coping and higher scores on Superstitious Thinking, Categorical Thinking, Esoteric Thinking, and Naive Optimism. Not surprisingly, Asian as compared to Caucasian Americans also reported lower scores on Global Constructive Thinking.

Again, although one might conclude from these findings that Asian Americans manifest poorer experientially based coping than their Caucasian counterparts, it first is necessary to look at how these coping styles relate to adjustment for the two ethnic groups. The correlations between the CTI scales with the SWLS and the BDI for Asian and Caucasian Americans are presented in Table 11.4. Consistent with CEST, Emotional Coping and Behavioral Coping both were related significantly to greater life satisfaction and lower depressive symptoms for Asian and Caucasian Americans. As one might expect, Global Constructive Thinking in both Asian and Caucasian Americans also was associated strongly with higher life satisfac-

Table 11.3 Mean Ethnic Differences Between Asian and Caucasian Americans on the Constructive Thinking Inventory (CTI)

| | Ethnic group | | |
CTI Scale	Asian	Caucasian	p
Global Constructive Thinking	92.08 (15.92)	98.17 (17.01)	<.05
Emotional Coping	73.39 (17.29)	79.18 (16.42)	<.05
Behavioral Coping	50.36 (6.70)	52.16 (7.05)	ns
Superstitious Thinking	20.23 (5.40)	17.36 (4.69)	<.001
Categorical Thinking	46.19 (7.62)	43.38 (7.89)	<.05
Esoteric Thinking	38.66 (7.11)	35.63 (9.59)	<.05
Naive Optimism	53.56 (6.68)	51.03 (6.04)	<.01

Note. For Asian Americans, $n = 64$; for Caucasian Americans, $n = 175$. Numbers in parentheses are standard deviations. ns = not significant.

Table 11.4 Relations Between Constructive Thinking and Life Satisfaction and Depressive Symptoms

CTI Scale	Life Satisfaction	Depressive Symptoms
Global Constructive Thinking	.46***	−.40***
	(.40***)	(−.50***)
Emotional Coping	.44***	−.35**
	(.39***)	(−.52***)
Behavioral Coping	.48***	−.28*
	(.36***)	(−.40***)
Superstitious Thinking	−.33**	.34**
	(−.47***)	(.47***)
Categorical Thinking	−.14	.27*
	(−.11)	(.22**)
Esoteric Thinking	−.03	.24
	(−.09)	(.22**)
Naive Optimism	.13	.06
	(.21**)	(−.13)

Note. For Asian Americans, $n = 64$; for Caucasian Americans, $n = 175$. Numbers in parentheses are for Caucasian Americans. CTI = Constructive Thinking Inventory.
*$p < .05$; **$p < .01$; ***$p < .001$.

tion and lower depressive symptoms. Some important exceptions, however, should be noted. For example, despite Asian Americans scoring higher on Esoteric Thinking, this was not associated with lower life satisfaction or greater depressive symptoms. In contrast, Esoteric Thinking was associated significantly with greater depressive symptoms for Caucasian Americans. Likewise, despite the higher scores on Naive Optimism among Asian Americans, this was not associated significantly with life satisfaction or depressive symptoms for this ethnic group. In contrast, for Caucasian Americans, Naive Optimism was associated with greater life satisfaction, but not significantly related to fewer depressive symptoms. This last finding fits well with a review showing that people's expression of positive illusions in the West is positively associated with adjustment (34).

Taken together, these findings again reveal that there not only are magnitudinal coping differences between Asian and Caucasian Americans, but there also are important relational differences in what is conceived as destructive coping elements.

D'Zurilla's Rational Coping Model

Although there are some differences and similarities between Asian and Caucasian Americans on measures of experientially based coping styles, such findings do little to illuminate potential differences and similarities between the two ethnic groups across their rational systems. To look at this issue, I now examine a final coping model, one that focuses on the rational system as it applies to the real word.

According to D'Zurilla and Nezu (35), *social problem solving* refers to problem solving as it occurs in the real world. More specifically, it is defined as the self-generated cognitive-affective-behavioral process by which a person attempts to discover effective ways of coping with daily problematic situations. Thus, stressful situations are synonymous with problems in living, and they require some sort of coping action. The importance of this multifaceted construct has been consistently documented in recent years when researchers have found a significant link between problem-solving deficits and maladjustment (36, 37). Moreover, in a growing number of studies examining suicidal risk in college populations, investigators have shown repeatedly that problem-solving deficits also are significantly associated with greater hopelessness and suicide ideation (15, 38).

According to D'Zurilla and his associates (39, 40, 41), social problem solving has been found to reflect five relatively distinct dimensions as measured by the Social Problem Solving Inventory-Revised (SPSI-R). If cultural differences influence the way in which Asian and Caucasian Americans cope, we should find that the social problem solving styles of these two ethnic groups are not identical.

Social Problem Solving Among Asian Americans

In the previously mentioned study in which the CSI was used (5), the SPSI-R also was administered. The SPSI-R is composed of five scales. Positive Problem Orientation involves constructive ways of thinking about a problem (e.g., "When I have a problem, I usually believe that there is a solution for it"). Negative Problem Orientation taps destructive ways of thinking about a problem, as well as the negative emotions that are associated with it (e.g., "I usually feel threatened and afraid when I have an important problem to solve"). Not surprisingly, these dimensions of social problem solving have been found to be related to, but not redundant with, dimensions of constructive and destructive thinking (39). Rational Problem Solving Style reflects the deliberate and systematic use of problem-solving skills to deal with a problem (e.g., "Before I try to think of a solution to a problem, I usually set a specific goal that makes clear exactly what I want to accomplish"). Implusivity/Carelessness Style involves problem solving efforts that are acted upon impulsively and without much deliberation (e.g., "When I am attempting to solve a problem, I usually go with the first good idea that comes to mind"). Avoidance Style gets at efforts to procrastinate and take little action in dealing with the problem at hand (e.g., "I usually go out of my way to avoid having to deal with problems in my life"). Of these dimensions, only Positive Problem Orientation and Rational Problem Solving are believed to reflect positive or adaptive problem-solving dimensions.

The mean differences on the SPSI-R scale scores for Asian and Caucasian Americans are presented in Table 11.5. We observe in this table that there was only one significant difference between Asian and Caucasian Americans. Specifically, Asian compared to Caucasian Americans reported more impulsively when attempting to solve or deal with a problem. This finding is consistent with those from another study in which Asian Americans reported higher Impulsivity/Carelessness than did Caucasian Americans (15).

Table 11.5 Mean Ethnic Differences Between Asian and Caucasian Americans on the Social Problem Solving Inventory-Revised (SPSI-R)

SPSI-R Scale	Ethnic Group		p
	Asian	Caucasian	
Positive Problem Orientation	12.16 (3.82)	11.78 (3.41)	ns
Negative Problem Orientation	19.78 (7.81)	17.43 (7.60)	ns
Rational Problem Solving Style	46.60 (11.43)	45.47 (14.11)	ns
Impulsivity/Carelessness Style	16.98 (7.54)	12.76 (6.97)	$<.01$
Avoidance Style	11.06 (5.15)	9.20 (5.70)	ns

Note. For Asian Americans, $n = 45$; for Caucasian Americans, $n = 49$. Numbers in parentheses are standard deviations. ns = not significant.

Table 11.6 Relations Between Social Problem Solving and Life
Satisfaction and Depressive Symptoms

SPSI-R Scale	Life Satisfaction	Depressive Symptoms
Positive Problem Orientation	.46***	−.47***
	(.24)	(−.30*)
Negative Problem Orientation	−.41**	.60***
	(−.36*)	.54***
Rational Problem Solving Style	.13	.08
	(.17)	(−.10)
Impulsivity/Carelessness Style	−.22	.17
	(−.14)	(.15)
Avoidance Style	−.24	.29
	(−.44***)	(.28*)

Note. For Asian Americans, $n = 45$; for Caucasian Americans, $n = 49$.
Numbers in parentheses are for Caucasian Americans. SPSI-R = Social
Problem-Solving Inventory-Revised.
* $p < .05$; ** $p < .01$; *** $p < .001$.

It is important to look again at the relationships of these five social problem
solving dimensions with adjustment. The correlations between the SPSI-R
scales with measures of adjustment are presented in Table 11.6, where it
can be seen that similarities and differences again were found to be independent of magnitudinal differences (or lack thereof) between two ethnic
groups. As shown in Table 11.5, there were no significant differences between the Positive Problem Orientation of Asians ($M = 12.16$) and Caucasians ($M = 11.78$). Yet, for Asian Americans, higher scores on Positive Problem Orientation were significantly correlated with greater life satisfaction
and lower depressive symptoms; for Caucasian Americans, however,
higher scores on Positive Problem Orientation were significantly correlated
with lower depressive symptoms only. Moreover, despite the fact that the
Asian compared to Caucasian Americans report significantly higher scores
on Impulsivity/Carelessness, this seemingly "maladaptive" problem solving style was not associated with significantly less life satisfaction, nor with
greater depressive symptoms.

Thus, although there were considerable similarities in the magnitude
and relational pattern of social problem solving, some differences also were
observed across Asian and Caucasian American coping styles.

Discussion

As noted earlier, Asian and Caucasian Americans come from differing cultural backgrounds. Whereas most Asian Americans interact with their
world from a collectivist frame of reference, Caucasian Americans typically

act from an individualist framework. Given these cultural differences, Asian Americans should cope with stress somewhat differently than Caucasian Americans. Of note, significant differences were found between these two ethnic groups when we examined three different models of coping. Moreover, even when magnitudinal differences were not found on a given coping dimension, relations with measures of adjustment sometimes differed for Asian and Caucasian Americans.

Perhaps the most interesting findings in this chapter are those pertaining to the considerable differences between Asian and Caucasian Americans on measures of experientially based coping. Recall, significant differences were found on all but one coping dimension measured by the CTI. In contrast, little difference was found on the SPSI-R, which has been considered a measure of rationally based coping. Insofar that constructive and destructive coping styles are influenced by experience (30), one could ask what types of experiences might differentiate Asian from Caucasian Americans. In that regard, several factors may be considered. For example, unlike Caucasian Americans, Asian Americans are delegated a minority status in the United States. Furthermore, Asian Americans are faced with a paradox in that they are viewed as a model minority (4), while also enduring racial prejudices. Likewise, the collectivism of most Asian Americans may pose a constant source of stress in an individualistic society (42). Lastly, differences in residency, language, ethnic identity, and cultural customs add to the stress experienced by Asians in America.

Future Directions in Studying Asian American Coping Behaviors: The Challenge Ahead

In this chapter, my goal was not to provide a definitive statement about the coping behaviors of Asian Americans. Rather, I aimed for a more modest goal—the preliminary examination of the coping behaviors of Asian Americans. To obtain a better understanding of how Asian Americans cope, several conceptual and methodological issues will need to be addressed in future research.

First, studies that involve large samples of Asian Americans are needed if we are to look at both between-group (e.g., comparisons with mainland Asians, Caucasian Americans) as well as within-group (e.g., Korean Americans compared with Chinese Americans) differences in coping behaviors. Unfortunately, as noted at the beginning of this chapter, studies on ethnic minorities in general have been the exception rather than the rule. In that regard, it is important for researchers to gain a greater appreciation for the value of testing their models and measures on a more representative sample of the diverse and ever-changing population living in the United States. In the absence of such efforts, what some might find to be a meaningful model for one group, unintentionally might be presented as a cultural standard for another group (43).

Relatedly, insofar as most of the coping models presented in the research literature have been based on the study of Caucasian Americans, it also would be valuable to develop models of coping behavior that are derived from an understanding of Asian Americans. For example, coping behaviors related to dealing with stresses associated with the experiences of racism, prejudice, or acculturation rarely are explored in research. Somehow, those in the mainstream of coping research seem to continue ignoring how Asian Americans, and other ethnic minorities, are stressed by the forces of racism, prejudice, and acculturation as they cope with living in America (44).

In addition, cultural differences do not necessarily have to influence coping behaviors via a direct path. In fact, culture can influence other factors such as personality characteristics which, in turn, can influence coping behaviors (45). For example, although no differences were found in the present examination of Asian and Caucasian Americans on measures of problem solving (e.g., as assessed by the Problem Solving scale of CSI), Chang (13) found that the heightened pessimism of Asian Americans was associated positively with their employment of greater problem solving coping strategies, whereas the reverse was true for pessimistic Caucasian Americans. Another important personality variable has been perfectionism (46, 47). Noteworthy, Chang (15) again found important similarities and differences in the relations between perfectionism and social problem solving between Asian and Caucasian Americans.

Another issue that will need to be addressed if we are to gain a better understanding of the coping behaviors of Asian Americans is the role of development. As Aldwin (48) has noted, researchers often have failed to consider how coping behaviors change across time. For example, certain types of coping behaviors, although appropriate and effective at one point in development, might be quite inappropriate and ineffective at another point, and conversely. To understand the coping behaviors of Asian Americans, therefore, long-term prospective studies are needed for examining their coping behaviors over the entire life span, including late adulthood (49).

At the microlevel, new and innovated studies using Experience Sampling Method (ESM), which assesses behavior several times a day, over a typical course of a week, promise to provide interesting information about coping behavior that is not captured by typical self-report coping measures (50). In that regard, use of ESM also might provide important insights into the coping behaviors of Asian Americans as compared to that of Caucasian Americans. For example, in a recent study looking at the studying habits of Asian and Caucasian American adolescents, Asakawa and Csikszentmihalyi (51) found that Asian as compared to Caucasian Americans reported greater positive feelings when studying. This finding suggests that one possible factor related to the high educational attainments of Asian Americans is their enjoyment of the studying process.

Lastly, if we are to obtain a better sense of what coping behaviors are "maladaptive" or "adaptive" for Asian Americans, studies also will need to be conducted so as to compare the coping behaviors of Asian Americans across different levels of adjustment. Although this sounds simple enough, problems arise in the classification and assessment of adjustment among Asian Americans (7, 52). For example, according to Beck's (53, 54) cognitive model of major depression, pessimism is an important antecedent and hallmark of clinical depression. Similarly, expressions of pessimism also are considered an important sign for making a diagnosis of major depression based on the fourth edition of the *Diagnostic and Statistical Manual of Mental Disorders* (55). In two studies involving normal (i.e., nonclinical) college students, however, Chang (13, 14) found that Asian as compared to Caucasian American students expressed a higher level of pessimism, but that elevated pessimism was *not* related to greater maladjustment (e.g., dysphoria) for the Asian American students. Hence, this finding raises the problem of distinguishing between those elements (e.g., pessimism) that are truly indicative of maladjustment and psychopathology, and those that do not necessarily represent a vulnerability factor for illness. Until such basic issues are resolved, it will remain difficult to distinguish adaptive from maladaptive coping behaviors in Asian Americans.

Conclusion

In the present chapter, I have examined different models of coping among Asian and Caucasian Americans through the lens of presumed cultural differences. As I indicated previously, there are numerous questions that will need to be addressed before a more definitive statement can be made about the coping behaviors of Asian Americans. It will suffice for now, however, to submit the summarizing view that the coping strategies and styles expressed by Asian Americans appear both similar to and different from those of Caucasian Americans. It is now time to raise our doubts and work on the challenging issues raised by this latter summary.

Acknowledgments
I would like to thank C. R. Snyder for his valuable feedback on earlier versions of the present chapter. I also would like to acknowledge Chang Suk-Choon and Tae Myung-Sook for their encouragement and support throughout this project.

References

1. Graham, S. (1992). "Most of the subjects were White and middle class": Trends in published research on African Americans in selected APA journals, 1970–1989. *American Psychologist, 47*, 629–639.
2. Root, M. (Ed.) (1992). *Racially mixed people in America*. Newbury Park, CA: Sage.

3. Sue, S., & Okazaki, S. (1990). Asian-American educational achievements: A phenomenon in search of an explanation. *American Psychologist, 45*, 913–920.
4. Yee, A. H. (1992). Asians as stereotypes and students: Misperceptions that persist. *Educational Psychology Review, 4*, 95–132.
5. Chang, E. C. (1992). Coping strategies and styles, life satisfaction, and depressive symptoms in Asians and Caucasians. Unpublished raw data.
6. Chang, E. C. (1993). Social problem solving, life satisfaction, and depressive symptoms in Asians and Caucasians. Unpublished raw data.
7. Uba, L. (1994). *Asian Americans: Personality patterns, identity, and mental health.* New York: Guilford Press.
8. Daniels, R. (1988). *Asian America: Chinese and Japanese in the United States since 1850.* Seattle: University of Washington Press.
9. Takaki, R. (1989). *Strangers from a different shore: A history of Asian Americans.* Boston: Little Brown.
10. Nagata, D. (1991). Transgenerational impact of the Japanese American internment: Clinical issues in working with children of former internees. *Psychotherapy, 28*, 121–128.
11. Abe, J. S., & Zane, N. W. S. (1990). Psychological maladjustment among Asian and White American college students: Controlling for confounds. *Journal of Counseling Psychology, 37*, 437–444.
12. Phinney, J. (1996). When we talk about American ethnic groups, what do we mean? *American Psychologist, 51*, 918–927.
13. Chang, E. C. (1996a). Cultural differences in optimism, pessimism, and coping: Predictors of subsequent adjustment in Asian American and Caucasian American college students. *Journal of Counseling Psychology, 43*, 113–123.
14. Chang, E. C. (1996b). Evidence for the cultural specificity of pessimism in Asians versus Caucasians: A test of a general negativity hypothesis. *Personality and Individual Differences, 21*, 819–822.
15. Chang, E. C. (1998a). Cultural differences, perfectionism, and suicidal risk: Does social problem solving still matter? *Cognitive Therapy and Research, 22*, 237–254.
16. Chang, E. C. (1999). *Cultural differences in the assessment of psychological disturbance in Asian and Caucasian American college students: Examining the role of cognitive and affective concomitants of distress.* Manuscript submitted for publication.
17. Brislin, R. (1993). *Understanding culture's influence on behavior.* Fort Worth, TX: Harcourt Brace and Jovanovich.
18. Hofstede, G. (1980). *Culture's consequences.* Beverly Hills: Sage.
19. Triandis, H. C. (1995). *Individualism and collectivism.* Boulder, CO: Westview Press.
20. Greenwald, A. G. (1980). The totalitarian ego: Fabrication and revision of personal history. *American Psychologist, 35*, 603–618.
21. Markus, H. R., & Kitayama, S. (1991). Culture and the self: Implications for cognition, emotion, and motivation. *Psychological Review, 98*, 224–253.
22. Weisz, J. R., Rothbaum, R. M., & Blackburn, T. C. (1984). Standing out

and standing in: The psychology of control in America and Japan. *American Psychologist, 39*, 955–969.

23. Roland, A. (1988). *In search of self in India and Japan: Toward a cross-cultural psychology.* Princeton: Princeton University Press.

24. Lazarus, R. S., & Folkman, S. (1984). *Stress, appraisal, and coping.* New York: Springer.

25. Suls, J., & Fletcher, B. (1985). The relative efficacy of avoidant and non-avoidant coping strategies: A meta-analysis. *Health Psychology, 4,* 249–288.

26. Tobin, L. D., Holroyd, K. A., Reynolds, R. V., & Wigal, J. K. (1989). The hierarchical factor structure of the Coping Strategies Inventory. *Cognitive Therapy and Research, 13*, 343–361.

27. Diener, E., Emmons, R. A. Larsen, R. J., & Griffin, S. (1985). The Satisfaction With Life Scale. *Journal of Personality Assessment, 49*, 71–75.

28. Beck, A. T., Ward, C. H., Mendelson, M., Mock, L., & Erbaugh, J. (1961). An inventory for measuring depression. *Archives of General Psychiatry, 4*, 561–571.

29. Epstein, S. (1973). The self-concept revisited, or a theory of a theory. *American Psychologist, 28*, 404–416.

30. Epstein, S. (1990). Cognitive-experiential self-theory. In L. A. Previn (Ed.), *Handbook of personality: Theory and research* (pp. 165–192). New York: Guilford Press.

31. Epstein, S., & Meier, P. (1989). Constructive thinking: A broad coping variable with specific components. *Journal of Personality and Social Psychology, 57*, 332–350.

32. Epstein, S. (1992). Coping ability, negative self-evaluation, and over-generalization: Experiment and theory. *Journal of Personality and Social Psychology, 62*, 826–836.

33. Epstein, S., & Katz, L. (1992). Coping ability, stress, productive load, and symptoms. *Journal of Personality and Social Psychology, 62,* 813–825.

34. Taylor, S. E., & Brown, J. D. (1988). Illusion and well-being: A social psychological perspective on mental health. *Psychological Bulletin, 103*, 193–210.

35. D'Zurilla, T. J., & Nezu, A. M. (1990). Development and preliminary evaluation of the Social Problem-Solving Inventory (SPSI). *Psychological Assessment, 2*, 156–163.

36. D'Zurilla, T. J. (1986). *Problem-solving therapy: A social competence approach to clinical intervention.* New York: Springer.

37. Nezu, A. M., Nezu, C. M., Perri, M. G. (1989). *Problem-solving therapy for depression: Theory, research, and clinical guidelines.* New York: Wiley.

38. D'Zurilla, T. J., Chang, E. C., Nottingham, E. J., IV, & Faccini, L. (1998). Social problem-solving deficits and hopelessness, depression, and suicidal risk in college students and psychiatric inpatients. *Journal of Clinical Psychology, 54*, 1–17.

39. D'Zurilla, T. J., & Chang, E. C. (1995). The relations between social problem solving and coping. *Cognitive Therapy and Research, 19,* 549–564.

40. D'Zurilla, T. J., & Maydeu-Olivares, A. (1995). Conceptual and methodological issues in social problem-solving assessment. *Behavior Therapy, 26*, 409–432.
41. D'Zurilla, T. J., Nezu, A. M., & Maydeu-Olivares, A. (in press). *Manual for the Social Problem-Solving Inventory-Revised.* North Tonawanda, NY: Multi-Health Systems.
42. Doi, T. (1973). *The anatomy of dependence.* Tokyo: Kodansha.
43. Prilleltensky, I. (1989). Psychology and the status quo. *American Psychologist, 44*, 795 802.
44. Fong, T. P. (1998). *The contemporary Asian American experience: Beyond the model minority.* Upper Saddle River, NJ: Prentice Hall.
45. Chang, E. C. (1998b). Dispositional optimism and primary and secondary appraisal of a stressor: Controlling for confounding influences and relations to coping and psychological and physical adjustment. *Journal of Personality and Social Psychology, 74*, 1109–1120.
46. Chang, E. C. (2000). Perfectionism as a predictor of positive and negative psychological outcomes: Examining a mediation model in younger and older adults. *Journal of Counseling Psychology, 47*, 18–26.
47. Chang, E. C., & Rand, K. L. (2000). Perfectionism as a predictor of subsequent adjustment: Evidence for a specific diathesis-stress mechanism among college students. *Journal of Counseling Psychology, 47*, 129–137.
48. Aldwin, C. M. (1994). *Stress, coping, and development: An integrative perspective.* New York: Guilford Press.
49. Wong, P. T. P., & Reker, G. T. (1985). Coping and well-being in Caucasian and Chinese. *Canadian Journal of Aging, 4*, 29–37.
50. Stone, A. A., Schwartz, J. E., Shiffman, S., Marco, C. A., Hickcox, & Paty, J. (1998). A comparison of coping assessed by ecological momentary assessment and retrospective recall. *Journal of Personality and Social Psychology, 74*, 1670–1680.
51. Asakawa, K., & Csikszentmihalyi, M. (1998). The quality of experience of Asian American adolescents in academic activities: An exploration of educational achievement. *Journal of Research on Adolescence, 8*, 241–262.
52. Sue, S., & Morishima, J. (1982). *The mental health of Asian Americans.* San Francisco: Jossey-Bass.
53. Beck, A. T. (1967). *Depression: Clinical, experimental and theoretical aspects.* New York: Harper & Row.
54. Beck, A. T. (1976). *Cognitive therapy and the emotional disorders.* New York: International Universities Press.
55. American Psychiatric Association. (1994). *Diagnostic and statistical manual of mental disorders* (4th ed.). Washington, DC: Author.

12

Aging and Coping: The Activity Solution

Gail M. Williamson
W. Keith Dooley

G rowing old involves physical, cognitive, and psychosocial changes that force people to either adapt or be overcome by stress. With the knowledge that the lives of people of all ages are disrupted by stressful events (1), psychologists and other health professionals, for many years, have been studying the effects of stress and the methods that people use to cope with it. Coping successfully is widely regarded as a sign of effective functioning in adulthood (2), and efforts to cope have important implications for physical and psychological well-being throughout the life span.

There are numerous emotional, cognitive, and behavioral elements involved in coping. In this chapter, we focus on a specific type of coping—maintaining normal activities—and the consequences of losing these activities in late life.

Stress and Coping—Background and Definitions

As yet, no single definition of stress is universally accepted. It has been defined as physiological and psychological reactions to either internal or external events (stressors) or, more comprehensively, as complex relations between stressors, responses, and additional mediating variables (e.g., 3, 4). For our purposes, we conceptualize stress as psychological reactions to stressors. We define stressors as situations that threaten, or are perceived as threatening, one's well-being.

Through major life events, as well as daily hassles, we experience stress and must cope. Through our coping efforts, we intend to avoid, reduce, or adapt to the threat or challenge. Adaptation involves behaving in ways that maintain psychological stability in the face of potentially stressful circumstances. Depending on the situation, however, some coping techniques are more adaptive than others. In other words, attempts to cope can be adaptive or maladaptive, effective or ineffective, healthy or unhealthy, and successful or unsuccessful.

Coping strategies thought to be maladaptive, ineffective, unhealthy, or unsuccessful are related to increased distress, typically in the form of depressive symptoms (5). To be effective (or adaptive), people should match their coping mechanisms to the demands of the situation (6). When a stressor is amenable to change, our use of active problem-solving strategies is likely to produce less psychological stress; on the other hand, when the stressor is not amenable to change, emotion-focused strategies may be more adaptive (6). Therefore, depending on the situation, both problem-focused and emotion-focused coping strategies may be useful.

Mediating variables intervene to alter relations between stressors and responses. Influenced by such factors, the person is able to either increase or decrease stress, and by identifying such mediating factors, scientists can understand why different people react in different ways to the same stressor (1). For example, imagine that several elderly women are confronting similar events—selling their homes and moving in with an adult child. Each may react quite differently, depending on her level of functional and financial independence, as well as a host of other factors. The woman who is physically capable of caring for herself but no longer can afford her own home may perceive this situation as extremely stressful. For a woman who is physically disabled but financially secure, moving in with a loved one may be seen as a blessing and a way to alleviate some of her stress. Still another woman may be able to acknowledge that she has both physical and financial limitations, but she experiences levels of stress that depend on other aspects of the situation—for example, the quality of her relationship with her adult child. Thus, depending on the circumstances surrounding an event, people have differing perceptions of the event as being stressful, and these perceptions strongly influence emotional adjustment.

Stress in Late Life

Most of us believe that old age is a time when highly stressful situations are most likely to occur. Researchers in the field of aging have debunked this and many other myths associated with aging. Still, we persist in perceiving elderly adults as sick, frail, and socially isolated people who have ceased most activities while waiting for their lives to end. Such stereotypes are supported, in part, by the fact that aging individuals *are* at greater risk for declining physical health, functional disability, and social isolation. But the picture is not that simple.

Elderly people experience as much stress as any other age group, but a critical difference is that they encounter different types of stressors. For example, younger adults are more stressed by financial, economic, and employment issues, whereas older adults report more hassles associated with social problems, home, and health (7). However, many of the most impactful events in life—death of a spouse, retirement, and chronic illness—do occur primarily in old age (8). Moreover, seniors must make some difficult decisions that younger adults are less likely to face—quandaries about retiring, whether to institutionalize a spouse or provide care at home, and how to distribute finances and assets in a will. Older adults also lose loved ones, possessions, and functional abilities at higher rates than do younger adults. Because of physical, cognitive, or financial problems, many seniors are forced to stop driving or must sell their homes. Elderly women frequently become widows, living, on average, about seven years longer than men. As more people live into old age, more elders will experience the death of a spouse, close friends, or even children. In addition, the opportunity for multiple and simultaneously occurring stressors increases with age and may overtax the coping resources of seniors.

Compared to younger individuals, elderly people also are more prone to experience an often overlooked, but important, stressor—understimulation or having nothing meaningful to do for long periods of time. Regardless of age, people perform best when environmental demands slightly exceed their abilities (9, 10). Consequently, stress is a two-edged sword in that it can (and does) result from environmental demands that are either too high *or* too low. Older adults, particularly those who live alone or in long-term care facilities, are highly susceptible to understimulation.

In sum, older people must cope with a variety of life changes. A complicated aspect of studying stress and coping is that many life events cannot be classified uniformly as either positive or negative. Rather, their effects vary greatly and depend on how one perceives the situation and available coping resources. For example, retiring from a lifelong career may be perceived by an older adult as highly stressful, a long-awaited release from responsibility, or anything between these extremes.

Coping in Late Life

Coping is complex at any age, but, for elderly people, changes in health, social status, physical environment, family composition, and social support are sources of stress and threats to adaptive coping. Elders often are subject to a variety of situations they have not encountered (or learned how to handle) earlier in life. Coupled with the increased likelihood of multiple stressors occurring simultaneously in late life, along with substantial declines in resources that facilitate coping, we might expect that the average older adult is less effective in dealing with stress than his or her younger counterpart. However, this does not appear to be the case. If health, economic, and social resources remain intact, there is little reason to expect that one's ability to cope with stress will decline with age (1).

Indeed, elders exhibit many effective coping behaviors, and they have been found to cope more effectively with stressful life events than do younger adults (11). With their many life experiences and successes in coping with a variety of stressors, elders may have adaptive attitudes and beliefs that generalize to coping with new stressors. This effective coping also may be attributable, in part, to less stigmatizing social and cultural roles in modern times for the senior citizens in this country. In addition, other societal changes may be implicated. For example, medical technology has improved dramatically in the past 20 years, allowing older people to live longer, healthier, and more active lives. Economic prosperity has created financial security for many older Americans, and they are using their money to pursue active lifestyles in retirement. Furthermore, based on advances in early detection of Alzheimer's disease and other forms of dementia, seniors and their families are able to plan proactively for future living arrangements and end of life decisions.

What Qualifies as Coping?

Coping is most often divided into two basic categories. *Problem-focused* coping involves actively trying to change a stressful situation, including obtaining information from external sources to facilitate more effective coping (4). An example is seeking counseling for marital difficulties. *Emotion-focused coping* involves using thoughts and behaviors to manage the negative emotions that often accompany stressors (4)—accepting that the situation has occurred and making the best of it. Most people use both types of coping, but because older adults typically must deal with less easily ameliorated stressors, they tend to use more emotion-focused strategies (e.g., 7). Reconceptualizing coping in their life span theory of control, Schulz and Heckhausen (12) propose that, regardless of age, people are motivated to exercise personal control over the important aspects of their lives. As people age, "primary" control (e.g., solving the problem) may become less feasible or, indeed, impossible (e.g., when a spouse becomes chronically ill or dies). Consequently, older adults may increase "secondary" control measures that focus on their emotional reactions (e.g., accepting the situation, functioning as normally as possible) in order to maintain or regain some sense of control. However conceptualized, coping dynamically changes to meet demands over the life span.

Still, there are dimensions of coping that remain remarkably stable throughout life and vary between individuals regardless of age and specific challenging events. That is, coping can be conceptualized as a stable internal personality trait (13). For example, many of us know someone who catastrophizes every event and whose major coping style involves complaining, an inability to take any sort of constructive action toward solving the problem, and dwelling on how much better things would be if the problem would just go away. At the other extreme are those people who handle every event with aplomb. They take appropriate action to ameliorate the situation, and when they have done all they can and the problem still persists, they accept it (often with a sense of humor) and get on with their lives. Most of us fall somewhere between these two extremes, and this is true for older as well as younger adults. Like other personality traits, dispositions toward coping in general tend to remain stable across the life span (13, 14). People who were neurotic-style copers in their 20's and 30's are highly likely to be neurotic-style copers in their 60's and 70's (15). And people who were adaptive copers early in life are likely to cope successfully with the losses that they encounter late in life.

In summary, there are aspects of coping that remain stable from young to old age. However, the changing demands of advancing age are likely to require that older adults adopt strategies that differ from those that were effective when they were younger. Does the conflict between disposition and situational requirements place older adults in an untenable position and predispose them to depression? If we consider the average elderly person, the answer is no. Clinically diagnosable depression is less prevalent in older than younger adults (1, 2). Given that older people are subject to levels of stress that are at least as high as those of younger people, we can infer that old age does *not* foster maladaptive coping. Again, however, we emphasize that reactions to stressors vary as widely among older as younger adults, with some young people being highly effective copers and some old people being highly ineffective copers. In other words, there is a group of people (e.g., the neurotic copers) who cope in maladaptive ways across all situations throughout their lives. In contrast, there are those with more flexible approaches to coping who deal with each problem as it presents itself. These nonneurotic copers are dispositionally inclined to face the situation, rationally evaluate possible solutions, seek help and information as appropriate and, if all else fails, accept that the problem has occurred, deal with their emotional reactions to it (perhaps with help from others), and make every effort to resume life as usual. *Herein lies the foundation of the Activity Restriction Model of Depressed Affect.*

The Activity Restriction Model of Depressed Affect

Activity restriction is the inability to continue normal activities (e.g., self-care, care of others, doing household chores, going shopping, visiting friends, working on hobbies, and maintaining friendships) in the face of stressful life events such as debilitating illness (16). From the standpoint of stress and coping models, activity restriction qualifies as a coping behavior whereby normal activities are curtailed in response to stress.

As proponents of the Activity Restriction Model of Depressed Affect, we have stated that, "the extent to which routine activities are restricted by a major life stressor plays a central role in psychological adjustment, with major disruptions in normal activities resulting in poorer mental health outcomes" (17, p. 327). Within this model, illness and disability are conceptualized as life stressors, depression as one of several possible reactions, and activity restriction as a mediator of the relation between stress and emotional responses. Stated simply, people are emotionally disturbed by stressors to the extent that they can no longer engage in their usual activities. Researchers have found support for this model in several studies (16, 18, 19, 20, 21, 22).

People, both young and old, vary widely in how well they adapt to stress (1). If we are to intervene in this process, it is critical to determine which variables enable us to best predict those who will cope successfully or who will not. Activity restriction is one such variable. Using the concept of activity restriction, researchers and lay people alike can better understand the relation between stress and mental health outcomes. In a model of stress, such as that proposed by Lazarus and Folkman (23), activity restriction qualifies as a direct consequence of stress, as well as a coping behavior that can produce negative emotional outcomes. For example, a person with a broken leg is realistically hampered in vigorous activities, but persistence in avoiding previously enjoyed activities after the leg is healed is maladaptive coping, particularly if it leads to depression.

The Early Activity Restriction Literature

The Activity Restriction Model of Depressed Affect originally was grounded in associations between pain, functional disability, and symptoms of depression. In previous research, it had been demonstrated that pain and depression are related, but the direction of causality (or even temporality) was far from clear. Intuitively, pain may cause people to become depressed. However, it also is possible that depressed people simply report more pain and other illness symptoms as a function of their generally negative approach to life (17). Short of extensive large-sample prospective research, one way to tease apart causal direction is to investigate temporally identifiable aspects of the situation. Among older adults, two such factors are illness severity and living environment. Differences between population samples in independently conducted studies provide such an opportunity. And it was precisely because of this set of circumstances that we initiated the program of research leading to the development of the Activity Restriction Model of Depressed Affect.

In 1991, Parmelee and colleagues reported that among institutionalized elderly persons, illness severity and functional disability did not account for the relation between pain and depression (24). In other words, regardless of how ill or disabled these patients were, the more pain they reported, the more depressed they were. Moreover, this effect was strongest when there had been a medical condition formally diagnosed that could justify their pain. Parmelee et al. interpreted their results as indicating that elderly people may more readily adopt a sick role in which they *expect* to experience both pain and depression.

Employing a very similar set of assessments, Williamson and Schulz (16) speculated that results might be quite different for community-residing older persons. Seniors who still reside in the community generally are less ill and disabled and more responsible for their own well-being than their institutionalized counterparts. Because restriction of normal activities may signal functional declines that can preclude independent living, those who still live independently should be more distressed when their usual activities become more difficult. Indeed, contrary to results for the Parmelee et al. institutionalized sample, most of the association between pain and depression was explained by the degree to which pain caused functional disability—that is, restriction of normal daily activities (16). In other words, activity restriction mediated the relation between pain and depression, indicating that "in community-residing older adults, the strongest effect of pain on depression may be the extent to which it results in the inability to engage in routine activities" (17, p. 329).

How do these findings relate to coping with painful, perhaps debilitating, illness conditions? Most people, particularly those who reside in the community, presumably have some control over how restricted their activities become as a result of physical pain or illness. Because activity restriction is so strongly related to depression, foregoing more activities than is medically necessary can be detrimental to emotional well-being. Conversely, continuing valued activities can promote emotional well-being.

Subsequent Activity Restriction Studies

To broaden applicability of the activity restriction findings, studies have been conducted in samples of several medically compromised populations, and a few of these will be highlighted here. For example, people who have undergone lower limb amputation face threats to their psychological well-being (25), are highly likely to be elderly adults, and are at high risk for functional disability. Findings from our limb amputation studies are remarkably consistent with our previous research. The less patients used a prosthesis, the more they restricted their activities, and the more depressed they became (21). More important, when ability to conduct routine daily activities is considered, prosthesis use no longer predicts depression. Therefore, effectively using a prosthetic limb appears to promote psychological well-being by facilitating normal activities.

The Activity Restriction Model applies to other populations as well. In one more example, data were collected at two points in time from patients with recurrent cancer (20). Analyses of these longitudinal data revealed that as pain increased over time, so did activity restriction, and, in turn, increased activity restriction predicted more depressed affect. Finding the same pattern of results both cross-sectionally and longitudinally not only increases confidence in the activity restriction effect, but it also has implications for intervention. Based on longitudinal results, in particular, it appears that if activity restriction can be alleviated, emotional-well-being is likely to improve as well. We further suggest that practitioners not only should focus on reducing both pain and depression but also target increasing participation in normal activities. More exactly, if older adults do not know how to constructively deal with pain and disability, they may limit their activities, responsibilities, and social interactions under the assumption that doing so will alleviate their symptoms. But, contrary to this popular belief, *activity restriction appears to determine whether pain leads to symptoms of depression.*

Are pain and severity of illness the only contributors to activity restriction? Given that various assessments of these variables explain relatively small portions of the variance in activity restriction—that is, from 7% to 31% (19), the answer would seem to be no. Drawing on the large stress and coping literature, we have begun investigating personal and environmental variables that also may foster activity restriction. Several psychosocial variables have been identified, many of which interact with each other or with indicators of illness severity to predict activity restriction.

Age is one such factor. Similar levels of pain are tolerated better by older than younger adults (26, 27). A common explanation here is that, through increasing exposure to pain and disabling conditions, older people habituate to these stressors and thus are better able to cope with them. Moreover, older adults tend to rely on emotion-focused coping strategies when faced with adapting to irreversible physical changes. Indeed, Williamson and Schulz (20) report that, when it comes to predicting activity restriction, age interacts with having multiple chronic health conditions. Younger patients (less than 65 years of age) with no other chronic conditions report the highest levels of activity restriction as a result of recurrent cancer. But activity restriction in younger patients with multiple chronic illness conditions is comparable to that of older (65 years of age and older) patients—that is, relatively low. The inference to be gleaned from these data is that experience, rather than chronological age, matters more in terms of predicting those who will use activity restriction as a coping mechanism. Data from a study of pediatric patients with chronically painful medical conditions confirm these findings (18). Like the younger adult cancer patients, depressed affect among younger children (5–12 years old) depends on how much their pain precludes normal activities. The older children (13–18 years old) in this study look much like the older adult cancer patients—that is, the extent to which pain predicts depression does not depend on how restricted their activities are. Thus, a history of illness or disability seems to help people habituate to functional declines. Or it may be that these individuals have learned through experience to use coping strategies that are more adaptive than restricting their usual activities.

Another potentially important contributor to activity restriction is financial resources. Although some researchers have reported that inadequate income interferes with normal activities in the presence of illness or disability (28), absolute dollar amounts of total household income often do not predict activity restriction. Examination of other data, however, leads to the conclusion that such discrepancies are best explained by differences in how income is measured (17). That is, absolute income may not be related to activity restriction, but when financial resources are *perceived* as less than adequate, participants report that their activities are more restricted. These results are logical in that, when resources are perceived as inadequate, individuals cope by cutting back on normal activities such as shopping, recreation, and hobbies.

Aside from demographic factors, aspects of the individual's personality also explain additional variance in activity restriction. Put simply, some people are more dispositionally inclined than others to forego their usual activities. Of particular relevance when the illness condition results in bodily disfigurement is public self-consciousness, a stable tendency to be highly concerned about aspects of the self that are evident to others and from which others form impressions (29). People who score high on this trait worry a great deal about their personal appearance and actively avoid disapproval and rejection from others. As would be expected, limb amputation patients high in public self-consciousness restrict their public activities (e.g., shopping, visiting friends) more than those who are low in public self-consciousness (30). Additionally, however, these more self-conscious individuals also restrict their nonpublic activities (e.g., household chores). Thus, giving up activities in the presence of others may generalize to private behaviors and foster disability. This finding is reminiscent of the Parmelee et al. (24) results for older adults in nursing homes. For example, when a disabling condition occurs, some people may cope by foregoing all usual activities because they have a justification for doing so. Is this an adaptive strategy? We strongly propose that it is not. The reason we take such an adamant position is that, even after controlling for a wide variety of other factors, activity restriction remains the most proximal predictor of depression (17).

We suspect that personality variables influence activity restriction via their impact on available social support. Those with less socially desirable or less socially proactive characteristics may have less supportive social ties as well. Based on a large literature, people who have stronger social support networks can cope better with all types of stressful life events. Moreover, when pain, illness, or disability are present, social support increases ability to perform routine activities (31, 32). Social support comes in many forms and typically involves behaviors that show people that they are loved, cared for, and valued members of a social network (33). That such social support can foster adaptive coping behaviors is explicitly recognized in the Activity Restriction Model. For example, less satisfaction with social contacts predicts more activity restriction (21), and the same is true when people perceive that social support is not available to the extent that it might be needed (34). As evidence of the importance of social support, the benefits of having supportive others remain even after controlling for demographics (e.g., age, financial resources), illness severity, and personality variables such as public self-consciousness (34).

To summarize our analysis of accumulating evidence, people consistently become depressed in the wake of stressful life events largely because those events disrupt their ability to go about life as usual. Depending on how comprehensively it is measured, illness severity explains, on average, about 20% of the variance in activity restriction, and psychosocial variables account for an average of 14% of the variance in activity restriction beyond the effects of illness severity (17). In addition to illness severity, younger age (or lack of experience with debilitating health problems), inadequate income, less social support, and higher public self-consciousness all contribute to more restricted activities. And *activity restriction consistently emerges as a highly proximal predictor of depressed affect* (16, 17, 18, 20, 22, 34).

Implications for Future Research and Intervention

When viewed through the Activity Restriction Model of Depressed Affect, we can see that coping with stress is a complex, multifaceted process that is influenced by numerous factors. Stressors vary in nature across the life span, with those faced by older adults being at least as threatening as those confronted by young adults. However, because sources of physical, psychological, and emotional stress differ (e.g., in terms of controllability) with increasing age, coping successfully may require replacing strategies that once were (but are no longer) adaptive with techniques that more adequately meet the demands of advancing age. Therefore, interventions are warranted to help older adults develop new coping techniques. Such interventions may require convincing these individuals that a shift from primary (problem-focused) to secondary (emotion-focused) control mechanisms is the way to go.

In our view, the Activity Restriction Model of Depressed Affect corresponds to, but is not subsumed by, a general model of stress and coping. Although the stress-activity restriction–mental health pathway can be mapped onto a stress and coping model (e.g., 23), doing so implies that the constructs are independent of each other and that the causal path is unidirectional—that is, that stress causes activity restriction which, in turn, causes negative affect. Without doubt, these implications are inadequate when it comes to describing the myriad facets of dealing with threatening life events.

First, components of the model are not so easily categorized. This is perhaps most evident in the ways that activity restriction has been studied in the past. Specifically, instruments designed to measure pain often include assessments of the extent to which patients' routine activities are restricted, supposedly as a consequence of pain (16). Much the same is true for assessing depression—that is, one indicator of depression is a decline in normal activities (35). Thus, activity restriction has been studied as a stressor (e.g., a component of pain and illness severity), a coping mechanism (e.g., a factor that influences adaptation to stress), and an affective outcome (e.g., a component of depression). When two or more of these measures are included in the same study, the results may be so confounded that accurate interpretation of their meaning is impossible.

To further complicate matters, psychosocial variables shown to predict increased activity restriction (e.g., poor social support, inadequate income) are independent sources of stress in their own right, but they also can be conceptualized as both coping mechanisms and outcomes. For instance, access to social support (or, more aptly, the perception of available support resources) is a major factor in dealing with stressful events, one that facilitates coping in multiple ways (e.g., 36, 37). Moreover, as an outcome of stressful events, social support resources can be severely taxed by life stress, particularly if it is ongoing. Most people will rally round an individual when a stressful event first occurs, but they tend to fade away as the situation becomes chronic—especially if the individual appears to be doing little to solve the problem or adapt to it (e.g., see 38). Our society tends to view all illnesses as acute rather than chronic, and the overwhelming expectation is for a patient to get well. Such a cognitive bias alone can be problematic for older adults whose health conditions overwhelmingly are chronic.

Similar to social support, financial resources have been viewed in multiple ways. As any of us who has ever worried about having enough money can testify, less than adequate income can be a source of stress. Financial resources also facilitate adaptation to (i.e., coping with) some of the most serious life-altering events. For example, one participant in a limb amputation study, a retired dentist who had never married, reported feeling fortunate that he was financially able to hire a companion. He stated that "money can make it easier to deal with almost any of life's difficulties" (21, p. 262). Finally, major life stressors (illness and disability, death of a spouse, retirement) can compromise income and perceived income adequacy. In other words, financial resources can be studied as precipitating, intervening, or resultant variables.

The point we want to make here is that the supposedly distinct constructs identified in any stress and coping model (and the Activity Restriction Model of Depressed Affect is one of these) are not as easily separated as we might prefer (or want to believe). Our second point is that, although these models propose unidirectional associations, complex bidirectional and reciprocal models will need to be tested extensively before a fuller understanding can be reached. Let's consider pain and depression as an example. Unidirectional models postulate that depression is an outcome resulting from an inability to adjust to a life that includes chronic pain, most likely due to inadequate or ineffective coping. Yet, substantial research suggests that depression can foster higher levels of reported pain (e.g., 39, 40). Similarly, the Activity Restriction Model of Depressed Affect can be turned on its head, and we can propose that, as clinicians have long known, being depressed causes people to forego many of their previously enjoyed activities. In fact, one of the better behavioral treatments for depression is to find ways to motivate patients to become more socially and physically active (41). There also are reasons to suspect that inactivity increases the level of experienced pain, an effect most likely due to both physiological (e.g., not using muscles, lack of neurological stimulation) and psychological (e.g., internal focus that increases attention to discomfort) factors. In sum, it is not our intent to propose that the Activity Restriction Model provides all the answers to questions relevant to the complex association between stress and adaptation.

We do strongly believe, however, that acknowledging depressed affect as a function of restricted normal activities means that interventions designed to reduce activity restriction can reduce depression (and the reciprocal effects thereof). But simply encouraging older adults to engage in more of their normal activities is probably not the best strategy. Rather, efforts to increase activity as a positive coping mechanism in older adults might take three (and, probably, several more) forms. First, therapists should carefully consider the (likely multiple) reasons that activities have become restricted and design their interventions accordingly. Second, they should target the individuals most at risk for poor adaptation as those most likely to need and benefit from early intervention. Third, identifying manageable activities and available resources means that programs can be implemented to engage aging adults in activities that meet their specific needs and fit their functional capacities.

Are older adults the ones who will benefit most from these interventions? Perhaps. But Williamson and Schulz (20) found that activity restriction plays a stronger part in the relation between pain and depression in younger (under 65 years) than older (over 65 years) adults. Researchers have reported parallel findings among pediatric patients (18), and we thus infer that this trend is attributable more to experience with illness than chronological age alone. In other words, it is likely that older people and those who have experience with chronic illness (regardless of age) cope by accepting pain and restricted activities as a routine part of life. Although most people adapt to even severe forms of disability over time (42), effective coping may be more challenging for individuals who have not reached an age at which functional limitation is expected or who have never experienced chronic illness and disability (for an interesting discussion of adjustment to "on-time" versus "off-time" stress, see 43). What does this imply for intervention? When an illness occurs, younger people who have had little or no experience with chronic pain or functional disability are likely to become depressed. These individuals should benefit most from interventions designed to increase activity or reduce activity restriction. The transition from acute to chronic illness, however, may warrant psychological intervention as well. We should not assume that "an individual knows how to adjust to an illness downturn because she or he has experienced it before" (44, p. 576).

As with younger adults, older adults' financial resources vary widely. While most of the older population is concentrated at the lower end of the national economic distribution, lifestyle changes (e.g., fewer dependents and no mortgage payments) may reduce seniors' perceptions of income inadequacy. On the other hand, higher costs for insurance and health care in late life have the potential to sap resources of even the most financially prepared seniors. Still, the impact of financial circumstances on activity restriction appears to depend on how income is measured. Specifically, assessing *perceived* income adequacy may be more useful than measuring actual dollar amounts (17). We repeatedly have observed that individuals with low incomes do not necessarily see their financial resources as being inadequate; likewise, those with higher incomes do not always report that their financial resources are adequate (19). Thus, it may be more worthwhile to focus on perceptions of income adequacy rather than actual dollar amounts. While financial losses due to illness and disability may prohibit many previously enjoyed activities, people can be encouraged to engage in less costly substitute activities. Older adults also need to be directed toward the social and recreational resources especially available to them at local and community levels.

In addition to evaluating demographic characteristics, such as age and financial resources, we advocate assessing relevant personality dimensions. Although most personality traits are quite stable across the life span (13, 15) and, consequently, should be difficult to change, identifying the traits that predispose people to choose inadequate coping strategies is still a worthwhile undertaking. In particular, differences in personality can help determine which older adults are at risk for poor adaptation. For example, when the condition involves body disfigurement (e.g., limb amputation and breast cancer surgery), patients high in public self-consciousness are vulnerable to increased activity restriction (30, 34). People who are highly concerned about the impression they make on others may voluntarily give up their usual activities in an effort to control their public images. These individuals can be targeted for interventions to improve their self-esteem and sense of efficacy such as hope enhancement (47; 53; 54), training in adaptive coping skills, and support groups.

Other personality traits also warrant consideration. Dispositional tendencies toward optimism, neuroticism, agency-mastery, and hopefulness are likely candidates. For instance, people high in optimism adjust better to illness and disability, cope in more effective ways (45), and, we suspect, are less likely to experience activity restriction. High levels of neuroticism are related to more maladaptive coping (13) and, we suspect, increased chances for activity restriction. Individuals who are more agentically oriented and those who have a strong sense of mastery probably find ways to continue some of their rewarding activities when faced with illness and disability (e.g., 41, 46). In addition, those who are high in the dispositional predeliction to hope for positive outcomes should be more likely to conceptualize multiple ways to continue (or replace) valued activities and to persist in their efforts to do so, even when one or more pathways to achieving these goals are blocked (e.g., 47). Thus, many aspects of personality are likely to determine coping styles and resources. Although research in this area is in its infancy, these traits should not be ignored—particularly when the goal is to identify those most at risk for poor adaptation to stress.

Social support, like personality traits and experience with illness, interacts with health-related variables to influence older individuals' choice of coping behavior. An elderly person with a chronic illness or disability will attend church and visit friends more often if other people help with walking, transportation, and words of encouragement. All else being equal, the more satisfying and supportive one's social support network is perceived to be, the less likely one is to cope with illness by restricting routine activities. Maintaining routine activities in the face of illness, disability, or other stressors, in turn, reduces the possibility of depression and other negative emotional responses. Thus, identifying community-residing older adults with deficits in social support is a good starting point for intervention.

To go a step further, it seems clear that interventions designed to increase social support (or the perceptions thereof) can help people continue performing more of the routine activities associated with independent living (19, 21, 34). It is important to specify which aspects of social support are absent or most distressing, however, because doing so has implications for treatment (32). Some older people may be depressed simply because they are not interacting enough with other people. Others may have concrete needs for assistance that are not being met (e.g., getting out of bed or grocery shopping). Still others may be exposed to extremely damaging exploitative or abusive social contacts (48, 49, 50, 51). Because interpersonal relationships are a prime area for clinical intervention (17), it will be important to increase our understanding of the antecedents and outcomes of less than optimal social interactions.

Concluding Comments

In the MacArthur Foundation Study (33), successful aging is defined as a combination of three elements: "avoiding disease and disease-related disability, maintaining high cognitive and physical functioning, and active engagement with life" (pp. 38–39). The investigators in this landmark study believe that these elements involve a common process that revolves around active behaviors (in other words, active attempts to cope). Research clearly indicates that the physiological changes associated with normal aging can be exacerbated by environmental stressors that place older adults at risk for immune system dysfunction (52). Therefore, successful aging, or aging without compromising quality of life, may critically depend on effectively coping with age-related life events.

In the Activity Restriction Model, we specify that people experience decrements in mental health in direct proportion to how these stressors interfere with their normal activities. Several demographic, personality, psychosocial, and health-related factors help to explain why disability and activity restriction increase the possibility of experiencing negative emotions. Still, many questions remain unanswered. For example, the list of variables studied thus far is by no means exhaustive, and other personal and social factors also bear investigation.

Conducting controlled experimental studies can help us fill remaining gaps by more definitively demonstrating that specific strategies designed to increase activity level in the presence of disability will produce changes in well-being. Through such controlled studies, we also could identify more exactly the physical, cognitive, and emotional effects of decreasing activity restriction. Finally, by differentiating seniors who will tolerate discomfort in order to continue engaging in meaningful activities from those who will not voluntarily make such efforts under similar levels of discomfort, we may come closer to producing successful applications for clinical, medical, and rehabilitation settings.

The emerging picture is that the association between stress and adjustment is multifaceted and complex. People always look for the simplest and most parsimonious answer, and we as researchers are no different in this respect. The more we study the relation between life stress and adjustment, however, the more we become convinced that, because older adults and their personal circumstances vary widely, simple solutions are unlikely to (a) adequately represent what really happens or (b) provide easy answers about ways to intervene. The Activity Restriction Model of Depressed Affect is a highly parsimonious representation, and we use it to state that when a stressful life event (illness and disability are good examples but certainly not all-inclusive) interferes with the ability to go about life as usual, people become distressed. On a more positive note, if methods can be found to help people continue at least some of their valued activities, distress should be greatly reduced. We also see added benefits of such interventions in terms of improved functional capacity and reduced need for assistance from others. In sum, we propose that increasing (or, at least, maintaining) activities that are meaningful and personally valued can promote both physical and psychological well-being. Indeed, activity maintenance may be a solution to many of the problems associated with aging.

Acknowledgments
Manuscript preparation was supported by the National Institute on Aging (AG15321, G. M. Williamson, principal investigator) and further facilitated by a fellowship to the first author from the Institute for Behavioral Research at The University of Georgia.

References

1. Schulz, R., & Ewen, R. B. (1993). *Adult development and aging: Myths and emerging realities* (2nd ed). New York: MacMillan.
2. Rybash, J. M., Roodin, P. A., & Hoyer, W. J. (1995). *Adult development and aging* (3rd ed). Madison, WI: Brown & Benchmark.
3. Lazarus, R. S. (1966). *Psychological stress and the coping process.* New York: McGraw-Hill.
4. Folkman, S. L., & Lazarus, R. S. (1980). An analysis of coping in a middle-aged community sample. *Journal of Health and Social Behavior, 21,* 219–239.
5. Rohde, P., Lewinsohn, P. M., Tilson, M., & Seeley, J. R. (1990). Dimensionality of coping and its relation to depression. *Journal of Personality and Social Psychology, 58,* 499–511.
6. Williamson, G. M., & Schulz, R. (1993). Coping with specific stressors in Alzheimer's disease caregiving. *The Gerontologist, 33,* 747–755.
7. Folkman, S. L., Lazarus, R. S., Plmley, S., & Novacek, J. (1987). Age differences in stress and coping responses. *Psychology and Aging, 2,* 171–184.
8. Hooyman, N., & Kiyak, H. A. (1996). *Social gerontology: A multidisciplinary perspective* (5th ed.). Boston: Allyn & Bacon.
9. Lawton, M. P. (1989). Behavior-relevant ecological factors. In K. W. Schaie & C. Schooler (Eds.), *Social structure and aging: Psychological processes* (pp. 57–78). Hillsdale, NJ: Erlbaum.
10. Lawton, M. P., & Nahemow, L. (1973). Ecology and the aging process. In C. Eisdorfer & M. P. Lawton (Eds.), *Psychology of adult development and aging* (pp. 619–674). Washington, DC: American Psychological Association.
11. McCrae, R. R. (1989). Age differences and changes in the use of coping mechanisms. *Journal of Gerontology, 44,* 161–164.
12. Schulz, R., & Heckhausen, J. (1996). A life-span model of successful aging. *American Psychologist, 51,* 702–714.
13. McCrae, R. R., & Costa, P. T., Jr. (1986). Personality, coping, and coping effectiveness in an adult sample. *Journal of Personality, 54,* 385–405.
14. Thomae, H. (1992). Emotion and personality. In J. E. Birren, R. B. Sloane, & G. D. Cohen (Eds.), *Handbook of mental health and aging* (2nd ed., pp. 355–375). New York: Academic Press.
15. Costa, P. T., & McCrae, R. R. (1993). Personality, defense, coping, and adaptation in older adulthood. In E. M. Cummings, A. L. Greene, & K. K. Karraker (Eds.), *Life span developmental psychology: Perspectives on stress and coping* (pp. 277–293). Hillsdale, NJ: Erlbaum.
16. Williamson, G. M., & Schulz, R. (1992). Pain, activity restriction, and symptoms of depression among community-residing elderly. *Journal of Gerontology, 47,* 367–372.
17. Williamson, G. M. (1998). The central role of restricted normal activities in adjustment to illness and disability: A model of depressed affect. *Rehabilitation Psychology, 43,* 327–347.
18. Walters, A. S., & Williamson, G. M. (1999). The role of activity restriction in the association between pain and depressed affect: A study of

pediatric patients with chronic pain. *Children's Health Care, 28,* 33–50.

19. Williamson, G. M., & Shaffer, D. R. (2000). The Activity Restriction Model of Depressed Affect: Antecedents and consequences of restricted normal activities. In G. M. Williamson, D. R. Shaffer, & P. A. Parmelee (Eds.), *Physical illness and depression in older adults: A handbook of theory, research, and practice* (pp. 173–200). New York: Plenum.

20. Williamson, G. M., & Schulz, R. (1995). Activity restriction mediates the association between pain and depressed affect: A study of younger and older adult cancer patients. *Psychology and Aging, 10,* 369–378.

21. Williamson, G. M., Schulz, R., Bridges, M., & Behan, A. (1994). Social and psychological factors in adjustment to limb amputation. *Journal of Social Behavior and Personality, 9,* 249–268.

22. Williamson, G. M., Shaffer, D. R., & Schulz, R. (1998). Activity restriction and prior relationship history as contributors to mental health outcomes among middle-aged and older caregivers. *Health Psychology, 17,* 152–162.

23. Lazarus, R. S., & Folkman, S., (1984). *Stress, appraisal and coping.* New York: Springer.

24. Parmelee, P. A., Katz, I. R., & Lawton, M. P. (1991). The relation of pain to depression among institutionalized aged. *Journal of Gerontology, 46,* 15–21.

25. Frank, R. G., Kashani, J. H., Kashani, S. R., Wonderlich, S. A., Umlauf, R. L., & Ashkanazi, G. S. (1984). Psychological response to amputation as a function of age and time since amputation. *British Journal of Psychiatry, 144,* 493–497.

26. Cassileth, B. R., Lusk, E. J., Strouse, T. B., Miller, D. S., Brown, L. L., Cross, P. A., & Tenaglia, A. N. (1984). Psychosocial status in chronic illness: A comparative analysis of six diagnostic groups. *New England Journal of Medicine, 311,* 506–511.

27. Foley, K. M. (1985). The treatment of cancer pain. *New England Journal of Medicine, 313,* 84–95.

28. Merluzzi, T. V., & Martinez Sanchez, M. A. (1997). Assessment of self-efficacy and coping with cancer: Development and validation of the Cancer Behavior Inventory. *Health Psychology, 16,* 163–170.

29. Scheier, M. F., & Carver, C. S. (1985). The Self-Consciousness Scale: A revised version for use with general populations. *Journal of Applied Social Psychology, 15,* 687–699.

30. Williamson, G. M. (1995). Restriction of normal activities among older adult amputees: The role of public self-consciousness. *Journal of Clinical Geropsychology, 1,* 229–242.

31. Mutran, E. J., Reitzes, D. C., Mossey, J., & Fernandez, M. E. (1995). Social support, depression, and recovery of walking ability following hip fracture surgery. *Journal of Gerontology, 50,* 354–361.

32. Oxman, T. E., & Hull, J. G. (1997). Social support, depression, and activities of daily living in older heart surgery patients. *Journal of Gerontology, 52,* 1–14.

33. Rowe, J. W., & Kahn, R. L. (1998). *Successful aging.* New York: Pantheon Books.

34. Williamson, G. M. (2000). Extending the Activity Restriction Model of Depressed Affect: Evidence from a sample of breast cancer patients. *Health Psychology, 19,* 339–347.

35. American Psychiatric Association. (1994). *Diagnostic and statistical manual of mental disorders* (4th ed., DSM-IV). Washington, DC: American Psychiatric Association.

36. Billings, A. G., & Moos, R. H. (1984). Coping, stress, and social resources among adults with unipolar depression. *Journal of Personality and Social Psychology, 46,* 877–891.

37. Cohen, S., & Wills, T. A. (1985). Stress, social support, and the buffering hypothesis. *Psychological Bulletin, 98,* 310–357.

38. Williams, H. A. (1993). A comparison of social support and social networks of black parents and white parents with chronically ill children. *Social Science Medicine, 37,* 1509–1520.

39. Lefebvre, M. F. (1981). Cognitive distortion and cognitive errors in depressed psychiatric and low back pain patients. *Journal of Consulting and Clinical Psychology, 49,* 517–525.

40. Mathew, R., Weinman, M., & Mirabi, M. (1981). Physical symptoms of depression. *British Journal of Psychiatry, 139,* 293–296.

41. Herzog, A. R., Franks, M. M., Markus, H. R., & Holmberg, D. (1998). Activities and well-being in older age: Effects of self-concept and educational attainment. *Psychology and Aging, 13,* 179–185.

42. Schulz, R., & Decker, S. (1985). Long-term adjustment to physical disability: The role of social support, perceived control, and self-blame. *Journal of Personality and Social Psychology, 48,* 1162–1172.

43. Neugarten, B. L. (1977). Personality and aging. In J. E. Birren & K. W. Schaie (Eds.), *Handbook of the psychology of aging* (pp. 626–649). New York: Van Nostrand Reinhold.

44. Erdal, K. J., & Zautra, A. J. (1995). Psychological impact of illness downturns: A comparison of new and chronic conditions. *Psychology and Aging, 10,* 570–577.

45. Carver, C. S., Pozo, C., Harris, S. D., Noriega, V., Scheier, M. F., Robinson, D. S., Ketcham, A. S., Moffat, F. L., Jr., & Clark, K. C. (1993). How coping mediates the effect of optimism on distress: A study of women with early stage breast cancer. *Journal of Personality and Social Psychology, 65,* 375–390.

46. Femia, E. E., Zarit, S. H., & Johansson, B. (1997). Predicting change in activities of daily living: A longitudinal study of the oldest old in Sweden. *Journal of Gerontology, 52,* 294–302.

47. Snyder, C. R. (1998). A case for hope in pain, loss, and suffering. In J. H. Harvey, J. Omarza, & E. Miller (Eds.), *Perspectives on loss: A sourcebook* (pp. 63–79). Washington, DC: Taylor and Francis.

48. Cohen, S., & McKay, G. (1983). Interpersonal relationships as buffers of the impact of psychosocial stress on health. In A. Baum, S. E. Taylor, & J. E. Singer (Eds.), *Handbook of psychology and health* (Vol. 4, pp. 253–267). Hillsdale, NJ: Erlbaum.

49. Suls, J. (1982). Social support, interpersonal relations, and health: Benefits and liabilities. In G. S. Saunders & J. Suls (Eds.), *Social psychology of health and illness* (pp. 255–277). Hillsdale, NJ: Erlbaum.

50. Wortman, C. B. (1984). Social support and the cancer patient. *Cancer, 53,* 2339–2360.
51. Williamson, G. M., Shaffer, D. R., & The Family Relationships in Late Life Project. (2000). Caregiver loss and quality of care provided: Pre-illness relationship makes a difference. In J. H. Harvey & E. D. Miller (Eds.), *Loss and trauma: General and close relationship perspectives* (pp. 307–330). Philadelphia: Brunner/Mazel.
52. Applegate, K. L., Kiecolt-Glaser, J. K., & Glaser, R. (in press). Depression, immune function, and health in older adults. In G. M. Williamson, D. R. Shaffer, & P. A. Parmelee (Eds.), *Physical illness and depression in older adults: A handbook of theory, research, and practice* (pp. 135–145). New York: Plenum.
53. McDemott, D., & Snyder, C. R. (1999). *Making hope happen.* Oakland, CA: New Harbinger Publications.
54. Snyder, C. R. (1984). *The psychology of hope: You can get there from here.* New York: Free Press.

13

Methods of Coping from the Religions of the World: The Bar Mitzvah, Karma, and Spiritual Healing

Kenneth I. Pargament
Margaret M. Poloma
Nalini Tarakeshwar

Long before there was a discipline of psychology, people were applying systems of belief and practice from the religions of the world to understand and come to terms with the most profoundly disturbing aspects of life. In response to questions about birth, death, accident, illness, suffering, and the meaning of life more generally, they drew on a variety of religious methods of coping that were developed and refined by the world's religions. Surprisingly, although psychologists often share many of the goals of organized religious systems, they have largely ignored the wisdom of age-old religious traditions. Writers have suggested many explanations for the neglect of the religious dimension by psychologists, including the emotional sensitivity of religious issues; competitiveness between organized religion and the field of psychology, which could be viewed as a "pseudoreligion" with its own beliefs, values, and practices; and lower levels of religiousness among psychologists than the general public (i.e., the "religiosity gap") and their associated underestimation of the importance of religion (1, 2).

Whatever the explanation for the oversight, there are several good reasons why psychologists should take a closer look at religious coping resources. First, religious coping is commonplace. In fact, some groups, such as the elderly and African-Americans, cite religion as the most frequently used resource for coping with major life stressors (e.g., 3, 4, 5). Second, religious coping can be effective. Methods of religious coping have been associated with a variety of positive outcomes, including better physical health, better mental health, and enhanced spiritual well-being; moreover, people have obtained such benefits when facing various critical life situations, including organ transplantation, serious medical illness, the loss of loved ones, natural disasters, and terrorism (e.g., 6, 7, 8). Third, individuals may profit by adding the special characteristics of religious coping to their coping repertoire. In several comparative studies, measures of religious coping have been found to predict adjustment to life crises beyond the effects of traditional secular coping measures (see 9 for review). What is this "something special" of religion? Religious methods of coping may be particularly well-suited to the problem of human insufficiency. On this point, the first author (9) has written:

> Try as we might to maximize significance through our own insights and experiences or through those of others, we remain human, finite, and limited. At any time we may be pushed beyond our immediate resources, exposing our basic vulnerability to ourselves and the world. To this most basic of existential crises, religion holds out solutions. The solutions may come in the form of spiritual support when other forms of social support are lacking, explanations when no other explanations seem convincing, a sense of ultimate control through the sacred when life seems out of control, or new objects of significance when old ones are no longer compelling. In any case, religion complements nonreligious coping, with its emphasis on personal control, by offering responses to the limits of personal powers. (p. 310)

We believe that psychologists have something to learn about, indeed *learn from*, the religions of the world. In fact, we lack an important factor when we try to understand and facilitate adaptive processes and people without an appreciation for the religious dimension. Fortunately, several psychologists, have begun to explore the resources of religious traditions. Much of this work has focused on mainline Christians in the United States. It is important to note, however, that the population of the United States is becoming increasingly pluralistic religiously (10). To work with heterogeneous communities, psychologists will need to better understand the resources of diverse religious groups. In this chapter, we follow our own advice by focusing on three relatively unstudied methods of religious coping from three relatively unstudied religions of the world: (1) the Bar Mitzvah among Jews, (2) karma among Hindus, and (3) healing among Pentecostal-Charismatic Christians. As a prelude, we offer a definition of religion and a framework for the analysis of these religious coping methods.

Defining Religion and Religious Coping

Religion as a Process

Among psychologists, the term religion often is associated with thoughts of church, cult, dogma, and ritual (11). Religion, however, is more than a static set of beliefs, practices, and institutions. It is a process, as Pargament (9) has put it, "a search for significance in ways related to the sacred" (p. 34). There are two important assumptions in this definition.

The first assumption is consistent with recent developments in motivation theory that stress the goal-directed character of human behavior (e.g., 12, 13, 14, 15). We assume that people seek significance. Objects of significance may be material, physical, psychological, social, or spiritual. They may be socially valued (e.g., loving relationships) or condemned (e.g., alcohol addiction). Certainly, individuals define significance differently. However significance is defined, we assume that virtually everyone tries to find things that matter to them (discovery), hold on to them (conservation), and let go and rediscover new things of value when necessary (transformation). It also is useful to think about the search for significance in terms of pathways and destinations—that is, means and ends.

What makes a search for significance religious? Our second assumption is that the defining quality of religion comes from peoples' involvement of the sacred in the search for significance. According to the Oxford English Dictionary, the sacred refers to the holy, those things "set apart" from the ordinary, worthy of veneration and reverence. The sacred includes ideas of the divine, the transcendent, and God (16). However, the sacred goes beyond concepts of higher powers by including objects sanctified by virtue of their association with, or representation of, the holy (17). Sacred objects can take several forms: time and space (Sabbath, cathedrals), events and transitions (births, funerals), materials (water, wine), cultural products (music, literature), people (saints, clergy), practices (prayer, confession), psychological attributes (self, meaning), social attributes (patriotism, compassion), and roles (marriage, work).

We call a person religious when he or she takes a pathway that somehow is connected to the sacred or seeks a sacred life destination (9). The sacred can be a part of the thoughts (e.g., religious beliefs, dogma), behaviors (e.g., practices, rituals), relationships (e.g., with fellow congregations, with clergy), and emotions (e.g., awe, fear) that, to a greater or lesser extent, define the individual's life path. These paths can lead to many ends. Psychologists and social scientists from Freud to Durkheim have articulated a number of goals or functions of religion, including the promotion of life meaning, emotional comfort, impulse control, intimacy and social solidarity, physical health, a sense of control, and a better world. It is important to note, however, that the sacred can also be an end in itself. Indeed, the search for the sacred represents the core function of religion and the essence of spirituality. "It is the ultimate Thou whom the religious person seeks most of all," psychologist Paul Johnson (18, p. 70) wrote. Furthermore, seemingly secular ends can take on a spiritual character by virtue of their association with the sacred. To seek justice, to make the world a better place, to love one another are, for many, profoundly religious goals.

There are myriad religious paths and religious destinations. Indeed, part of the staying power of the world's great religious traditions may lie in the fact that adherents experience a variety of ways of being religious. Even beneath some of the same religious roofs, individuals with different temperaments, strengths, needs, and goals conceivably can find places to stay.

Part of the durability of religion also may lie in its ability to respond to the to the greatest life challenges.

Religious Coping

For many people religion is a way of life, an overarching orientation that directs their thoughts, feelings, actions, relationships, and values in every-day living as well as more stressful moments. In short, religion is more than a way of coping. Religion does, however, offer specific methods to help people understand and come to terms with life stressors. Religious coping methods are designed to conserve or transform significance in the face of difficult life situations.

Psychologists have long noted the connection between religion and times of stress. However, they have tended to view religion in limited, stereotyped, and negative terms. Religion has been called a defense, avoidant, passive, irrational, and a form of escapism and denial (e.g., 19, 20). A closer look at the roles of religion in stressful periods, though, reveals a more complex picture. It is true that religion can serve defensive roles. Examples of religiously based denial, passivity, and avoidance are found easily. However, religion takes on other guises in coping as well—assertive as well as defensive, active as well as passive (see Table 13.1 for illustrations).

For example, Pargament and his colleagues (21, 22) distinguished among four religious approaches to achieving a sense of control in coping. The first type, deferring, reflects the form of religion that is so often criticized by social scientists. This style of religious coping places the responsibility for problem solving on God. Solutions are believed to emerge through the active efforts of God alone and, as a result, the individual responds to stressors with a passive coping stance. In sharp contrast, the second type, self-directing religious coping, assumes that God gives the individual the skills and resources to solve problems. The responsibility for problem solving then rests on the individual's shoulders alone. In the third type, pleading, the individual asks God to intercede in the situation on his or her behalf. Here, the individual attempts to achieve control indirectly through petitions to God. Finally, collaborative religious coping assumes that God and the individual share the responsibility for problem solving. This fourth type of coping is experienced as a partnership in which both God and the individual work actively together to resolve crises. Thus, religious coping methods run the gamut from passive to active strategies.

Researchers have begun to examine other religious coping methods in more detail, including spiritual support (23), congregational support (24), purification and confession (25), and religious appraisals (26). Different forms of religious coping appear to have different implications for adjustment to critical life events (see 6). For example, with respect to the control-oriented forms of religious coping, collaborative and self-directing approaches have been associated with higher levels of mental health (21, 27, 28). In contrast, the deferring and pleading approaches have been tied to

Table 13.1 Illustrative Methods of Religious Coping

Deferring Religious Coping: Passively waiting for God to control the situation.

Self-Directing Religious Coping: Seeking control through individual initiative rather than help from God.

Pleading Religious Coping: Seeking control indirectly through petitions to God for help.

Collaborative Religious Coping: Seeking control through a partnership with God in problem-solving.

Benevolent Religious Reappraisal: Redefining the stressor through religion as benevolent and potentially beneficial.

Punishing God Reappraisal. Redefining the stressor as a punishment from God for the individual's sins.

Demonic Reappraisal: Redefining the stressor as the act of the Devil.

Reappraisal of God's Powers: Redefining God's powers to influence the stressful situation.

Seeking Spiritual Support: Searching for comfort and reassurance through God's love and care.

Spiritual Discontent: Expressing confusion and dissatisfaction with God.

Seeking Congregational Support: Searching for comfort and reassurance through the love and care of congregation members and clergy.

Interpersonal Religious Discontent: Expressing confusion and dissatisfaction with congregation members and clergy.

Religious Purification: Searching for spiritual cleansing through religious actions.

Religious Forgiving: Looking to religion for help in letting go of anger, hurt, and fear associated with an offense.

Rites of Passage: Participating in rituals to facilitate the transition from one phase of life to another.

Religious Conversion: Shifting from a life oriented around self-centered concerns to a life oriented toward the transcendent.

---

lower levels of mental health. Interestingly, however, some researchers have found that the value of the collaborative, deferring, and self-directing approaches may also depend on the controllability of the situation. In one study of adult church members, higher levels of collaborative and deferring and lower levels of self-directing religious coping were associated with less depression in uncontrollable situations (29); the reverse held true for controllable situations.

Many religious coping methods are conservational in nature. They are designed to help people maintain or hold on to an object of significance in stressful situations, be it a sense of control, a sense of meaning and purpose in life, or emotional comfort. However, through the mechanisms of religion, people also can replace old objects of significance with new ones. Rites of passage assist people in the transition from one phase of life to another.

Through forgiveness, individuals replace anger and bitterness with tolerance and compassion (30). Religious conversion fosters a transformation from a life oriented around self-centered concerns to a life oriented around transcendent values (31).

In sum, short-hand descriptions of religion as a defense, a passive form of coping, or a form of denial underestimate the complexity of religious life. Researchers are beginning to learn about the rich variety of religious coping methods. Although much of this initial work has focused on mainline Christian groups, there are many other important religious traditions and they too represent potentially rich resources for coping. In the remainder of this chapter we consider three of these relatively neglected forms of religious coping.

Coming of Age: The Bar Mitzvah as a Rite of Passage

Our movement through the life span is not simply linear. It is marked by sharp changes—births, coming of age, marriages, deaths—periods of rapid qualitative shift from one phase of life to another. The religions of the world have long provided their adherents with rites of passage that announce these radical transitions and shepherd people through them. There are many types of rites of passage, but they share a common function and structure; they are designed to mark and facilitate the transition through these "hinges of time" (32, p. 164). Rites of passage have a dual nature; they are both conservational and transformational, encouraging continuity and change (9). Cushioned by the reassurance of an on-going relationship with the sacred, and by an on-going membership in a community, the individual is nurtured through a major change in role status and identity.

Although births, marriages, and funerals continue to be embedded in religious rites of passage (e.g., baptism, church wedding, church funeral) in Western culture, the period of transition from childhood to adulthood—the coming of age—no longer is generally shrouded in religious sacrament (e.g., initiation, puberty rites). This is a noteworthy omission given that adolescence is a time of dramatic change involving psychological, sexual, and cognitive maturation, with new expectations and the need for a clear identity. An important exception to this rule is the Bar Mitzvah. Even though only a small percentage of the world's population is Jewish, the Bar Mitzvah remains a central rite of passage for even secularized Jews.

Describing the Bar Mitzvah

The words "Bar Mitzvah" mean "son of the commandments," and indicate that the 13-year-old boy is now obligated to follow Jewish laws. For girls, this transition is called a Bat Mitzvah. Typically, girls celebrate it at the age of 13, although according to Jewish law, girls become Bat Mitzvah at 12.

We will focus on the Bar Mitzvah here, because it has traditionally received more attention, particularly within Orthodox Judaism.

Two commandments are particularly noteworthy for the Bar Mitzvah boy. If he is observant, he begins to put on *tefillin*, two small black boxes with straps attached to them, before his prayers on weekday mornings. Wearing the *tefillin* symbolizes the covenant between God and Israel, God's presence, and reminds the individual of God's commandments (33). The Bar Mitzvah is also the occasion of the boy's first *aliyah* (meaning "going up"), in which he makes a physical and spiritual ascension to the altar to recite a blessing over the Torah before it is read. Reserved for transitions in the life cycle and special life events, the *aliyah* is one of the greatest honors to be accorded the synagogue member.

In the United States, the Bar Mitzvah has come to be associated with a more elaborate religious ceremony and celebration (some have called it a major industry). Here the boy is expected to stand in front of family, friends, and teachers at the synagogue and read the entire Torah portion for the week or chant the *Haftorah*, a smaller selection from the prophetic books of the Bible. This is no easy task. The *Haftorah* is written in Hebrew and must be sung according to prescribed musical notes. It takes time and effort to prepare for the ritual. It is common for the Bar Mitzvah boy to begin his lessons several months prior to the ceremony.

Far from a simple religious ritual, the Bar Mitzvah demonstrates the boy's learning, poise, and readiness to take on adult responsibilities. The ritual provides the boy with the opportunity to conquer his doubts, stand up in front of others, and show off his newfound power. As one rabbi put it, this is a "process of doing rather than sitting back and worry. . . . In this experience [the Bar Mitzvah boy] is pushed through to producing, to taking command of the situation" (34, p. 120).

In some ways, the Bar Mitzvah is as much a rite of passage for the family as it is for the boy. Not only must the Bar Mitzvah boy show that he can begin to assume the mantle of adulthood, but also the family must show that it can begin to "let go" of their child and support his emerging autonomy. And together, the boy and his family also must reaffirm their commitments to each other, to God, and to the Jewish people. Thus, the Bar Mitzvah boy and family make this passage together.

Unfortunately, neither the Bar Mitzvah nor its impact on the young man and his family have received much empirical scrutiny. A few observational studies, however, have been conducted. Judith Davis (35) presents a rich account of three families' passage through this rite. Following the conceptual framework of anthropologist van Gennep (36), she divides the Bar Mitzvah into three phases: preparation, ceremony, and aftermath.

Preparation   The year before the Bar Mitzvah ceremony is a peculiar "never-never land." No longer a child but not yet an adult, the boy has entered a period of clouded identity, embodied by the paradoxical adult/child title of "Bar Mitzvah boy." In this time, a "sacred space" is created around the family to sustain it through the transition (35). As the boy begins to rehearse his *Haftorah* and the family starts planning for the ceremony and celebration, they take on a special status in their own eyes and in the eyes of the community.

One of the most important tasks of the preparation phase, Davis notes, is the prevention of conflicts that threaten to defile the sacred occasion and disrupt the family order. For instance, one divorced family, in which parents shared custody of their son, went to great lengths to ensure that the tensions between the parents did not spoil the event. While planning for the Bar Mitzvah, both sides agreed to set aside other potentially divisive issues, such as finances and visitation. "It was as if everyone had implicitly agreed to use the time for consolidating and nurturing the system's strengths before tackling the next set of difficult issues" (35) p. 181). Although money was limited, all sides agreed to share the expense of a hospitality suite where the extended families could come together to meet and relax in between the weekend's ceremonies and events. The hospitality suite became a metaphor that expressed the family's desire to wrap the Bar Mitzvah in sacred time and place.

Ceremony   As the Bar Mitzvah ceremony comes nearer, pressures mount on the boy and his family. Friends and family ask the boy whether he "knows his *Haftorah*," and the family wonders whether the celebration will go smoothly. The ceremony itself provides the culminating moment. Here the escalating tensions come to a head and are resolved as the individual and family make a symbolic leap from one status to another. The Bar Mitzvah boy, now center-stage, reveals to family and friends his social poise, intellectual mastery, and commitment to his faith. The immediate family sits close to the stage or on it as a sign that they support him and that they too are going through a passage. The prayers, sermons, and benedictions of the service acknowledge that something momentous is taking place, and the congregation as a whole murmurs its approval.

Toward the end of the ceremony, or at the celebrations that follow over the weekend, the boy is given further opportunities to remind himself and others that he is ready to assume the adult role. A speech on the altar or a toast at the celebration provides additional evidence that the boy is maturing into a man. At the same time, the messages themselves reassure the audience that, even as he becomes more independent, he remains connected to family and religion. Listen to one Bar Mitzvah toast from a boy who had immigrated from the former Soviet Union:

> I want to thank you all for coming to my Bar Mitzvah. Especially I want to thank [my mother]. If not for her, I would never have had this Bar Mitzvah and this wonderful party. If not for her, I would never have come to America. If not for her, I would never have been born. (35, p. 192)

Relatives also may give speeches. Some are melancholy, reflecting a mixture of pride in the accomplishments of the Bar Mitzvah boy, sadness in the loss of his childhood, and deep appreciation of the continuity between this occasion, generations past, and generations to come.

> Barely choking back the tears, Ken presented his son with his deceased father's *tallis* [prayer shawl] and *tefillin* and with his prayer book in which four or five generations of Bar Mitzvahs had been recorded. As he handed over each item, Ken talked about what his father would have wished for his grandson had he been alive on this day. "What I think he would say is that you should . . . live your life to the fullest . . . and always do what you think is right. . . . And what my father gave me above all else was a feeling that I was always loved. That I was always good and the world was a safe place. And if I could give you anything, it would be that." (35, p. 182

Through their tears, applause, and shouts of Mazel Tov (congratulations), the congregation welcomes the child into the adult community and congratulates the family for its role in this transformation.

Aftermath   After the Bar Mitzvah ceremony, the young man reenters the everyday world with a new status. Childhood behind him, he is expected to take on greater responsibilities in the family and, in turn, receive treatment from others befitting his new position. Although the young man has become more autonomous, he is expected to remain connected to the larger Jewish community by participating in the synagogue, passing on his heritage to his children, and living a life of ethics and compassion. Here is how one young man put it: "It's a lot of bull if you [are Bar Mitzvahed] and then you go out and do nothing for Judaism for the rest of your life" (34, p. 126).

The twin threads of continuity and change run through this rite of passage. In each phase of the Bar Mitzvah, individuals and families are sustained as they undergo a transformation of significance. Davis (35) captures the essence of this multilevel paradoxical process in her summary:

> It is both a ritual of transition and ritual of continuity. In the context of the family, it is a ritual of elevation (i.e., transition), and in the context of the larger system, a ritual of consecration (i.e., continuity). It helps the child's movement away from the nuclear family at the same time that it binds him closer to that family through its larger past; it is a vehicle for separating the parents from the child while simultaneously moving them closer to each other and to their own parents; it celebrates the child's movement while mourning his loss; it strengthens boundaries while making them more flexible. (p. 201)

In short, the Bar Mitzvah illustrates a rite of passage that encourages, celebrates, and cushions the shock of the youth's coming of age.

Conclusions

How effective is the Bar Mitzvah? As noted, this rite of passage has received very little empirical attention. In one exception to this rule, children who receive a Jewish education, confirmation, and Bar/Bat Mitzvah have been shown to be more likely to participate in Jewish life as adults and less likely to marry someone outside the faith (e.g., 37). However, many questions remain about the short-term and long-term effects of the Bar Mitzvah. Critics have noted that, at least for some, the Bar Mitzvah has become an expensive consultant-dominated industry that disconnects people from the underlying psychological, social, and spiritual power of the ritual itself (38).

The descriptions and narrative accounts presented previously, however, suggest that this rite of passage may be at least partly successful in attaining its dual goals: facilitating the transition of the celebrant and his family to a new status, and cementing the individual's commitment to his family and the Jewish community. Furthermore, without rituals of this kind, some writers have suggested that we are vulnerable to a "flattening of time" (cf. 39); that is, a feeling that there is no difference between past and present and between present and future. Without rites of passage, we may lose the special, transcendent character of particular life moments. Likewise, perhaps, the difficulties experienced by many adolescents (e.g., alcohol use, drug use, violence, suicidality) are, in part, a result of our culture's failure to provide children with rites of passage that facilitate the coming of age, encouraging them to change within a cushion of community and culture.

Karma: Cosmic Meaning and Control in Coping

Hinduism, one of the world's most ancient religions, is practiced by more than 750 million people worldwide. Furthermore, over 16 million people in the world practice Sikhism, greater than 8 million observe Jainism, and more than 3 million people adhere to Buddhism (40). After the passing of the Hart-Celler Act of 1965 which relaxed the restrictions imposed on Asian immigration by earlier laws, the number of Asian immigrants to the United States belonging to each of these four religious groups has been growing at a steady rate (41). Buddhism, Jainism, and Sikhism stand apart from Hinduism in explicitly rejecting the scriptural authority of the Vedas. The Vedas form the core of the sacred literature in Hinduism and include the hymns, rituals, and sacrifices performed by Hindus. However, all four religious groups accept the doctrine of karma as one of the basic tenets of their religion (42).

Karmic doctrine is widely and deeply diffused in the Indian culture (43, 44, 45), and applies especially to people dealing with major stressors. The term "karma" also has made its way into popular Western culture (e.g., good and bad karma). Few, however, know what it means or how it is applied in its religious context. The doctrine of karma embodies a causal explanation for events that defy human understanding and provides a method of gaining control over the future by focusing on present actions. In this section, we elucidate karma as a common way of coping throughout the world. Toward this end, we consider theological writings and evidence, a modest amount of empirical research on Hindus, and interviews of a small American Hindu group who use karma for coping.

The Doctrine of Karma

In the Upanishads the doctrine of karma appears in clearly recognizable, albeit esoteric form (46, 47). The following is a quote from the *Mundaka Upanishad* in the Vedas:

> Brahman willed that it should be so, and brought forth out of himself the material cause of the universe; From this came the primal energy, and from the primal energy mind, from mind the subtle elements, From the subtle elements the many worlds, and from the acts performed by beings in the many worlds, The chain of cause and effect— the reward and punishment of works. . . . . .Living in the abyss of ignorance, the deluded think themselves best Attached to works, they know not God. Words lead them only to heaven, whence, to their sorrow, their rewards quickly exhausted, they are flung back to earth. . . . . .But, wise, self-controlled, and tranquil souls who are contented in spirit, and who practice austerity and meditation in solitude and silence, are freed from all impurity, and attain by the path of liberation to the immortal, the truly existing, the changeless self. (48, pp. 43–44)

According to the doctrine of karma, moral life is not chaos; people are reflections of their past deeds and, furthermore, present actions will shape their future (49). Karma has a multifaceted character, with different philosophers highlighting different aspects. There are however, several key elements of karma theory.

First, the law unifies time by connecting current events with the past and future. Within the physical universe, every effect must have a cause; the karmic law extends this notion to the moral realm. It implies that the individual's present condition is the result of the cumulation of past personal actions, and that the future can be shaped by righteous deeds in the present life. There appears to be no equivalent to the doctrine of karma in Western religions.

Second, although karma may seem to be a deterministic doctrine, there is a place for free will. Though the results of past actions have to be experienced in the present life (called *prārabdha karma*), an individual can develop tendencies and dispositions to act in a righteous manner (42, 50). Furthermore, a portion of the results of past actions is still suspended (known as *sañcita karma*). A person also can invoke the grace of God to prevent or mitigate the effects of bad actions. Finally, by performing actions without selfish motive (referred to as *niṣkāma karma*), an individual is freed of karmic effects (51, 52).

Third, some actions may produce immediate effects, while others may produce delayed reactions. In fact, one lifetime may be insufficient to reap the fruits of all actions. As a result, the theory of reincarnation of the same soul in different bodies forms another crucial aspect of the doctrine (44). The nature and circumstances of an individual's soul are said to depend on past deeds. For example, having previously performed many good actions, that person would be born in benevolent circumstances and vice versa (53).

Finally, the doctrine of karma alludes to the ultimate purpose of humankind—liberation from the misery and suffering that accompanies the rebirth cycle. When this liberation is achieved, the individual can realize the ultimate goal of eternal bliss in which the soul becomes one with the immortal, Supreme *Brahman* (48). This state can be attained when the person has exhausted accumulated karma through the accumulation of good deeds and freed him or herself from ignorance, desire, and self-interest. Thus, karma offers a preliminary route to spiritual liberation (47).

Karma as a Conservational Method of Coping

In our coping framework, karma represents a conservational method of coping that serves several functions.

Conservation of Comfort   The theory of karma provides a sense of comfort and hope that, ultimately, the cycle of life and death can be broken and *moksha* or spiritual liberation can be achieved. The doctrine also is comforting to the sufferer of ill fortune. Although sins in past lifetimes are responsible for present situations, these sins are committed by remote selves that are "differently constituted" from the individual's current identity (54). As a result, the person is spared the intense onus of blame. It cannot be known why an individual has a particular karmic destiny. However, an individual's present circumstances can be traced to the past, and that past has to be accepted. Thus, the stoic acceptance of personal destiny may help people cope with the most difficult life situations. One Hindu father, inteviewed for this chapter by Nalini Tarakeshwar, had experienced tremendous pain when his daughter was very ill. He shared a remark his daughter made that was most comforting to him: "Dad, my *samsara* (cycle of birth, death, and rebirth due to actions or karma) will determine when I will die. You might try a lot within your capacity, your skills, and your resources to save my life. But, if I am destined to die, you cannot hold me back."

Conservation of Meaning and Faith in a Just World   As a theory of causation, the doctrine of karma provides convincing explanations for human misfortune (44, 55). Another Hindu, inteviewed for this chapter, described how karma helped him understand the tragic loss of his brother. He said "my brother was killed when I was 11 years old. All the villagers asked us to place a complaint with the police. My mother told me that it is our fate. It is not within our control. We have committed sins in our past." In locating the cause of the loss in a distant past, karma provided the family with a compelling and benevolent explanation for a seemingly nonsensical event.

The karmic principle of moral order within a law-abiding universe also reinforces an individual's faith in a just world. Because the future can be reshaped by present behavior, whatever the present circumstances, the ultimate goal of liberation from the chain of life and death is available to all. This appeared to provide one Hindu interviewee with a sense of ultimate fairness and accompanying peace of mind. He stated, "Knowing that I cannot escape the results of my actions, I know that doing good deeds will help me. If I see good things happen to bad people, I know that s/he will not be able to escape from the consequences of bad actions. I can rest peacefully." It is important to note that karma does not function independently of other causal attributions. Other explanations of negative events are common in India, such as the malice of some other person, an angry deity, or other immediate agencies (54). In his work in central India, Babb (55) also found a healthy appreciation among villagers for the role of practical effort in avoiding pain and suffering. Karmic explanations of misfortune, he argued, functioned as explanations of a last resort, when the negative event could not be explained by a lack of ability or a lack of practical effort.

Conservation of a Benevolent View of God   The belief that misfortunes reflect past personal deeds conserves the view of God as the benefactor of human beings. In a study of patients who had recovered from psychoses, Narayanan et al. (45) found that 51% indicated that God was not responsible for their illness. A statement by another Hindu captures the essence of this karmic function: "Surely all the bad things that happen to people is because they must have done some bad things in the past. God is not a cruel person. He has to punish bad actions and teach us a lesson." For another interviewee, the role of God in the doctrine of karma was to mitigate bad deeds and encourage good behavior on earth. She claimed, "The best thing is to become a devotee of God. Though we have suffered from a lot of misfortunes in the past 15 years, our children have done well for themselves. That is because our faith in God kept us from choosing the wrong path, and our children have had the benefit of our good karma."

Conservation of a Sense of Control   The karma theory conserves the believer's sense of control. The locus of control is both internal and external. According to this doctrine, the individual's personal destiny is shaped by his or her response to difficult situations. Thus, the locus of control for the future is internal. With respect to the present and past, however, the locus of control has a mixed character. As noted earlier, the individual has some capacity to mitigate the effects of past actions. Thus, there is some opportunity for personal control over immediate events. The individual's present status also can be attributed to actions committed by a self from the past. However, the past self that is responsible for current conditions may have been a very different kind of self, a self "external" to the present self. In any event, the theory of karma provides the individual with the knowledge that life operates according to an underlying set of orderly principles and the assurance that control can be found in life, through external or internal focus.

Outcomes of Belief in Karma

Unfortunately, the relationship between belief in karma and mental and physical health has received scant empirical attention. Given the functions of karma, we might expect to find it related to at least two different outcomes. First, by providing benevolent explanations of misfortunes and a sense of control, individuals' beliefs in karma may lead to positive mental health. Consistent with this view, Dalal and Pande (56) found that psychological recovery among permanently and temporarily disabled Hindu patients was positively correlated with causal attributions to karma ($r = .37$). In this vein, one Hindu interviewee described how belief in the theory provided him with "peace of mind": "Since good actions will definitely lead to good outcomes in one of our many lives on earth, I have the moral confidence to withstand suffering and feel mentally prepared to try my best while being ready for the worst. I do not feel scared to take responsibility."

Second, karma permits both active and passive interpretations. Whether beliefs in karma lead to helplessness or hopefulness may depend on the ways in which it is understood. In a study comparing Tibetan with native Hindu priests residing in Himachal Pradesh in north India, Fazel and Young (57) reported that the Tibetans displayed greater life satisfaction than the Hindus. The difference between the two groups was explained by their varying interpretations of karma. The Hindus viewed karma as rigidly unalterable, while the Buddhists adopted a more flexible perspective. Other researchers also have found Hindus to be particularly concerned about the constraints that karma placed on their freedom of action. Buddhists, on the other hand, reportedly speculate more about karmic "prospects" than about karmic "retrospects" (58).

Finally, consistent with the passive view of karma, some sociologists argue that beliefs in the doctrine have helped perpetuate the caste system in India (59, 60). Though there are several castes and subcastes, four are important: *Brahmin* (religious scholars), *Kshatriya* (warrior class), *Vaisya* (business class), and *Sudra* (the class which supports the other three by doing the lower jobs—cleaning toilets, picking up garbage, becoming paid servants in the houses of the above three castes, etc.) (53, 61). Omprakash (60) conducted extensive interviews with 60 members of the lower caste and concluded that belief in the karmic doctrine promotes an acceptance of their exploitation and, in turn, other lower caste-affirming negative attributes (low self-esteem, low need for achievement).

Conclusions

The doctrine of karma offers its believers a resource to comprehend and assume a sense of control of challenging situations. In extending the principle of cause and effect to the cosmic realm, the law provides individuals with a unique way to understand and experience life's tragic moments. Available research suggests that, though they recognize that the effects of past deeds have to be experienced, individuals remain hopeful that righteous actions in the present life may mitigate harmful effects and, more important, lead to a better future. Some researchers, however, assert that beliefs in karma may encourage passive acceptance of current misfortunes and perpetuate the social oppression of the lower castes. Many questions obviously remain about karma and its part in coping. Studies especially are needed to address the potential costs and benefits to doctrinal adherents for coping with the vicissitudes of life

From Cure to Healing: Coping with Illness and Disease Among Pentecostal-Charismatics

The rise of allopathic medicine in the twentieth century has been both a blessing and a challenge. Vaccinations and pharmaceuticals have given humans unprecedented protection from many once-lethal diseases; biomedicine has allowed feats with transplants, human reproduction, and surgical procedures not dreamed possible in an earlier era; and medical technology has enabled precise diagnoses (often without promise of a cure) of problems that would astound their predecessors. Fear seems to be spreading, however, that the search for cures often leaves patients both uncured and unhealed. The hegemony of allopathic medicine is being increasingly challenged by the rise of alternative or complementary medical practices, many of which are more interested in healing the total person than in partial remedies. While acknowledging the vast contributions of allopathic medicine, the adherents of alternative medical practices point to the increase of chronic diseases with no known cure as signals of the limitations of a medical system in which the human spirit has been exorcised from the physical body.

The best-publicized proponents of a return of the spirit to medicine are the New Age gurus, whose books line the shelves of large bookstores, who appear on television talk shows, and whose faces grace the covers of national magazines. Their popularity, however, is eclipsed by another major stream of alternative healing whose history is as old as Christianity, with tenets about a unity of mind, body, and spirit that have much in common with the healing beliefs and practices of other premodern civilizations which inspire much New Age thought. Though rooted in different traditions, both New Age and Christian healing practitioners share a suspicion of post-Enlightenment empiricism, materialism, rationalism, and scientism; the former roots its medical philosophy in Eastern thought, while the latter centers its philosophy in an often literal interpretation of the Christian New Testament.

The Christian perspective on healing is exemplified principally in the Pentecostal-Charismatic movement, commonly dated to the Azusa Street Revival (1906–1909) led by William Seymour in Los Angeles and to Charles Parham's Zion City Revival (1906) outside Chicago. Together, the participants of these two revivals launched the Pentecostal denominations and independent charismatic churches that promote a religious experience known as Spirit-baptism (62). Citing biblical examples (e.g., John the Baptist's proclamation that he "baptized with water" but one was coming after him who would "baptize with the Spirit" [Luke 3:16], Pentecostal-Charismatic believers expect a second transforming experience to complement being baptized in water. Although different groups may emphasize different outward signs of Spirit-baptism, they agree that it will be accompanied by paranormal experiences, including glossolalia (speaking in tongues), healing, demonic deliverance, and miracles.

Through extensive missionary activity, the Pentecostal-Charismatic worldview spread throughout the United States and to other continents during the twentieth century (63, 64, 65). One in four Christians worldwide are thought to be part of this movement, crossing denominational as well as geographical boundaries (66, 67). It is estimated that some 12% of all Americans are Spirit-baptized, with a majority found in classical Pentecostal churches, newer independent Charismatic sects, as well as Roman Catholicism and all Protestant denominations (68).

The Pentecostal-Charismatic movement is about a distinctive Christian worldview (rather than a particular denomination, set of doctrines, or precisely defined ritual practices). This worldview blends premodern miracles, modern technology, and post modern mysticism in which the natural merges with the supernatural (69). In the words of the late John Wimber, founder of the Vineyard, a newly emerging denomination contributing to the reinvention of American Protestantism, Christianity is "supernaturally natural" (70, 71). Believers expect to experience as "normal" events, the Spirit of God through healing, miracles, prophecy, deliverance, and other paranormal happenings. Pentecostal-Charismatic Christians almost universally believe in healing. The vast majority know someone who has been healed through prayer, and many have personally experienced such divine healing. Testimonies about healing are given in most Pentecostal-Charismatic churches, prayer for healing is a regular part of church rituals, and healing testimonies and prayer are featured on Pentecostal-Charismatic television, all working together to maintain what sociologist Peter Berger has termed a "plausibility structure" to support the belief in divine healing.

Although Pentecostal-Charismatic Christians believe in and expect cures to take place, it should be emphasized that the normative focus is on holistic healing—spirit (soul), mind, and body. As with many other alternative healing systems, Pentecostal-Charismatic Christians seek more than a mechanistic solution to physical problems; they seek to make sense of affliction and instill a sense of ultimate hope (72, 73, 74). This search for meaning and hope in the face of illness, disability, and disease offers a unique window to view the Pentecostal-Charismatic. Divine healing, we believe, is a transformational coping form, wherein people adopt the goal of a closer relationship with God. In the next sections, we provide an actual account of this transformative process which includes a cure, a shaken worldview, and finally, a terminal illness and death. Although we see one person's struggle with illness in "Karen's Story," this transformational process is a widely applicable form of coping for Pentecostal-Charismatics.

Karen's Story

Some years ago, while working on a major research project on the Assemblies of God, the largest white Pentecostal denomination with over 2 million members in the United States and 20 million worldwide, I (Margaret Poloma) was introduced to Karen by an usher at the local assembly. Karen was a new visitor to the church who had a story—a narrative in postmodern terminology—a testimony, to tell in charismatic parlance. As Karen began to share her testimony, I quickly connected her story with a news article appearing in the local paper a few months earlier. This 40-year-old woman was "allergic" to the modern world, with allergies so severe that, even with the best of medical treatment, she was unable to live normally. In a desperate search for a cure, her husband sent her to a hospital in Dallas known for treating cases of severe allergic reactions. As Karen continued sharing her narrative, she introduced me to Ann, a Messianic Jew and charismatic Christian with professed gifts of both healing and prophecy, who often visited the Dallas hospital in search of people who sought prayer for healing. With Karen's permission, Ann had prayed with Karen. Karen said she "knew" immediately that she had been healed and quickly embraced the charismatic faith modeled by Ann.

Neither Karen nor her husband were Christian believers (both claimed to be agnostic at the time of the healing), and Karen's husband, a former Protestant minister, understandably refused to accept that his wife had actually been cured. He instructed Karen to return home only when there was solid evidence that she no longer suffered from the severe allergic reactions making it impossible to live in their new home. Karen used her husband's skepticism to remain with Ann in Dallas for a few weeks, and she became more familiar with her new Christian charismatic faith. I met Karen a week after she returned home. Karen's cure, later followed by a diagnosis of terminal cancer and finally her death, can be described in three stages, each of which has significance for understanding healing as a transformative coping strategy.

Stage 1: Searching for a Cure   As already noted, Karen was an agnostic when Ann appeared in her hospital room, prayed with her, and proclaimed her cured. For those like Karen who are not part of the Pentecostal-Charismatic community, the experience of such a cure can set them on a totally new pathway. Karen was unfamiliar with her new journey, and she welcomed the extra time with Ann to get grounded in her new faith before returning home. Once she returned home, she immediately sought support for her new beliefs, in a Pentecostal church.

The first stage of Karen's healing process emphasized curing rather than the possibility of a deeper healing through pain and affliction. She found the plausibility structure and hope she was seeking in a new group that taught a more extreme form of "faith healing," inspired by the teachings of Tulsa evangelist Kenneth Hagin's Word-Faith movement. Pentecostal-Charismatic critics commonly refer to this stream of the charismatic movement as "name-it-and claim-it," reflecting the belief that once one asks for something in Jesus' name, the person already has received it. The failure to have the gift (whether it be health, money, or some other desired resource) materialize supposedly is due to a lack of faith (75, 76, 77).

While many come seeking healing gifts (e.g., physical cure, new job, repair of broken relationships), mainstream Pentecostal-Charismatic theology admonishes converts to seek the Giver rather than the gifts—to seek the Baptizer rather than the baptism. Sooner or later, however, a prayer seems unanswered, a prophecy fails, or a sick person dies. The believer is then thrust into a second stage, being forced to struggle with a shaken worldview. In Karen's case, the onset of this second stage came about through her development of terminal cancer.

Stage Two: A Shaken Worldview   Nearly two years after I first met her, I received a phone call from Karen's husband. Karen had developed an incurable form of lymphatic cancer. When I expressed my concern, her husband, who had embraced Karen's faith after her return from Dallas, responded: "Oh, we are not worried. Karen is already healed. Ann prayed with her over the telephone and prophesied that God was healing her. We all believe that Karen is healed." Being less certain of the outcome than Karen's husband, I once again entered Karen's life. She shared with me the letter she had obtained from her physician about her first healing (which enabled her to appear and share her testimony on Christian television some months earlier), as well as lab reports and a letter with the dismal prognosis regarding her current medical condition.

Karen had decided to decline the prescribed chemotherapy and radiation, not because she rejected modern medicine, but because the best the physicians could promise was that the treatment might prolong her life by six months or so. While continuing to profess being healed, Karen also spoke realistically about issues relating to the "quality of life and death." She insisted that declining the treatment would increase the quality of her time remaining. I listened to her carefully and made a resolution to visit her regularly. Karen was very clear on one issue; if she were in fact dying, she wanted to die at home. Within a couple of short months, Karen's deteriorating physical and then mental condition made it impossible for her to believe that she would receive the physical cure she once expected.

It was during this time that Karen's shaken faith caused her to abandon the more extreme Word-Faith perspective in favor of the more moderate position adhered to by the larger Pentecostal-Charismatic movement. At one point, Karen struggled with doubts about God's love for her and began to question what she had done to deserve this "punishment from God." In line with Word-Faith teaching, Karen initially affirmed the Pentecostal-Charismatic belief that the demonic is the source of illness. When a cure was not forthcoming, however, Karen faced the dilemma of choosing between believing in a God who did not have power over Satan or in a God who was deliberately allowing Satan to kill her. The shaking of Karen's worldview opened up the opportunity for a transformation into a deeper relationship with God. This is the goal of spiritual healing within the Pentecostal Charismatic community.

Stage Three: From Cure to Healing   At this point, a friend gave Karen a copy of Hannah Hurnard's (78) devotional allegory *Hinds' Feet on High Places*, which served as a model for further transformation. Hurnard's book described the inner change of an allegorical character ("Much Afraid") from paralyzing fear to glorious confidence as she climbed a treacherous mountain with the Shepherd (Jesus) as her guide. At the end of the allegory, the Shepherd gave Much Afraid a new name, Grace and Glory, to symbolize the transformation that had taken place during the climb. As Karen read, reflected on, and talked about the allegory, she experienced fresh assurance about God's faithful love that empowered her to abandon herself to the mystery of life and death confronting her. Similar to the biblical character in the Book of Job, Karen's fear was replaced with an abandonment to a perceived divine will only dimly understood—a surrender that moved her from seeking a cure to preparing for the "final healing" (as Pentecostal-Charismatic Christians often refer to death).

I continued to visit Karen as the cancer metastasized to her brain, took away her speech, and eventually left her paralyzed. Although no longer able to communicate in words, she seemed to have a new sense of peace. Within four months after my initial visit, Karen died. Her funeral was held in the local charismatic Episcopal church which she attended infrequently, where healing was believed and practiced but in a more moderate form than in the Word-Faith groups that Karen had originally favored. In these last months before she had died, Karen was able to redefine healing from being a *cure* to a final transformation of *union with God*.

Discussion and Conclusions

Despite the fervent belief in miraculous healing, curing is not the heart of Pentecostal-Charismatic faith. Most believers, even those in the forefront of the healing movement, are reluctant to explain why a particular cure does not take place. In the words of a Presbyterian minister who has prayed for thousands of persons who have received healings during his 40 years of an active healing ministry, "I have not been called to explain; I have been called to proclaim that Jesus heals today" (79). This worldview, which commonly makes a distinction between "curing" and "healing," allows persons to believe in and have hope for being cured; but even when such a cure is not forthcoming, they can point to other ways in which they have been healed by God.

Healing in the Pentecostal-Charismatic tradition appears to be a form of transformational coping. In response to poor health, the individual experiences a fundamental shift in the meanings of health and healing. The coping functions of healing receive additional support from two survey projects—a random sample of residents of Akron, Ohio (77) and a Gallup Poll (80)—in which those who reported miraculous healings were significantly more likely to be in poorer physical health. While there is no evidence from either of these surveys that religiosity actually promotes better physical health, there is evidence that it does promote a sense of spiritual well-being (see 81) and, perhaps, a sense of hope (82). What we have described here is the process by which transformational coping takes place in light of the Pentecostal-Charismatic worldview. Karen's story of her transformation from curing to healing provides an illustration of a process that is repeated time and again within the lives of many Pentecostal-Charismatic believers.

Final Thoughts

Over thousands of years, the religions of the world have evolved a variety of mechanisms designed to help people come to terms with the most fundamental problems of living. Are these mechanisms effective? At this time, empirical research on the short-and long-term effects of these and other religious coping methods is limited. Researchers are, however, finding that methods of religious coping are significant predictors of psychological, social, and spiritual well-being (9). Even if we were to disregard this initial evidence, however, the sheer staying power of the world's religions and their religious coping methods suggests that we take them seriously. In fact, psychologists may have something not only to *learn about* but also to *gain from* the solutions religions offer to life's most baffling, intractable problems.

In this chapter, we have taken a closer look at three relatively unexplored methods of religious coping—the Bar Mitzvah, karma, and spiritual healing. Each of these methods, we believe, is noteworthy for psychological theory and practice. The doctrine of karma and the practice of spiritual healing represent ingenious solutions to the problems raised by seemingly unfathomable, uncontrollable situations. Psychology in the United States, with its focus on the here-and-now and the extension of human control, should take note of these very different approaches. For example, we can learn from the notion in karma theory that there is a great cosmic causal order. We can learn how healing sometimes comes from a surrender of control to a higher power and a transformation from a focus on survival and cure to a greater transcendent value. Additionally, American psychology and society more generally should take note of religious rites of passage, as illustrated by the Bar Mitzvah, designed to facilitate the transition of people through critical "hinges of time."

It is unfortunate that psychology as a discipline has generally overlooked the resources of religious traditions, because the worlds of psychology and religion share an interest in understanding and enhancing the human condition. Moroover, the two disciplines have something to offer each other in the pursuit of common goals. Ultimately, with greater interaction and better understanding, we may be able to move toward a closer integration of psychological and religious thought and practice in our efforts to facilitate adaptive coping processes. Promising examples of collaborative, integrative "psychoreligious" programs and interventions already have been implemented (see 83, 84, 85, 86, 87) The time appears right for psychological and religious communities to begin learning more about and from each other. By pooling our resources, we may be able to unleash the power of the coping process and, in turn, enhance the psychological, social, and spiritual well-being of people.

References

1. Bergin, A. E. (1980). Psychotherapy and religious values. *Journal of Consulting and Clinical Psychology, 48*, 95–105.
2. Shafranske, E. P., & Malony, H. N. (1990). Clinical psychologists' religious and spiritual orientations and their practice of psychotherapy. *Psychotherapy, 27*, 72–78.
3. Conway, K. (1985–1986). Coping with the stress of medical problems among black and white elderly. *International Journal of Aging and Human Development, 21*, 39–48.
4. Koenig, H. G. (1988). Religious behaviors and death anxiety in later life. *Hospice Journal, 4*, 3–24.
5. Manfredi, C., & Pickett, M. (1987). Perceived stressful situations and coping strategies utilized by the elderly. *Journal of Community Health Nursing, 4*, 99–100.
6. Pargament, K. I., Koenig, H. G., & Perez, L. (2000). The many methods of religious coping: Development and initial validation of the RCOPE. *Journal of Clinical Psychology, 56*, 519–543.
7. Park, C. L., & Cohen, H. (1993). Religious and nonreligious coping with the death of a friend. *Cognitive Therapy and Research, 17*, 561–577.
8. Tix, A. P., & Frazier, P. A. (1998). The use of religious coping during stressful life events: Main effects, moderation, and mediation. *Journal of Consulting and Clinical Psychology, 66*, 411–422.
9. Pargament, K. I. (1997). *The psychology of religion and coping: Theory, research, practice.* New York: Guilford.

10. Roof, W. C., & McKinney, W. (1987). *American mainline religion: Its changing shape and future.* New Brunswick, NJ: Rutgers University Press.
11. Zinnbauer, B. J., Pargament, K. I., & Scott, A. B. (1999). The emerging meanings of religiousness and spirituality: Problems and prospects. *Journal of Personality, 67,* 889–919.
12. Emmons, R. A. (1986). Personal strivings: An approach to personality and subjective well-being. *Journal of Personality and Social Psychology, 51,* 1058–1068.
13. Ford, D. H. (1987). *Humans as self-constructing living systems: A developmental perspective on behavior and personality.* Hillsdale, NJ: Erlbaum.
14. Karoly, P. (1993). Mechanisms of self-regulation: A systems view. *Annual Review of Psychology, 44,* 23–52.
15. Snyder, C. R. (1994). *The psychology of hope: You can get there from here.* New York: Free Press.
16. Pargament, K. I. (1999). The psychology of religion *and* spirituality? Yes and no. *International Journal for the Psychology of Religion, 9,* 3–16.
17. Mahoney, A., Pargament, K. I., Jewell, T., Swank, A. B., Scott, E., Emery, E., & Rye, M. (1999). Marriage and the spiritual realm: The role of proximal and distal religious constructs in marital functioning. *Journal of Family Psychology, 13,* 321–338.
18. Johnson, P. E. (1959). *Psychology of religion.* Nashville, TN: Abingdon Press.
19. Ellis, A. (1986). *The case against religion: A psychotherapist's view and the case against religiosity.* Austin: American Atheist Press.
20. Freud, S. (1927/1961). *The future of an illusion.* New York: Norton.
21. Pargament, K. I., Kennell, J., Hathaway, W., Grevengoed, N., Newman, J., & Jones, W. (1988). Religion and the problem-solving process: Three styles of coping. *Journal for the Scientific Study of Religion, 27,* 90–104.
22. Pargament, K. I., Cole, B., Vandecreek, L., Belavich, T., Brant, C., & Perez, L. (1999). The vigil: Religion and the search for control in the hospital waiting room. *Journal of Health Psychology, 4,* 327–341.
23. Maton, K. I. (1989). The stress-buffering role of spiritual support: Cross-sectional and prospective investigations. *Journal for the Scientific Study of Religion, 28,* 310–323.
24. Krause, N., Ellison, C. G., & Wulff, K. M. (1998). Church-based emotional support, negative interaction, and psychological well-being: Findings from a national survey of Presbyterians. *Journal for the Scientific Study of Religion, 37,* 725–741.
25. Pennebaker, J. W., & Beall, S. (1986). Confronting a traumatic event: Toward an understanding of inhibition and disease. *Journal of Abnormal Psychology, 95,* 274–281.
26. Mickley, J. R., Pargament, K. I., Brant, C. R., & Hipp, K. (1999). God and the search for meaning among hospice caregivers. *Hospice Journal, 13,* 1–18.
27. Hathaway, W. L., & Pargament, K. I. (1990). Intrinsic religiousness, religious coping, and psychosocial competence: A covariance struc-

ture analysis. *Journal for the Scientific Study of Religion, 29,* 423–441.

28. McIntosh, D. N., & Spilka, B. (1990). Religion and physical health: The role of personal faith and control. In M. L. Lynn and D. O. Moberg (Eds.), *Research in the social scientific study of religion,* Vol. 2 (pp. 167–194). Greenwich, CT: JAI Press.

29. Bickel, C. O., Ciarrocchi, J. W., Scheers, N. J., Estadt, B. K., Powell, D. A., & Pargament, K. I. (1998). Perceived stress, religious coping styles, and depressive affect. *Journal of Psychology and Christianity, 17,* 33–42.

30. McCullough, M. E., Worthington, E. L., Jr., & Rachal, K. C. (1997). Interpersonal forgiving in close relationships. *Journal of Personality and Social Psychology, 73,* 321–336.

31. Zinnbauer, B. J., & Pargament, K. I. (1998). Spiritual conversion: A study of religious change in college students. *Journal for the Scientific Study of Religion, 37,* 161–180.

32. Friedman, E. H. (1985). *Generation to generation: Family process in church and synagogue.* New York: Guilford Press.

33. Donin, H. H. (1980). *To pray as a Jew: A guide to the prayer book and the synagogue service.* New York: Basic Books.

34. Zegans, S., & Zegans, L. S. (1979). Bar Mitzvah: A rite for a transitional age. *Psychoanalytic Review, 66,* 115–132.

35. Davis, J. (1988). Mazel tov: The Bar Mitzvah as a multigenerational ritual of change and continuity. In E. Imber-Black, J. Roberts, & R. Whiting (Eds.), *Rituals in families and family therapy* (pp. 177–208). New York: W. W. Norton and Company.

36. van Gennep, A. (1960). *The rites of passage* (M. B. Vizedom & G. L. Caffee, Trans.). Chicago: University of Chicago Press.

37. Lazerwitz, B., Winter, J. A., Dashefsky, A., & Tabory, E. (1998). *Jewish choices: American Jewish denominationalism.* Albany: State University of New York Press.

38. Imber-Black, E., & Roberts, J. (1992). *Rituals for our times: Celebrating, healing, and changing our lives and our relationships.* New York: Harper Perennial.

39. Eisenstadt, S. N. (1965). Archetypal patterns of youth. In E. H. Erikson (Ed.), *The challenge of youth* (pp. 29–50). New York: Doubleday-Anchor.

40. Breuilly, E., O'Brien, J., & Palmer, M. (1997). *Religions of the world: The illustrated guide to origins, beliefs, traditions, and festivals.* New York: Transedition Limited and Fernleigh Books.

41. Tweed, T. A. (1999). General introduction. In T. A. Tweed & S. Prothero (Eds.), *Asian religions in America: A documentary history* (pp. 1–12). New York: Oxford University Press.

42. Sharma, A. (1996). *Hinduism for our times.* New Delhi: Oxford University Press.

43. Dalal, A. K., & Singh, A. K. (1992). Role of causal and recovery beliefs in the psychological adjustment to a chronic disease *Psychology and Health, 6,* 193–203.

44. Hiriyanna, M. (1996). *Essentials of Indian philosophy.* London: Diamond Books.

45. Narayanan, H. S., Mohan, K. S., & Radhakrishnan, V. K. (1986). The karma theory of mental illness. *NIMHANS Journal, 4*, 61–63.

46. Lipner. J. (1994). *Hindus: Their religious beliefs and practices.* New York: Routledge.

47. Reichenbach, B. R. (1990). *The law of karma: A philosophical study.* Honolulu: University of Hawaii Press.

48. Prabhavananda, S., & Manchester, F. (1975). *The Upanishads: Breath of the eternal.* New York: New American Library.

49. Mahadevan, T. M. P. (1946). *Whither civilization and other broadcast talks.* Madras, India: Central Arts Press.

50. Mahadevan T. M. P. (1962). Indian ethics and social practice. In C. A. Moore (Ed.), *Philosophy and culture east and west: East-West philosophy in practical perspective* (pp. 476–493). Honolulu: University of Hawaii Press.

51. Rao, P. N. (1968). Trends in contemporary Indian philosophy. In R. J. Singh (Ed.), *World perspectives in philosophy, religion, and culture: Essays presented to Professor Dhirendra Mohan Datta* (pp. 291–298). Patna, India: Bharati Bhavan.

52. Singh, B. (1971). *Foundations of Indian philosophy.* New Delhi: Orient Longmans.

53. Chennakesavan, S. (1974). *A critical study of Hinduism.* New Delhi: Asia Publishing House.

54. Sharma, U. (1973). Theodicy and the doctrine of karma. *Man, 8*, 347–364.

55. Babb, L. A. (1983). Destiny and responsibility: Karma in popular Hinduism. In C. F. Keyes & E. V. Daniel (Eds.), *Karma: An anthropological inquiry* (pp. 163–181). California: University of California Press.

56. Dalal, A. K., & Pande, N. (1988). Psychological recovery of accident victims with temporary and permanent disability. *International Journal of Psychology, 23,* 25–40.

57. Fazel, M. K., & Young, D. M. (1988). Life quality of Tibetans and Hindus. *Journal for the Scientific Study of Religion, 27*, 229–242.

58. Leichter, D., & Epstein, L. (1983). Irony in Tibetan notions of the good life. In C. F. Keyes & E. V. Daniel (Eds.), *Karma: An anthropological inquiry* (pp. 223–259). California: University of California Press.

59. Karnik, S. J., & Suri, K. B. (1995). The law of karma and social work considerations. *International Social Work, 38*, 365–377.

60. Omprakash, S. (1989). The doctrine of karma: Its psychosocial consequences. *American Journal of Community Psychology, 17,* 133–145.

61. Raju, P. T. (1985). *Structural depths of Indian thought.* New Delhi: South Asian Publishers.

62. Hunter, H. D. (1983). *Spirit-Baptism. A Pentecostal alternative.* Lanham, MD: University Press of America.

63. DeArteaga, W. (1992). *Quenching the spirit.* Lake Mary, Fl: Creation House.

64. Hytatt, E. L. (1996). *2000 years of charismatic Christianity.* Tulsa, OK: Hyatt International Ministries.

65. Synan, V. (1997). *The holiness-Pentecostal tradition.* Grand Rapids, MI: William B. Eerdmans.

66. Barrett, D. B. (1982) (Ed.). *World Christian encyclopedia*. New York: Oxford University Press.

67. Cox, H. (1995). *Fire from heaven*. Reading, MA: Addison-Wesley.

68. Green, J. C., Guth, J. L., Smidt, C. E., & Kellstedt, L. A. (1997). *Religion and the culture wars*. Lanham, MD: Rowman and Littlefield.

69. Poloma, M. M. (1999). The 'Toronto blessing' in postmodern society: Manifestations, metaphor and myth. In M. Dempster, B. Klaus, & D. Peterson (Eds.) *The globalization of Pentecostalism: A religion made to travel* (pp. 365–385). Irvine, CA: Regnum Books International.

70. Miller, D. E. (1997). *Reinventing American Protestantism*. Berkeley, CA: University of California Press.

71. Wimber, J. & Springer, K. (1987). *Power healing*. San Francisco, CA: HarperCollins.

72. Csordas, T. J. (1994). *The sacred self: A cultural phenomenology of charismatic healing*. Berkeley, CA: University of California Press.

73. Good, B., & Good, Mary-Jo, D. G. (1981). The meaning of symptoms: A cultural hermeneutical model for clinical practice. In L. Eisenberg & A. Kleinman (Eds.), *The relevance of social science for medicine* (pp. 165–196). Dordrecht, Holland: D. Reidel.

74. McGuire, M. B. (1988). *Ritual healing in suburban America*. New Brunswick, NJ: Rutgers University Press.

75. Poloma, M. M. (1982). *The Charismatic movement: Is there a new Pentecost?* Boston, MA: Twayne Publishers.

76. Poloma, M. M. (1989). *The assemblies of God at the crossroads*. Knoxville, TN: University of Tennessee Press.

77. Poloma, M. M. (1991). A comparison of Christian science and mainline Christian healing ideologies and practices. *Review of Religious Research, 32*, 337–358.

78. Hurnard, H. (1997). *Hinds' feet on high places*. Wheaton, IL: Tyndale House.

79. Barrow, D. W. (in press). *Yes, Virginia, there is a God who heals today*. Canton, OH: Wholeness Publications.

80. Poloma, M. M., Sutherland-Bindas, J., & Benson, H. (1998). *Examining a twisted knot: Healing, health, spirituality and religion*. Paper presented at the Annual Meeting of the Association for the Sociology of Religion, San Francisco, California.

81. Poloma, M. M., & Hoelter, L. (1998). The 'Toronto blessing': A holistic model of healing. *Journal for the Scientific Study of Religion, 37*, 257–272.

82. Snyder, C. R., Cheavens, J., & Michael, S. T. (1999). Hoping. In C. R. Snyder (Eds.), *Coping: The psychology of what works* (pp. 205–251). New York: Oxford University Press.

83. Cole, B., & Pargament, K. I. (1999). Re-creating your life: A spiritual/psychotherapeutic intervention for people diagnosed with cancer *Journal of Psycho-Oncology, 8*, 395–407.

84. Miller, W. R. (Ed.) (1999). *Integrating spirituality into treatment: Resources for practitioners*. Washington, DC: American Psychological Association.

85. Propst, L. R. (1988). *Psychotherapy in a religious framework: Spirituality in the emotional healing process.* New York: Human Services Press.
86. Richards, R. S., & Bergin, A. E. (1997). *A spiritual strategy for counseling and psychotherapy.* Washington, DC: American Psychological Association.
87. Shafranske, E. P. (Ed.), (1996). *Religion and the clinical practice of psychology.* Washington, DC: American Psychological Association.

14

Copers Coping with Stress:
Two Against One

C. R. Snyder
Kimberley Mann Pulvers

In chapter 1, we presented our model of coping. In this model, in which we were inspired by the ideas of Dr. Seuss, people are viewed as "coping machines" who deal with life stressors by traversing either avoidance or approach routes. To reiterate this model briefly, when an individual is confronted with a stressor, he construes the stressor and appraises his possible responses. This appraisal is a critical juncture because it is here that either an avoidance or an approach route is implemented. When a person takes the avoidance track of the coping cycle, she will characteristically pass through four iterative phases: (1) submitting to reactive avoidance strategies; (2) experiencing hyperattention to the stressor; (3) having an intensified self-focus; and (4) experiencing an increase in disruptive thoughts and emotions. When an individual embarks on her coping journey using an approach route, she will pass through two general phases: (1) selecting active approach strategies; and (2) using environment- and/or self-directed strategies to cope with a given stressor. In both the avoidance and approach routes, an individual will cycle back and forth between phases. Furthermore, we posit that each of these coping machines is equipped with an individual differences repertoire of stress response styles that may predispose him or her to react to the stressors by taking the adaptive approach route or the less adaptive avoidance route; moreover, these individual differences may impact any one of the steps in either the avoidance or approach routes. Finally, contrary to views held by some researchers in this area, we hold that coping is an everyday process; it occurs either within or below consciousness and involves stressors of varying magnitudes (including seemingly "small" ones).

In our reading of the chapters in this volume, both adaptive and maladaptive coping styles emerge. To examine the shared ideas as they relate to our coping model, in the first section of this chapter we will explore factors undermining effective coping processes and develop these ideas within the avoidance route in our model. In the second section, we will discuss factors enhancing the coping process, and we will evaluate these from an approach viewpoint. Lastly, we will consider a broader context for coping, make recommendations for improving coping, and provide brief concluding statements about this research area.

Factors Impeding the Coping Process

Many of the ideas shared by the chapter authors fit within the category of avoidant coping. We provide a closer look at these processes in this section.

Rumination

In chapter 9, "Self-Focused Attention and Coping: Attending to the Right Things," Hamilton and Ingram propose that automatic thinking plays a central role in shaping persons' coping-related reactions to stressors. Thus, it is not the event, per se, that is stressful; rather, it is the negative, internal dialogues and appraisals of events that engender negative stress. Hamilton and Ingram propose that rumination compounds stressful experiences and their sequelae. Consistent with this logic, other researchers have found that rumination maintains negative emotional states which, in turn, often portend more entrenched psychological problems (1, 2).

In McCullough's "Forgiving" chapter, rumination is implicated as impeding the adaptive forgiving process. Researchers using cross-sectional methods have reported that rumination, as well as efforts to suppress these intrusive thoughts, were associated with more avoidance and revenge-motivation—the very processes that are antithetical to forgiveness (3, 4). Persons who rely on problem-solving strategies that involve revenge often have difficulty in maintaining relationships. Likewise, a lack of forgiveness and a drive for revenge are linked to destructive interpersonal behaviors and a host of societal level problems (5, 6, 7, 8). On the other hand, those who ruminate and suppress *less* have a greater capacity to forgive (3, 4). Overall, if the goal is to enhance coping by teaching forgiveness, a prime target would be to decrease persons' ruminations about the sources of the transgressions made against them.

In our coping model, rumination is located on the avoidance track. It may be viewed as hyperattention to a stressor that occurs when one attempts to suppress thoughts about that stressor. Typically, the more that one tries *not* to think about something, the more that one will be compelled to think about that very thing (9, 10).[1] Thus, coping efforts at avoiding the stressor often backfire so as to increase the intrusion of unwanted thoughts into awareness, with an ensuing cycle of rumination. This pattern leads to an intensification of self-focused attention, which we describe next.

Focusing Attention on Self

In Hamilton and Ingram's chapter, they define self-focused attention as an emphasis on information from one's internal world of thoughts and beliefs, as opposed to cues from the external world. They suggest that through this self-focused attentional style, a person has limited access to positive information and therefore focuses overwhelmingly on negative information; in turn, the person experiences an overall pattern of emotional distress and maladaptive coping.

Our model contains a midcycle component on the avoidance track titled "Intensified self-focus." Here, in addition to the counterproductive processes described in the previous paragraph, a person using avoidance coping becomes so acutely aware of his own negative internal experiences that he feels certain that other people must be aware of the very distress that he wishes to conceal. This further exacerbates the avoidant coper's negative self-focus, as well as the experience of disruptive thoughts and emotions.

Procrastinating

Procrastination provides a classic example of avoidant coping. As defined by Ferrari in chapter 2, procrastination is "the negative and purposeful delaying of the start of completion of a task as a form of avoidance." It is theorized that avoidant procrastinators delay beginning or finishing tasks because they fear the aversiveness of tasks, as well as probable failures associated with them.

Faulty cognitive analyses may well be at the heart of procrastination. In our coping model, after construing a stressor and appraising the possible responses, an individual too quickly yields to a reactive avoidance strategy by procrastinating. Historical and individual characteristics impact these construal and appraisal processes and propel the individual toward an avoidance rather than an approach response. Metaphorically, procrastination is a psychological act of hiding, but the reality is that one *cannot* hide forever. The procrastinator knows this latter verity all too well, and this knowledge probably evokes hyperattentive, as well as unpleasant self-focused thoughts and emotions.

Experiencing Hostility

In chapter 7 by Williams and Williams, they describe hostility as a tendency to harbor cynical thoughts and angry feelings. This personality style carries a number of physical and psychological costs, including a heightened incidence of coronary heart disease, depression, anxiety, and social isolation. These, in turn, compound the risk of illness, along with lower levels of happiness and well-being. It also can be inferred from prospective (11) and cross-sectional (12) studies that, as hostility increases, so too do the maladaptive coping behaviors that pose health risks—cigarette smoking, alcohol consumption, body-mass index, 24-hour caloric intake, and cholesterol/ HDL ratio.

We contend that a complex of individual differences characteristics and environmental experiences shape an individual's proclivity toward being hostile. Central to such chronic hostility, however, is a sense of being blocked in getting what one wants in life (see 13, 14). Fixated on constant thoughts of revenge and derogation (see 15), however, the person often cannot act toward the source of the goal blockage. Instead, this person is left with what may seem a paradoxical state of hypervigilance *and* self-focus, as well as the ruminative negative thoughts and feelings that typify avoidant coping. Indeed, because hostile individuals are often ensnared in a cycle of negative appraisal, rumination, and disruptive thoughts and emotions, their access to productive goals and positive outcomes remains blocked. (In a later section, we will discuss Williams and Williams' Life-Skills approach to improving coping behaviors.)

For a substantial minority of chronically hostile persons experiencing goal blockage, lashing out at the source of the blockage occurs. Having done this, however, *they still harbor their original counterproductive thoughts and feelings*, and they evidence even further intensified sensitivities to the previous and future perceived goal blockages. Thus, for those chronically hostile persons who act toward the perceived source of the goal blockage, they only solidify their counterproductive patterns of thinking and have actually avoided addressing the underlying stressors—their hypersensitivity to goal blockages. Therefore, while the lashing out at the source of the blockage may appear to exemplify approach coping, in reality it may well reflect avoidance of the more powerful stressor—a sense of repeatedly being impeded by others. (For a similar argument that is buttressed by empirical findings, see our discussion of how hostile humor aimed at others does not confer benefits.)

Factors Enhancing the Coping Process

A number of factors that enhance the coping process are evident in various chapters of this book. We turn to those in this section.

Obtaining Social Support

Overall, social support commonly involves information from other persons about one's value and importance in a network of people. Emotional, informational, and appraisal support may be involved, as well as tangible assistance (16). Any of these modes of support can help to buffer the impact of life stressors.

Several researchers have recognized the many psychological and health benefits enjoyed by individuals with supportive social networks (e.g., 17,

18, 19, 20, 21, 22, 23). Not surprisingly, many of the authors in this volume also invoke social support as an adaptive mechanism.

In Lefcourt's chapter, "The Humor Solution," he describes research in which humor helped individuals to obtain social support (24, 25). Persons who displayed humor were perceived as better adjusted and happier than those who did not evince humor. Individuals who showed signs of enjoyment and amusement through their facial expressions had fewer grief symptoms 14 and 25 months after the loss of a spouse (24). Such outward displays can be interpreted as a desire to interact with others; similarly, others may be more willing to interact with and maintain support of persons displaying friendly qualities. In a sense, then, humor is a means for gaining social support, which is known to buffer the effects of stress.

In Williamson and Dooley's "Aging and Coping" chapter, increased activity restriction in the wake of illness or disability is advanced as being one of the best predictors of depression (26). These authors maintain that individuals who believe that they have a satisfying network of social support, however, will be less likely to cope with physical adversity by restricting their routine physical activities. Maintaining such activities throughout illness or disability is known to reduce the likelihood of negative affective outcomes. Therefore, interventions to increase social support and assist people in independent living activities should be extremely valuable in coping effectively with depression.

In the "Forgiving" chapter, McCullough describes how a capacity for forgiveness is associated with better interpersonal relationships. Indeed, forgiveness is a prosocial behavior that increases the likelihood of harmonious interpersonal interactions. Interestingly, forgiveness also appears to have an adaptive, survival value. Primates are social creatures, and they possess strong drives to maintain positive relations with others. Thus, forgiveness fosters supportive interpersonal relationships when the inevitable human fallibilities arise (27, 28).

In chapter 10 titled "Dealing with Secrets," Kelly defines a secret as information that is deliberately hidden from other people (29). She notes that, by necessity, secrets exist within a social context, and that they are meaningful only in relation to the person or persons from whom information is being concealed. Secret keeping strains social relationships because the secret keepers may withdraw more and more from ordinary social outlets and interactions. This withdrawal, in turn, often leads to feelings of isolation from one's social support network.

In Neimeyer and Levitt's chapter, "Coping and Coherence: A Narrative Perspective on Resilience," finding meaning through telling stories of adverse life events serves multiple purposes. One such purpose is the solicitation of social support. From yet another perspective, telling stories about encounters with the vicissitudes of life draws both the storyteller and the listeners into a common pride about human coping capabilities. The apparent reasoning applied in such circumstances is the following: If the storyteller copes, the listeners conclude that they also could cope with similar stressors. In this process, the human collective sense of coping is maintained as people are drawn together by the tales of facing life stressors. Relatedly, the oral histories of families typically are woven around themes of facing and overcoming extreme hardships. Indeed, our interpretation of the phrase that a person "lived to tell about it" is that the recounting of the ordeal is an important *social* ritual.

We view the seeking of social support as approach coping. Members of a social network assist copers with strategies directed toward the environment, such as providing tangible assistance and acting directly on the stressor. Social network members also assist by providing emotional support aimed at helping the person to muster positive, emotion-focused coping. Therefore, social support truly is a flexible resource, and this may be a major reason that it is such an effective coping strategy.

Finding Meaning

Finding meaning plays a prominent role in an individual's adjustment to negative events. In the aftermath of stressful situations, people want to understand what caused the events to happen, as well as determine the impacts of the events on their lives (30). The belief that the world is meaningful is a fundamental assumption that people hold steadfastly, so much so that they actively reformulate their beliefs to accommodate life-changing traumatic events (31).

Neimeyer and Levitt, in their chapter, "Coping and Coherence: A Narrative Perspective on Resilience," assert that humans ascribe meaning to their experiences by constructing personal stories or narratives. The same event, of course, could be construed differently based on each person's unique interpretation of it. Neimeyer and Levitt contend that the meanings given by individuals to their experiences are central to the coping process. In telling their stories, people may gain insight into their emotional patterns and characteristic ways of coping, thereafter formulating alternative and potentially more adaptive styles of coping (see 32). Also, through this process of reflection, an individual may become more aware of his or her coping repertoire and incorporate this into a sense of both personal identity and empowerment to deal with subsequent stressors.

In "Coping with the Inevitability of Death: Terror Management and Mismanagement," Strachan, Pyszczynski, Greenberg, and Solomon assert that the construction of meaning and the ascription of cultural significance to events are both designed to ward off fear and anxiety related to an awareness of one's mortality. As such, one way to enhance persons coping with their anxieties is to facilitate their finding meaning in their experiences.

Lastly, in chapter 13 by Pargament and his colleagues, we see a meaning-making theme running through the tenets and practices of various religions and related practices that they describe. As we will discuss in more detail later in this chapter, the study of religion appears to have been a taboo subject matter for coping researchers. Perhaps the recent emergence of interest among coping researchers in the meaning-finding process will open doors to the further study of religion.

By ascribing meaning to stressful events, whether by constructing personal narratives or otherwise, people are using approach coping to effectively act on their experiences. In our coping model, finding meaning is a strategy directed toward the self, and successful copers gain a sense of mastery and hope over what otherwise would be construed as uncontrollable and overwhelming events (33).

Using Humor

In Lefcourt's chapter, "The Humor Solution," he views humor as a form of emotion-focused coping. According to Lazarus and Folkman (34), situations that are uncontrollable are most effectively dealt with by emotion-focused coping, in which an individual regulates his or her feelings about a situation. Numerous researchers have reported that humor is a moderator of stress and health outcomes, such as pain and mood disturbance (35, 36, 37, 38). Humor also has been linked to surviving traumatic stress. On this latter point, Viktor Frankl wrote about the role of humor in his concentration camp survival experience: "Humor was another of the soul's weapons in the fight for self-preservation. . . . I practically trained a friend of mine who worked next to me on the building site to develop a sense of humor. I suggested to him that we would promise each other to invent at least one amusing story daily, about some incident that could happen one day after our liberation" (39, p. 54).

Lefcourt also notes that there are different types of humor, and that some may be more effective than others for coping with stress. According to Vaillant (40), self-deprecating humor—laughing at oneself in the midst of stress—is quite adaptive. On the other hand, hostile humor involves asserting control by directing humor toward other people who are experiencing stress, and it is not associated with benefits. In this regard, there appear to be gender differences in how humor is used, with women being more apt to use self-deprecating humor, and men being more likely to use hostile humor.

In Williamson and Dooley's chapter, they discuss aging and its associated stressors—chronic illnesses and death of a loved one (41). After trying to modify a negative situation related to the aging process, an ability to accept life circumstances with a sense of humor in one's later years is an adaptive coping response.

We view humor as a form of approach coping, where one's strategy is directed toward the self. The use of humor makes the stressor more palatable; in turn, a person can deal more effectively with that stressor. Likewise, as we have noted previously in this chapter, humor is a means of attracting social support in coping with stressors. Lastly, taking these strategies together, it appears that those persons with high hostility could improve their coping skills by learning how to use self-deprecating humor.

Comparing with Others

In chapter 8 by Wills and Sandy, they define social comparison-oriented coping as "a cognitive process of comparing one's attributes with those of another person, thereby improving subjective well-being." They also theorize that this improved well-being facilitates individuals actively dealing with their problems. In downward social comparison, better feelings result from comparing one's own circumstances to those worse off. Based on the results of several studies of downward social comparison, this process does appear to be an effective coping strategy (42, 43, 44, 45).

We view social comparison as an active approach coping strategy that entails, at times, self-directed strategies *and then* environment-directed strategies. That is to say, the social comparison process first trades on appraising oneself relative to relatively less well-off comparison others, whereafter the person is energized to act on his or her stressor; moreover, this person may gain tips about dealing with the stressor in the process of comparing with others.

Revealing Secrets

In Kelly's chapter, she explains that under certain circumstances revealing secrets is a good coping strategy because it reduces the distress caused by the harboring of such secrets. Kelly offers coping guidelines for dealing with secrets and asserts that, most important, one must confide in someone who is discrete, nonjudgmental, and able to provide new insights into one's secret (46, 47). The act of suppressing such troubling secrets, however, can cause secret holders to experience rumination and negative thoughts and feelings—core characteristics of avoidance coping. Thus, dealing with secrets apparently enables the individual to move from an avoidance to an approach coping track. Moreover, as we have noted earlier, by disclosing a secret, the person has actively reached out to one or more people in her social support network.

Remaining Active

In Williamson and Dooley's chapter, they present activity as a key element in coping effectively with aging and its associated pains, illnesses, and disabilities. More specifically, *lack* of activity leads to depression and other negative outcomes (26). By remaining active, however, the person not only is receiving the benefits of goal-directed thinking and actions (see 48, 49), but also is distracted from the pain (50, 51). Although invoked initially for older persons, this principle may be applied to persons of any age who are dealing with pain or chronic medical conditions.

By its very nature, activity is an action-oriented, approach coping strategy. In this regard, Williamson and Dooley recommend that people need to be aided in identifying those activities in which they can participate, and then encouraged for their pursuits of these activities. On this latter point, they note that support groups may improve the self-esteem and confidence of individuals who have removed themselves from activities because of self-consciousness related to perceived inadequacies. Therefore, this activity-based coping also may involve self-focused approach activities.

Learning Distraction and Mindfulness Meditation

In Hamilton and Ingram's chapter, they provide antidotes for counterproductive self-focused attention. They discuss two ways to reduce maladaptive attentional self-focus: external distraction (52, 53) and mindfulness meditation (54). In brief, external distraction is an active strategy in which one engages in cognitively challenging activities. Such engagement does not leave enough mental energy for the person to become consumed with self-focused attention. Similarly, mindfulness meditation involves a shift from an attentional self-focus to an ongoing focus on sensory, affective, and cognitive awareness. Again, mindfulness meditation works by tying up enough cognitive resources so as to preclude the emergence of counterproductive and evaluative ruminative processes.

We believe that both distraction and mindfulness mediation are self-directed strategies that are part of the approach coping track in our model. While at first glance they may appear to be avoidance strategies that resemble suppression, we would hold that they are active techniques in which people engage in proactive behaviors and advocate adaptive solutions to difficult, entrenched problems.

Forgiving

McCullough describes forgiveness as an adaptive coping strategy in his chapter. Greater forgiveness is linked with increased psychological well-being and life satisfaction (55) and relational well-being (56, 57, 58, 59). Certainly, the desire to forgive is something for which people seek psychological services, and individual psychotherapy can be useful in helping people to achieve this goal (60, 61).

We consider forgiveness to be an approach coping behavior. In this regard, Snyder and Yamhure (28) have proposed a theory of forgiveness, based on the notion that the act of forgiving enables a person to break the ruminative, angry thoughts that continue to link that person to the source of the transgression. Having been freed of this "bond" to the transgression source, the person then can use his or her time in the pursuit of productive and satisfying life goals. In a temporal sense, therefore, forgiveness is first represented as a self-focused approach coping strategy that, once effectively implemented, allows the instillation of environmental approach strategies.

A Broader Context for Coping

In Chang's chapter, "A Look at the Coping Strategies and Styles of Asian Americans" and in Pargament, Poloma, and Tarakeshwar's chapter, "Methods of Coping from the Religions of the World," the authors' explicit take-home messages are that the scope of the coping literature needs to be broadened. They convincingly write that current coping researchers have focused on Western culture and largely ignored differences in coping that stem from culture and religion.

Chang outlines ways in which Asian Americans and Caucasians differ in their choice of coping strategies, and how certain strategies that are adaptive for members of one cultural group are not effective for those persons in another. Additional research with a variety of cultural groups is greatly needed so that we can understand the coping processes among populations of ethnic "minority" groups. Interestingly, many of us doing research on the topic of coping seem to ignore the fact that "minorities" already form a large portion of our American society, and that they will become the majority as we move further into the twenty-first century. In conducting research with people of diverse ethnic backgrounds, we probably will need new models of coping. Our own coping model, for example, is based on the presently available coping research conducted with mostly Caucasian Western populations. As such, our model may not apply to other racial groups. On this count, let us be the first to provide a major caveat about the questionable applicability of our coping model across racial groups.

In Pargament, Poloma, and Tarakeshwar's chapter, they make a compelling case for the place of religion in the coping literature, both as it is used around the world and across cultures. Their description of karma fits best with current conceptualizations of coping, as they state that karma provides a way for individuals to gain control, create meaning, and to believe in a just world. Similar principles are recognized by numerous coping researchers as necessary components of successful coping (31, 30). Indeed, the practice of religion is one of the oldest known methods of extracting meaning, control, and justice from an otherwise unpredictable world. In the field of psychology more generally, the study of religions has been virtually ignored, perhaps with the misguided thinking that to study religion somehow would be "unscientific." In the extent to which stress and coping researchers have bought into this more general view, which appears to be the case, we also have removed the possibility of gaining important insights. We would suggest that coping researchers should cast aside this purposeful neglect of studying religion, thereby serving as a positive example for the wider field of psychology.

By expanding our research so as to explore coping in diverse racial and cultural groups, as well as including religions and spirituality as worthy topics of investigation, our theories will at once become more inclusive and more accurate. These latter two principles are part of the foundation of the scientific approach.

Methods for Improving Coping

In recent years, coping has become a popular topic of study. Having amassed a large body of information concerning what is and what is not adaptive coping (e.g., 62), we still are left with questions concerning how to improve our coping efforts. Several of the chapter authors in this volume address this issue at length, and we make only brief observations here. For more information on coping interventions, we refer the interested reader to Folkman et al. (63); moreover, for a detailed exploration of the various psychological change interventions more generally, the reader is directed to Snyder and Ingram (48).

In general, behavioral interventions that target the acquisition of adaptive coping skills have received substantial empirical support (64, 65, 66, 67, 68, 70, 71, 72). These interventions have been used for a variety of problems, including coronary heart disease, cancer, and other chronic medical conditions. Williams and Williams, in the subtitle of their chapter "The LifeSkills Approach," focus on developing coping skills that are central to self-awareness and relationship-building (communication skills and empathy training) and skills for effective behavior (problem solving and assertion). We strongly agree that the building and managing of interpersonal relationships is crucial for coping with a variety of life stressors. Moreover, the group setting as compared to the individual setting may provide more power for enhancing coping skills. Indeed, the bulk of our coping activities are aimed at addressing stressors that have arisen in the context of real or imagined other people. In short, coping often occurs as part of our social commerce (73). Thus, it makes sense to increase our coping intervention efforts with group approaches.

Conclusions

Although there are no "hard and fast" rules when it comes to coping, we believe that approach coping generally is more adaptive than avoidance coping. We cannot and do not wish to say, however, that one type of approach strategy is better than another across different situations. There is an interplay between historical factors, situational factors, and individual differences characteristics that determines a person's best course of coping in any given situation. To the extent that an individual can choose approach coping strategies, remain motivated to use them, and be flexible in implementing courses of action, we would say that this person is using the basic tenets underlying adaptive coping.

In our approach-avoidance coping model, we maintain that appraisal occurs either at or below the level of awareness, and that coping involves stressors ranging from seemingly small daily hassles to major traumas. In expressing these views, we differ from those advocates of previous coping models in which coping is conceived as strictly a conscious activity applied to stressors of a large magnitude. Many of the stressors and coping strategies discussed in this book—aging, dealing with secrets, forgiving, etc.—would not fit well within the former, more circumscribed coping models. In our model, we also have ascribed equal efficacy to self-directed coping strategies (e.g., emotion-focused) and environment-directed strategies (e.g., problem-solving). Thus, we have eschewed the previous view that emotion-focused coping is bad. Indeed, we have placed emotion-focused coping on the adaptive approach path of our model. Lastly, we would suggest that individual differences variables are strongly involved as moderators of the stress and coping process, as well as being implicated in perhaps every phase of the avoidance and approach cycles. Together, individual differences and coping processes join forces in waging battles against the stressors that threaten to invade our lives (thus, the chapter subtitle "Two Against One").

Overall, therefore, we have purposefully widened the definition of that which falls under the rubric of coping. In doing this, we believe that a broader, more inclusive definition may serve as an invitation for theoreticians, researchers, and practitioners to consider coping processes in their work. As such, the topic of coping may be embraced by more people as we step into the twenty-first century of stressors.

Note

1. In the realm of persons coming to psychotherapy, however, practitioners sometimes report that their clients (a small percentage) truly have blocked aversive stressors from their awarenesses. Based on the available research that falls under the long-studied rubric of self-deception, which is classically defined as the purposeful pushing of an unpleasant self-referential thought *totally* out of awareness in favor of more positive thoughts, there does not appear to be empirical support for such clinical observations (74, 75). However, if one defines self-deception as the weighing of two negative self-referential thoughts, and placing the more negative thoughts lower in awareness than the more positive ones, there is some support for clinical lore (74, 75, 76, 77). It should be emphasized, however, that for the overwhelming majority of persons attempting *not* to think about a stressor, this results in *more* thoughts about those very stressors.

References

1. Teasdale, J. D. (1983). Negative thinking in depression: Cause, effect, or reciprocal relationship. *Advances in Behaviour Research and Therapy, 5*, 3–25.
2. Teasdale, J. D., & Barnard, P. J. (1993). *Affect, cognition, and change: Re-modeling depressive thoughts.* Hillsdale, NJ: Erlbaum.
3. McCullough, M. E., Bellah, C. G., Kilpatrick, S. D., & Johnson, J. L. (1999). *Vengefulness: Relationships with forgiveness, rumination, well-being, and the Big Five.* Manuscript submitted for publication.

4. McCullough, M. E., Rachal, K. C., Sandage, S. J., Worthington, E. L., Jr., Brown, S. W., & Hight, T. L. (1998). Interpersonal forgiving in close relationships II: Theoretical elaboration and measurement. *Journal of Personality and Social Psychology, 75,* 1586–1603.

5. Caprara, G. V. (1986). Indicators of aggression: The dissipation rumination scale. *Personality and Individual Differences, 7,* 763–769.

6. Collins, K., & Bell, R. (1997). Personality and aggression: The dissipation-rumination scale. *Personality and Individual Differences, 22,* 751–755.

7. Pfefferbaum, B., & Wood, P. B. (1994). Self-report study of impulsive and delinquent behavior in college students. *Journal of Adolescent Health, 15,* 295–302.

8. Stuckless, N., & Goranson, R. (1992). The vengeance scale: Development of a measure of attitudes toward revenge. *Journal of Social Behavior and Personality, 7* (1), 25–42.

9. Wegner, D. M. (1994). Ironic processes of mental control. *Psychological Review, 101,* 34–52.

10. Wegner, D. M., Schneider, D. J., Carter, S. R., & White, T. L. (1987). Paradoxical effects of thought suppression. *Journal of Personality and Social Psychology, 53,* 5–13.

11. Siegler, I. C., Peterson, B. L., Barefoot, J. C., & Williams, R. B. (1992). Hostility during late adolescence predicts coronary risk factors at midlife. *American Journal of Epidemiology, 136,* 146–154.

12. Scherwitz, K. W., Perkins, L. L., Chesney, M. A., Hughes, G. H., Sidney, S., & Manolio, T. A. (1992). Hostility and health behaviors in young adults: The CARDIA study. Coronary Artery Risk Development in Young Adults Study. *American Journal of Epidemiology, 136,* 136–145.

13. Snyder, C. R. (1994). *The psychology of hope: You can get there from here.* New York: Free Press.

14. Rodriguez-Hanley, A., & Snyder, C. R. (2000). The demise of hope: On losing positive thinking. In C. R. Snyder (Ed.), *Handbook of hope: Theory, research, and applications* (pp. 39–56). Orlando, FL: Academic Press.

15. Snyder, C. R., Crowson, J. J., Jr., Houston, B. K., Kurylo, M., & Poirier, J. (1997). Assessing hostile automatic thoughts: Development and validation of the HAT Scale. *Cognitive Therapy and Research, 4,* 477–492.

16. Taylor, S. E., & Aspinwall, L. G. (1996). Mediating and moderating processes in psychosocial stress: Appraisal, coping, resistance, and vulnerability. In H. B. Kaplan (Ed.), *Psychosocial stress: Perspectives on structure, theory, life-course, and methods* (pp. 71–110). San Diego: Academic Press.

17. Cohen, S., & Wills, T. A. (1985). Stress, social support, and the buffering hypothesis. *Psychological Bulletin, 98,* 310–357.

18. Dunkel-Schetter, C., & Wortman, C. B. (1981). Dilemmas of social support: Parallels between victimization and aging. In S. B. Kiesler, J. N. Morgan, & V. K. Oppenheimer (Eds.), *Aging: Social change* (pp. 349–381). New York: Academic Press.

19. Glick, I. O., Weiss, R. S., & Parkes, C. M. (1974). *The first year of bereavement.* New York: Wiley.

20. House, J. S., Umberson, D., & Landis, K. R. (1988). Structures and processes of social support. *American Review of Sociology, 14*, 293–318.
21. Kessler, R. C., & McLeod, J. D. (1985). Social support and mental health in community samples. In S. Cohen & S. L. Syme (Eds.), *Social support and health* (pp. 219–240). Orlando, FL: Academic Press.
22. Kulik, J. A., & Mahler, H. I. M. (1989). Social support and recovery from surgery. *Health Psychology, 8*, 221–238.
23. Taylor, S. E. (1995). *Health psychology* (3rd ed.). New York: McGraw-Hill.
24. Bonanno, G. A., & Keltner, D. (1997). Facial expressions of emotion and the course of conjugal bereavement. *Journal of Abnormal Psychology, 106*, 126–138.
25. Keltner, D., & Bonanno, G. A. (1997). A study of laughter and dissociation: Distinct correlates of laughter and smiling during bereavement. *Journal of Personality and Social Psychology, 73*, 687–702.
26. Williamson, G. M. (1998). The central role of restricted normal activities in adjustment to illness and disability: A model of depressed affect. *Rehabilitation Psychology, 43*, 327–347.
27. Baumeister, R. F., & Leary, M. R. (1995). The need to belong: Desire for interpersonal attachments as a fundamental human motivation. *Psychological Bulletin, 117*, 497–529.
28. Snyder, C. R., & Yamhure, L. (2000). *Forgiveness theory and the Heartlands Forgiveness Scale*. Unpublished manuscript. University of Kansas, Lawrence.
29. Margolis, G. J. (1974). The psychology of keeping secrets. *International Review of Psycho-Analysis, 1*, 291–296.
30. Taylor, S. E. (1983). Adjustment to threatening events: A theory of cognitive adaptation. *American Psychologist, 28*, 1161–1173.
31. Janoff-Bulman, R. (1999). Rebuilding shattered assumptions after traumatic life events: Coping processes and outcomes. In C. R. Snyder (Ed.), *Coping: The psychology of what works* (pp. 305–323). New York: Oxford University Press.
32. Snyder, C. R., McDermott, D., Cook, W., & Rapoff, M. (1997). *Hope for the journey: Helping children through the good times and the bad*. Boulder, CO, San Francisco, CA: Westview/HarperCollins.
33. Feldman, D. B. & Snyder, C. R. (2000). Hope for the many: An empowering social agenda. In C. R. Snyder (Ed.), *Handbook of hope: Theory, research, and clinical application* (pp. 389–412). Orlando, FL: Academic Press.
34. Lazarus, R. S., & Folkman, S. (1984). *Stress, appraisal, and coping*. New York: Springer.
35. Carver, C. S., Pozo, C., Harris, S. D., Noriega, V., Scheier, M. F., Robinson, D. S., Ketcham, A. S., Moffat, F. L., & Clark, K. C. (1993). How coping mediates the effect of optimism on distress: A study of women with early stage breast cancer. *Journal of Personality and Social Psychology, 65*, 375–390.
36. Kuiper, N. A., Martin, R. A., & Dance, K. A. (1992). Sense of humor and enhanced quality of life. *Personality and Individual Differences, 13*, 1273–1283.

37. Lefcourt, H. M., Davidson, K., Shepherd, R. S., Phillips, M., Prka-
    chin, K., & Mills, D. (1995). Perspective-taking humor: Accounting
    for stress moderation. *Journal of Social and Clinical Psychology, 14,*
    373–391.
38. Rotton, J., & Shats, M. (1996). Effects of state humor, expectancies and
    choice on post-surgical mood and self-medication: A field experiment.
    Journal of Applied Social Psychology, 26, 1775–1794.
39. Frankl, V. E. (1992). *Man's search for meaning: An introduction to lo-
    gotherapy* (4th ed.). Boston: Beacon Press.
40. Vaillant, G. E. (1977). *Adaptation to life.* Toronto: Little, Brown & Co.
41. Hooyman, N., & Kiyak, H. A. (1998). *Social gerontology: A multidisci-
    plinary perspective* (5th ed.). Boston: Allyn & Bacon.
42. Affleck, G., & Tennen, H. (1991). Social comparison and coping with
    major medical problems. In J. Suls & T. A. Wills (Eds.), *Social com-
    parison: Contemporary theory and research* (pp. 369–393). Hillsdale,
    NJ: Erlbaum.
43. Carver, C. S., Scheier, M. F., & Weintraub, J. K. (1989). Assessing cop-
    ing strategies: A theoretically-based approach. *Journal of Personality
    and Social Psychology, 56,* 267–283.
44. Gibbons, F. X., & Gerrard, M. (1991). Downward social comparison and
    coping with threat. In J. Suls & T. A. Wills (Eds.), *Social comparison:
    Contemporary theory and research* (pp. 317–345). Hillsdale, NJ: Erl-
    baum.
45. Wills, T. A. (1991). Similarity and self-esteem in downward social
    comparison. In J. Suls & T. A. Wills (Eds.), *Social comparison: Contem-
    porary theory and research* (pp. 51–78). Hillsdale, NJ: Erlbaum.
46. Kelly, A. E. (1999). Revealing personal secrets. *Current Directions in
    Psychological Science, 8,* 106–109.
47. Kelly, A. E., & McKillop, K. J. (1996). Consequences of revealing per-
    sonal secrets. *Psychological Bulletin, 120,* 450–465.
48. Snyder, C. R., & Ingram R. E. (Eds.) (2000). *Handbook of psychological
    change: Psychotherapy processes and practices for the 21st century.*
    New York: Wiley.
49. Snyder, C. R., Cheavens, J., & Michael, S. T. (1999). Hoping. In C. R.
    Snyder (Ed.), *Coping: The psychology of what works* (pp. 205–231).
    New York: Oxford University Press.
50. Snyder, C. R. (1998). A case for hope in pain, loss, and suffering. In
    J. H. Harvey, J. Omarzu, & E. Miller (Eds.), *Perspectives on loss: A
    sourcebook* (pp. 63–79). Washington, DC: Taylor & Francis.
51. Snyder, C. R. (In press). The hope mandala: Coping with the loss of a
    loved one. In Jane Gillham (Ed.), *Optimism and hope.* Radnor, PA:
    Templeton Foundation/Washington, DC: American Psychological As-
    sociation.
52. Erber, R. (1996). The self-regulation of moods. In L. L. Martin & T. Abra-
    ham (Eds.), *Striving and feeling: Interactions among goals, affect, and
    self-regulation* (pp. 251–275). Hillsdale, NJ: Erlbaum.
53. Erber, R., & Tesser, A. (1992). Task effort and the regulation of mood:
    The absorption hypothesis. *Journal of Experimental Social Psychology,
    30,* 319–337.

54. Kabat-Zinn, J. (1982). An outpatient program in behavioral medicine for chronic pain patients based on the practice of mindfulness meditation. *General Hospital Psychiatry, 4*, 31–47.
55. Poloma, M. M., & Gallup, G. H. (1991). *Varieties of prayer.* Philadelphia: Trinity Press International.
56. Holeman, V. T., & Myers, R. W. (1998). Effects of forgiveness of perpetrators on marital adjustment for survivors of sexual abuse. *The Family Journal: Counseling and Therapy for Couples and Families, 6*, 182–188.
57. Nelson, M. K. (1993). *A new theory of forgiveness.* Unpublished doctoral dissertation, Purdue University, West Lafayette, IN.
58. Woodman, T. (1991). *The role of forgiveness in marital adjustment.* Unpublished doctoral dissertation, Fuller Graduate School of Psychology, Pasadena, CA.
59. Rackley, J. V. (1993). *The relationships of marital satisfaction, forgiveness, and religiosity.* Unpublished Dissertation, Virginia Polytechnic Institute and State University, Blacksburg, VA.
60. Coyle, C. T., & Enright, R. D. (1997). Forgiveness intervention with post-abortion men. *Journal of Consulting and Clinical Psychology, 65*, 1042–1046.
61. Freedman, S. R., & Enright, R. D. (1996). Forgiveness as an intervention goal with incest survivors. *Journal of Consulting and Clinical Psychology, 64*, 510–517.
62. Snyder, C. R. (Ed.) (1999). *Coping: The psychology of what works.* New York: Oxford University Press.
63. Folkman, S., Chesney, M., McKusick, L., Ironson, G., Johnson, D. S., & Coates, T. J. (1991). Translating coping theory into an intervention. In J. Eckenrode (Ed.), *The social context of coping* (pp. 239–260). New York: Plenum Press.
64. Blumenthal, J. A., Jiang, W., Babyak, M., Krantz, D. S., Frid, D. J., Coleman, R. E., Waugh, R., Hanson, M., Appelbaum, M., O'Conner, C. M., & Morris, J. J. (1997). Stress management and exercise training in cardiac patients with myocardial ischemia. *Archives of Internal Medicine, 157*, 2213–2223.
65. Blumenthal, J. A., O'Connor, C., Hinderliter, A., Fath, K., Hedge, S. B., Miller, G., Puma, J., Sessions, W., Sheps, D., Zakhary, B., & Williams, R. B. (1997). Psychosocial factors and coronary disease. A National Multicenter Clinical Trial (ENRICHD) with a North Carolina focus. *North Carolina Medical Journal, 58*, 802–808.
66. Cummings, N. A., Pallak, M. S., Dorken, H., & Henke, C. W. (1991). The impact of psychological intervention on health care costs and utilization. The Hawaii Medicaid Project. *HCFA Contract Report #11-C-983344/9.*
67. Fawzy, F. I., Fawzy, N. W., Hyun, C. S., Elashoff, R., Guthrie, D., Fahey, J. L., & Morton, D. L. (1993). Malignant melanoma: Effects of an early structured psychiatric intervention, coping, and affective state on recurrence and survival six years later. *Archives of General Psychiatry, 50*, 681–689.
68. Friedman, M., Thoresen, C. E., & Gill, J. J. (1986). Alteration of type A behavior and its effect on cardiac recurrences in post myocardial in-

farction patients: Summary results of the Recurrent Coronary Prevention Project. *American Heart Journal, 112,* 653–665.

69. Spiegel, D., Bloom, J. R., Kraemer, H. C., & Gottheil, E. (1989). Effect of psychosocial treatment on survival of patients with metastatic breast cancer. *Lancet, 2,* 888–890.

70. Williams, R. B., & Chesney, M. A. (1993). Psychosocial factors and prognosis in established coronary artery disease: The need for research on interventions. *Journal of the American Medical Association, 270,* 1860–1861.

71. Williams, R. B., & Williams, V. P. (1993). *Anger kills: Seventeen strategies for controlling the hostility that can harm your health.* New York: Times Books/Random House.

72. Williams, V. P., & Williams, R. B. (1997). *LifeSkills: Eight simple ways to build stronger relationships, communicate more clearly and improve your health.* New York: Times Books/Random House.

73. Snyder, C. R., Cheavens, J., & Sympson, S. C. (1997). Hope: An individual motive for social commerce. *Group Dynamics: Theory, Research, and Practice, 1,* 107–118.

74. Snyder, C. R. (1985). Collaborative companions: The relationship of self deception and excuse-making. In M. Martin (Ed.), *Essays in self-deception* (pp. 35–51). Lawrence, KS: Regents Press of Kansas.

75. Snyder, C. R., & Higgins, R. L. (1997). Reality negotiation: Governing one's self and being governed by others. *General Psychology Review, 4,* 336–350.

76. Snyder, C. R., & Higgins, R. L. (1988). From making to being the excuse: An analysis of deception and verbal/nonverbal issues. *Journal of Nonverbal Behavior, 12,* 237–252.

77. Snyder, C. R., Higgins, R. L., & Stucky, R. J. (1983). *Excuses: Masquerades in search of grace.* New York: Wiley-Interscience.

Index

303